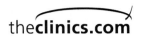

CHILD AND ADOLESCENT PSYCHIATRIC CLINICS OF NORTH AMERICA

Treating Autism Spectrum Disorders

GUEST EDITORS
David J. Posey, MD, MS
Christopher J. McDougle, MD

CONSULTING EDITOR
Harsh K. Trivedi, MD

October 2008 • Volume 17 • Number 4

SAUNDERS

An Imprint of Elsevier, Inc.
PHILADELPHIA   LONDON   TORONTO   MONTREAL   SYDNEY   TOKYO

W.B. SAUNDERS COMPANY

A Division of Elsevier Inc.

Elsevier Inc. • 1600 John F. Kennedy Boulevard • Suite 1800 • Philadelphia, Pennsylvania 19103-2899

http://www.childpsych.theclinics.com

CHILD AND ADOLESCENT PSYCHIATRIC CLINICS	**Volume 17, Number 4**
OF NORTH AMERICA	**ISSN 1056–4993**
October 2008	**ISBN-13: 978-1-4160-6278-3**
Editor: Sarah E. Barth	**ISBN-10: 1-4160-6278-5**

Child and Adolescent Psychiatric Clinics of North America (ISSN 1056-4993) is published quarterly by Elsevier Inc., 360 Park Avenue South, New York, NY 10010-1710. Months of issue are January, April, July, and October. Business and Editorial Offices: 1600 John F. Kennedy Boulevard, Suite 1800, Philadelphia, PA 19103-2899. Customer Service Offices: 6277 Sea Harbor Drive, Orlando, FL 32887-4800. Periodicals postage paid at New York, NY and additional mailing offices. Subscription prices are $220.00 per year (US individuals), $344.00 per year (US institutions), $113.00 per year (US students), $250.00 per year (Canadian individuals), $406.00 per year (Canadian institutions), $136.00 per year (Canadian students), $279.00 per year (international individuals), $406.00 per year (international institutions), and $136.00 per year (international students). International air speed delivery is included in all *Clinics* subscription prices. All prices are subject to change without notice. **POSTMASTER:** Send address changes to *Child and Adolescent Psychiatric Clinics of North America*, Elsevier Periodicals Customer Service, 6277 Sea Harbor Drive, Orlando, FL 32887-4800. **Customer Service: 1-800-654-2452 (US). From outside the United States, call 1-407-563-6020. Fax: 1-407-563-8521. E-mail: JournalsCustomerService-usa@elsevier.com.**

Reprints. For copies of 100 or more of articles in this publication, please contact the Commercial Reprints Department, Elsevier Inc., 360 Park Avenue South, New York, New York, 10010-1710; Tel.: (+1) 212-633-3813, Fax: (+1) 212-462-1935, and E-mail: reprints@elsevier.com.

Child and Adolescent Psychiatric Clinics of North America is covered in *MEDLINE/PubMed (Index Medicus)*, *ISI, SSCI, Research Alert, Social Search, Current Contents,* and *EMBASE/Excerpta Medica*.

Printed in the United States of America.

CONSULTING EDITOR

HARSH K. TRIVEDI, MD, Director of Adolescent Services and Site Training Director, Bradley Hospital; Assistant Professor of Psychiatry and Human Behavior (Clinical), Brown Medical School; President, Rhode Island Council of Child and Adolescent Psychiatry; Consulting Editor, Child and Adolescent Psychiatric Clinics of North America; East Providence, Rhode Island

CONSULTING EDITOR EMERITUS

ANDRÉS MARTIN, MD, MPH

FOUNDING CONSULTING EDITOR

MELVIN LEWIS, MBBS, FRCPsych, DCH

GUEST EDITORS

CHRISTOPHER J. MCDOUGLE, MD, Albert E. Sterne Professor and Chairman, Department of Psychiatry, Christian Sarkine Autism Treatment Center, Indiana University School of Medicine, Indianapolis, Indiana

DAVID J. POSEY, MD, MS, Associate Professor; and Chief, Christian Sarkine Autism Treatment Center, Department of Psychiatry, Indiana University School of Medicine, Indianapolis, Indiana

CONTRIBUTORS

MICHAEL G. AMAN, PhD, Professor, Department of Psychology; Professor, Department of Psychiatry; and Director of Research, The Nisonger Center UCEDD, Ohio State University, Columbus, Ohio

L. EUGENE ARNOLD, Med, MD, Professor Emeritus of Psychiatry, Department of Psychiatry; and Interim Director, The Nisonger Center UCEDD, Ohio State University, Columbus, Ohio

SCOTT BELLINI, PhD, Assistant Professor, and Assistant Director, Indiana Resource Center for Autism, Indiana University, Bloomington, Indiana

CRAIG A. ERICKSON, MD, Assistant Professor, Department of Psychiatry, Christian Sarkine Autism Treatment Center, Indiana University School of Medicine, Indianapolis, Indiana

CRISTAN A. FARMER, MA, Research Associate, The Nisonger Center UCEDD; and Doctoral Student, Intellectual and Developmental Disability Psychology Program, Ohio State University, Columbus, Ohio

RICHARD M. FOXX, PhD, Professor of Psychology, Psychology Program, Penn State University Harrisburg, Middletown; and Clinical Adjunct Professor of Pediatrics, Penn State University School of Medicine, Hershey, Pennsylvania

ERIC HOLLANDER, MD, Esther and Joseph Klingenstein Professor and Chair; and Director, Seaver & New York Autism Center of Excellence, Department of Psychiatry, Mount Sinai School of Medicine, New York, New York

JILL HOLLWAY, MA, Research Associate, The Nisonger Center UCEDD; and Doctoral student, Intellectual and Developmental Disability Psychology Program, Ohio State University, Columbus, Ohio

SUSAN L. HYMAN, MD, Associate Professor, Department of Pediatrics, University of Rochester School of Medicine, Golisano Children's Hospital at Strong, Rochester, New York

KYLE P. JOHNSON, MD, Associate Professor, Departments of Psychiatry and Pediatrics, Oregon Health & Science University; and Co-Medical Director, Oregon Health & Science University Sleep Disorders Program, Portland, Oregon

JESSICA KIARASHI, BA, Clinical Research Coordinator, Department of Psychiatry, One Gustave L. Levy Place, Seaver & New York Autism Center of Excellence, Mount Sinai School of Medicine, New York, New York

TIFFANY KODAK, Munroe-Meyer Institute, University of Nebraska Medical Center, Omaha, Nebraska

PATRICIA KORZEKWA, MS, Autism Special Education Liaison, HANDS in Autism Program, Christian Sarkine Autism Treatment Center, Indiana University School of Medicine, Riley Hospital for Children, Indianapolis, Indiana

SUSAN E. LEVY, MD, Clinical Professor, Department of Pediatrics, University of Pennsylvania School of Medicine, The Children's Hospital of Philadelphia, Philadelphia, Pennsylvania

BETH A. MALOW, MD, MS, Professor, Department of Neurology, Vanderbilt University Medical Center; and Medical Director, Vanderbilt Sleep Disorders Center, Nashville, Tennessee

CHRISTOPHER J. MCDOUGLE, MD, Albert E. Sterne Professor and Chairman, Department of Psychiatry, Christian Sarkine Autism Treatment Center, Indiana University School of Medicine, Indianapolis, Indiana

NOHA F. MINSHAWI, PhD, Assistant Professor of Clinical Psychology in Clinical Psychiatry, Indiana University School of Medicine and; Christian Sarkine Autism Treatment Center, James Whitcomb Riley Hospital for Children, Indianapolis, Indiana

RHEA PAUL, PhD, Professor, Yale Child Study Center, New Haven, Connecticut

JESSICA K. PETERS, MS, Graduate Student, School of Education, Indiana University, Bloomington, Indiana

CATHLEEN C. PIAZZA, Munroe-Meyer Institute, University of Nebraska Medical Center, Omaha, Nebraska

DAVID J. POSEY, MD, MS, Associate Professor; and Chief, Christian Sarkine Autism Treatment Center, Department of Psychiatry, Indiana University School of Medicine, Indianapolis, Indiana

LATHA SOORYA, PhD, Assistant Professor, Department of Psychiatry, One Gustave L. Levy Place, Seaver & New York Autism Center of Excellence, Mount Sinai School of Medicine, New York, New York

KIMBERLY A. STIGLER, MD, Assistant Professor of Psychiatry, Department of Psychiatry, Indiana University School of Medicine, Indianapolis, Indiana

MELISSA STUART, MS, Behavioral Research Specialist, HANDS in Autism Program, Christian Sarkine Autism Treatment Center, Indiana University School of Medicine, Riley Hospital for Children, Indianapolis, Indiana

NAOMI SWIEZY, PhD, HSPP, Alan H. Cohen Family Scholar of Psychiatry; Associate Professor of Clinical Psychology in Clinical Psychiatry; Clinical Director, Christian Sarkine Autism Treatment Center; and Program Director, HANDS in Autism Riley Hospital for Children and IU School of Medicine, Indianapolis, Indiana

Cover artwork Courtesy of Socorro Rivera G., Mexico City, Mexico

CONTENTS

including aggression, self-injurious behavior, and tantrums. Research to date supports the use of the atypical antipsychotics as a first-line pharmacologic treatment for this target symptom domain in PDDs. Currently, the atypical antipsychotic risperidone is the only medication approved by the US Food and Drug Administration for irritability in youth with autism. Additional large-scale, placebo-controlled studies of other medications are needed to determine their efficacy for the treatment of irritability in this diagnostic group.

This article provides an overview of psychopharmacological treatments for repetitive behaviors in autism spectrum disorders (ASDs) in the context of current conceptualizations of this understudied core symptom domain. The available literature on the widely used selective serotonin reuptake inhibitors (SSRIs), including fluvoxamine, fluoxetine, citalopram, escitalopram, and sertraline, are reviewed. In addition to SSRIs, research on effects of other pharmacologic interventions such as divalproex sodium, risperidone, and the neuropeptide oxytocin are presented. To date, data are mixed for interventions commonly prescribed in clinical practice and suggest several areas of investigation in advancing research on the medication management of repetitive behaviors.

Like children with other developmental disabilities, children with autism spectrum disorders suffer with sleep problems at a higher rate than do typically developing children. There is a growing recognition that addressing these sleep problems may improve daytime functioning and decrease family stress. Presented here is a discussion of the sleep problems experienced by children with autism spectrum disorders, focusing on appropriate assessment and pharmacologic treatment.

There are many challenges to studying drug effects on core social and language impairment in autism. Drugs such as fenfluramine, naltrexone, and secretin do not appear to be efficacious for these core symptoms. Risperidone has led to improvement in some aspects of social relatedness when used to treat irritability in autism. More research is needed on the utility of selective serotonin reuptake inhibitors, cholinergic drugs, glutamatergic drugs, and oxytocin for core autistic symptoms.

Complementary and alternative medical (CAM) treatments are commonly used for children with autism spectrum disorders. This review discusses the evidence supporting the most frequently used treatments, including categories of mind-body medicine, energy medicine, and biologically based, manipulative, and body-based practices, with the latter two treatments the most commonly selected by families. Clinical providers need to understand the evidence for efficacy (or lack thereof) and potential side effects. Some CAM practices have evidence to reject their use, such as secretin, whereas others have emerging evidence to support their use, such as melatonin. Most treatments have not been adequately studied and do not have evidence to support their use.

The treatment of individuals with autism is associated with fad, controversial, unsupported, disproven, and unvalidated treatments. Eclecticism is not the best approach for treating and educating children and adolescents who have autism. Applied behavior analysis (ABA) uses methods derived from scientifically established principles of behavior and incorporates all of the factors identified by the US National Research Council as characteristic of effective interventions in educational and treatment programs for children who have autism. ABA is a primary method of treating aberrant behavior in individuals who have autism. The only interventions that have been shown to produce comprehensive, lasting results in autism have been based on the principles of ABA.

Children with autism benefit from intensive, early intervention that focuses on increasing the frequency, form, and function of communicative acts. Available evidence shows that highly structured behavioral methods have important positive consequences for these children, particularly in eliciting first words. However, the limitation of these methods in maintenance and generalization of skills suggests that many children with autism will need to have these methods supplemented with less adult-directed activities to increase communicative initiation and carry over learned skills to new settings and communication partners. Providing opportunities for mediated peer interactions with trained peers in natural settings seems to be especially important in maximizing the effects of this intervention.

Social skill deficits are a pervasive and enduring feature of autism spectrum disorders (ASD). As such, social skills training (SST) should be a critical component of programming for youth with ASD. A number of SST strategies exist, including those employing social stories, video modeling interventions, social problem solving, pivotal response training, scripting procedures, computer-based interventions, priming procedures, prompting procedures, and self-monitoring. This article summarizes each intervention strategy and provides results from several research studies. Social skills assessment is a crucial first step to SST, and a number of assessment measures are described. Meta-analytic reviews of the research provide further recommendations for successful SST programs.

Self-injurious behaviors (SIB) are common in individuals who have autism and related developmental disabilities. When an individual engages in SIB, these behaviors frequently become the primary treatment target because of the potential for injury. A thorough behavioral assessment aimed at determining the function of the behaviors is the first step to developing a treatment plan. This article presents a brief background of SIB and a discussion of the behavioral assessment and treatment of these behaviors to familiarize readers with the behavioral perspective on SIB in individuals who have autism and other developmental disabilities.

Children diagnosed with autism or autism spectrum disorders (ASD) are more likely than other children to exhibit behaviors characteristic of a feeding or sleeping disorder. Parents of children with these disorders may be extremely concerned about the health and safety of their child. Sleeping and feeding problems can cause a great deal of stress to parents and other family members. Behavioral assessment and treatment procedures have been developed to address behavior problems related to sleeping and feeding disorders. This article reviews the literature about assessment and treatment, and provides recommendations regarding services to family members of individuals diagnosed with ASD and feeding or sleeping disorders.

The basis for the need for improved training and collaboration models in the field of autism is supported through historical background and literature in related fields. Ultimately, training specific to autism spectrum disorders and related evidence-based practices is proposed as necessary for all care providers having influence on programming related to this special population. It is also posited that the most effective avenue for training is through models incorporating more intensive and interactive training processes such as hands-on learning activities with opportunities for coaching, modeling, practice and feedback. Effective collaboration across systems (including home, medical, educational, and community settings) is emphasized to facilitate consistency in implementation of strategies for ultimate program success.

FORTHCOMING ISSUES

RECENT ISSUES

ELSEVIER
SAUNDERS

Child Adolesc Psychiatric Clin N Am
17 (2008) xiii–xiv

CHILD AND
ADOLESCENT
PSYCHIATRIC CLINICS
OF NORTH AMERICA

Foreword

Treating That Which We Now Know...

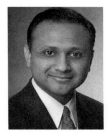

Harsh K. Trivedi, MD
Consulting Editor

Much progress has occurred in our ability to identify and differentially diagnose children and adolescents who are "in the spectrum." Even among providers who do not specialize in treating these youth, there has been an emerging appreciation for the many phenotypes of autism spectrum disorders (also known as pervasive developmental disorders). The early identification of these children has improved so much over recent years that there are some who are calling this an "autism epidemic." Without entering into the issue of whether these are new cases, or rather a better appreciation for what was already there, the focus of this issue is intentionally something quite different.

With many more youths being diagnosed as having autism spectrum disorders, the reality is that neither the number of treatment providers nor the availability of specialized services has increased dramatically. Certainly, any modest gains are not sufficient to meet the current need. Practically, what many of us have probably noticed in our own clinical work is that we find ourselves being referred and treating some of these affected youth.

Instead of creating an issue on the entire topic of autism spectrum disorders, a conscious effort has been made to focus this issue on treatment. Much is known at this time regarding treatments, both psychopharmacologic and psychotherapeutic, to help these youths. There is no doubt that significant advances will be made with autism spectrum disorders, as will occur in many other parts of our field. The intention here, however, was to create an issue that would serve as a resource for the current state of the art regarding treatments for autism spectrum disorders.

1056-4993/08/$ - see front matter © 2008 Elsevier Inc. All rights reserved.
doi:10.1016/j.chc.2008.08.001   *childpsych.theclinics.com*

I am grateful to David J. Posey and Christopher J. McDougle for creating such a thorough yet concise review of the major treatment modalities for autism spectrum disorders. I also thank each of the outstanding contributors for sharing their expertise and creating articles that are not only richly educational but also clinically invaluable. I have no doubt that we will get better at diagnosing and treating these youths as our research guides us forward. Let us focus our attention, however, on treating that which we now know.

Harsh K. Trivedi, MD
Bradley Hospital
Brown Medical School
1011 Veterans Memorial Parkway
East Providence, RI 02915, USA

E-mail address: harsh_trivedi@brown.edu

ELSEVIER
SAUNDERS

Child Adolesc Psychiatric Clin N Am
17 (2008) xv–xviii

CHILD AND
ADOLESCENT
PSYCHIATRIC CLINICS
OF NORTH AMERICA

Preface

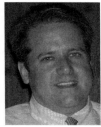 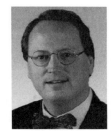

David J. Posey, MD, MS   Christopher J. McDougle, MD
Guest Editors

This issue of *Child and Adolescent Psychiatric Clinics of North America* is on the treatment of autism spectrum disorders (ASDs), also known as pervasive developmental disorders (PDDs). Typically diagnosed in childhood, these disorders cause lifelong and characteristic impairment in socialization, communication, and behavior. A number of specific "core" symptoms are found to varying degrees. These can include poor eye contact, deficits in other nonverbal behavior, social withdrawal, impairment in social interaction, echolalia, stereotypies, intense and circumscribed interests, and a preoccupation with parts of objects instead of the whole. These core impairments can range from mild to disabling. Autistic disorder (autism) is frequently associated with mental retardation, which contributes to impairment in functioning. Asperger's disorder and PDD not otherwise specified are less frequently associated with mental retardation. These three disorders represent the majority of patients seen clinically.

The increased prevalence of individuals receiving a diagnosis of an ASD has received widespread public attention and has led to occasional alarm about the emerging autism epidemic. Recent epidemiologic studies put prevalence rates at 0.6% for all ASDs, which is much higher than was thought to be 20 years ago [1]. Many experts in epidemiology believe that much of the increase can be accounted for by broadening or shifting diagnostic concepts, although this is not universally agreed upon. In essence, we may be diagnosing children who went undiagnosed or misdiagnosed in previous decades. This is underscored by some evidence suggesting that the most common

1056-4993/08/$ - see front matter © 2008 Elsevier Inc. All rights reserved.
doi:10.1016/j.chc.2008.07.001   *childpsych.theclinics.com*

ASD is actually PDD not otherwise specified [1]. Nevertheless, the high prevalence of these disorders makes it imperative that all physicians become aware of them so that they can make appropriate referrals for diagnosis, treatment, and services.

Child and adolescent psychiatrists and other mental health professionals will increasingly be called upon to provide treatment for children and adolescents with ASD. This may present challenges, as services for persons with developmental disabilities have frequently been administered and funded separately from those provided to persons with mental illness. Because there are often fewer resources for adults with ASDs, many child and adolescent psychiatrists continue to treat these individuals into adulthood.

The cause of autism is unknown. Evidence from twin and family studies indicates that autism is highly heritable. However, no single autism susceptibility gene has been consistently demonstrated to be important in a majority of cases [2]. Neurochemical investigations have identified abnormalities in monoamines, glutamate, gamma-amino hydroxybutyrate, and neuropeptides [3]. Functional neuroimaging studies are beginning to demonstrate differences between the brains of persons with autism and controls [4]. Brain regions potentially involved in ASDs are diverse and include the cerebellum [5], fusiform gyrus [6], amygdala [7], and prefrontal cortex [8,9].

This issue on ASDs is unique in that it is largely focused on treatment and less on the comprehensive characteristics and underlying neurobiology of autism. The reader interested in learning more on these topics may want to consult books by Volkmar and colleagues [10] and Moldin and Rubenstein [11], respectively. Instead, this issue delves into what we know about treating ASDs. It focuses on approaches to core symptoms and common behavioral problems and should serve as a resource for what treatments have been studied and what an appropriate treatment plan might include. The first six articles discuss various symptoms or aspects of autism that may be addressed with pharmacologic and medical approaches. The last six articles discuss behavioral and psychosocial interventions aimed at improving core deficits or problematic behaviors.

Drug treatments are not always necessary for every individual with an ASD. However, they frequently enhance the person's ability to benefit from educational and psychosocial interventions and can improve the quality of life for the individual and family [12]. Aman and colleagues [13] begin the issue with a review of medication treatments for inattention, overactivity, and impulsiveness. Surveys suggest that these "attention-deficit/hyperactivity disorder-like" symptoms are the most common problematic behaviors affecting youth with ASDs. Stigler and McDougle then review the research literature on the use of medications for irritability and associated aggression and self-injurious behavior. This research was integral in leading to Food and Drug Administration approval of the first medication specifically indicated for treating symptoms associated with autism, namely risperidone.

Interfering repetitive behaviors may also benefit from drug treatments. Soorya and colleageues describe these approaches in detail. Johnson and Malow then provide background on the characteristics of disordered sleep in autism and outline assessment and treatment principles. Posey and McDougle review challenges associated with conducting clinical trials of medication for social and communication impairment, as well as trials conducted for these core symptoms. Given the lack of effective treatments for the core symptoms of autism, it is little wonder that alternative treatments flourish. Finally, Levy and Hyman review the limited research literature on various alternative medical treatments that are so commonly sought by families.

Prior to considering medications for behavioral problems, clinicians should always attempt to implement behavioral therapy. Behavioral, educational, and psychosocial interventions are the cornerstone of treatment for individuals with ASDs. Experts in behavioral intervention are a crucial part of the multidisciplinary approach to autism. However, the dearth of suitably-trained behavioral therapists makes treatment planning difficult. Foxx reviews the principles of applied behavioral analysis, which are central to behavioral therapy and many other psychosocial interventions in autism.

The majority of children with ASDs will also need intensive and regular therapies aimed at improving their communication and socialization. Paul provides an overview of speech and language approaches aimed at improving communication in autism. Bellini and Peters describe the use of social skills training, which is especially helpful for individuals with higher-functioning ASDs.

Some behavioral problems in autism respond less well to drug interventions, making behavioral treatments even more necessary when addressing these problems. Self-injurious behavior (SIB) sometimes improves with medications aimed at reducing irritability, but many of our patients continue to exhibit severe SIB despite optimal medication use. Minshawi presents an article on the behavioral treatment of SIB that will be useful for all clinicians managing this difficult problem. Kodak and Piazza then provide behavioral approaches to treating disorders of feeding and sleeping.

One of the main challenges to quality treatment for children, adolescents, and adults with ASDs are the lack of professional care providers who have expertise in this area. Many families struggle with long waiting lists for appointments and lack of insurance reimbursement for particular treatments. The closing article by Swiezy and colleagues provides background and a hands-on model of training professional care providers that is both collaborative and practical.

This issue of the *Clinics* provides up-to-date reviews by experts in the area of ASDs treatment. It presents both psychopharmacologic and nonpharmacologic approaches. It dissects the myriad of problems individuals with ASD may present with into specific symptom areas that can be addressed through various treatment modalities. These symptom areas can then be addressed with an approach that is tailored to the specific situation of the individual.

It also will serve as a resource for child and adolescent psychiatrists and mental health professionals who treat these challenging disorders.

David J. Posey, MD, MS
Christian Sarkine Autism Treatment Center
Department of Psychiatry
Indiana University School of Medicine
Riley Hospital for Children, Room 4300
702 Barnhill Drive
Indianapolis, IN 46202, USA

E-mail address: dposey@iupui.edu

Christopher J. McDougle, MD
Christian Sarkine Autism Treatment Center
Department of Psychiatry
Indiana University School of Medicine
PB 2nd Floor, 1111 West 10th Street
Indianapolis, IN 46202-4800, USA

E-mail address: cmcdougl@iupui.edu

References

[1] Chakrabarti S, Fombonne E. Pervasive developmental disorders in preschool children: confirmation of high prevalence. Am J Psychiatry 2005;162(6):1133–41.
[2] Muhle R, Trentacoste SV, Rapin I. The genetics of autism. Pediatrics 2004;113(5):e472–86.
[3] McDougle CJ, Erickson CA, Stigler KA, et al. Neurochemistry in the pathophysiology of autism. J Clin Psychiatry 2005;66(Suppl. 10):9–18.
[4] Di Martino A, Castellanos FX. Functional neuroimaging of social cognition in pervasive developmental disorders: a brief review. Ann N Y Acad Sci 2003;1008:256–60.
[5] Allen G, Muller RA, Courchesne E. Cerebellar function in autism: functional magnetic resonance image activation during a simple motor task. Biol Psychiatry 2004;56(4):269–78.
[6] Schultz RT, Gauthier I, Klin A, et al. Abnormal ventral temporal cortical activity during face discrimination among individuals with autism and Asperger syndrome. Arch Gen Psychiatry 2000;57(4):331–40.
[7] Sweeten TL, Posey DJ, Shekhar A, et al. The amygdala and related structures in the pathophysiology of autism. Pharmacol Biochem Behav 2002;71(3):449–55.
[8] Luna B, Minshew NJ, Garver KE, et al. Neocortical system abnormalities in autism: an fMRI study of spatial working memory. Neurology 2002;59(6):834–40.
[9] Murphy DG, Critchley HD, Schmitz N, et al. Asperger syndrome: a proton magnetic resonance spectroscopy study of brain. Arch Gen Psychiatry 2002;59(10):885–91.
[10] Volkmar FR, Paul R, Klin A, editors. Handbook of Autism and Pervasive Developmental Disorders. Third ed. Hoboken, NJ: Wiley; 2005.
[11] Moldin SO, Robenstein JLR, editors. Understanding Autism: From Basic Neuroscience to Treatment. Boca Raton, FL: CRC Press; 2006.
[12] McDougle CJ. Psychopharmacology. In: Cohen DJ, Volkmar FR, editors. Handbook of Autism and Pervasive Developmental Disorders. Second edition. New York: John Wiley & Sons; 1997. p. 707–29.
[13] Lecavalier L. Behavioral and emotional problems in young people with pervasive developmental disorders: relative prevalence, effects of subject characteristics, and empirical classification. J Autism Dev Disord 2006;36(8):1101–14.

ELSEVIER
SAUNDERS

Child Adolesc Psychiatric Clin N Am
17 (2008) 713–738

CHILD AND
ADOLESCENT
PSYCHIATRIC CLINICS
OF NORTH AMERICA

Treatment of Inattention, Overactivity, and Impulsiveness in Autism Spectrum Disorders

Michael G. Aman, PhD[a,b,c,*], Cristan A. Farmer, MA[c,d],
Jill Hollway, MA[c,d], L. Eugene Arnold, Med, MD[b,c]

[a]Department of Psychology, Ohio State University, 225 Psychology Building,
1835 Neil Avenue, Columbus, OH 43210, USA
[b]Department of Psychiatry, Ohio State University, 1670 Upham Drive,
Columbus, OH 43210, USA
[c]The Nisonger Center UCEDD, Ohio State University, 1581 Dodd Drive,
Columbus, OH 43210-1296, USA
[d]Intellectual and Developmental Disability Psychology Program, The Nisonger Center,
McCampbell Hall, 1581 Dodd Drive, Columbus, OH 43210, USA

Research has shown that children with pervasive developmental disorders (PDDs) (autistic disorder, pervasive developmental disorder not otherwise specified [PDD-NOS] and Asperger's disorder) have very high rates of inattention, impulsivity, and overactivity, referred to here as attention-deficit/hyperactivity disorder (ADHD) symptoms. For example, Lecavalier [1] surveyed parents and teachers of 487 Ohio school children with the Nisonger Child Behavior Rating Form (NCBRF) [2], an instrument for assessing problems in young people with developmental disabilities. The percentages reported as displaying ADHD symptoms at moderate or severe levels were as follows:

Difficulty concentrating was a problem for 49% of children, according to parents, and 50% of children, according to teachers.
Prone to being easily distracted was a problem for 60% of children, according to parents, and 59% of children, according to teachers.
Fidgeting, wiggling, and squirming were problems for 42% of children, according to parents, and 43% of children, according to teachers.

This work was supported in part by Grant No. U10MH66768 from the National Institute of Mental Health.

* Corresponding author. The Nisonger Center, Room 175, Ohio State University, 1581 Dodd Drive, Columbus, OH 43210-1296.

E-mail address: aman.1@osu.edu (M.G. Aman).

childpsych.theclinics.com

Overactivity was a problem for 41% of children, according to parents, and 29% of children, according to teachers.

High energy levels were problems for 44% of children, according to parents, and 30% of children, according to teachers.

Short attention spans were problems for 54% of children, according to parents, and 47% of children, according to teachers.

Most impressively, these children did not represent a clinical sample, but were unselected children identified in the schools as having an autism spectrum disorder.

In this review, we summarize some of the key research that has been done in children with PDDs and ADHD symptoms. We conducted searches of Medline and PsycINFO using the following terms to capture reports on children with PDDs and ADHD symptoms: autism, PDD, Asperger's disorder, hyperactivity, and ADHD. We combined these terms with overarching drug categories, such as antidepressants, selective serotonin reuptake inhibitors (SSRIs), and individual examples of generic drugs belonging to the medication group (eg, imipramine, fluoxetine, venlafaxine). We then worked through the prominent groups of psychotropic agents with possible effects on ADHD symptoms. These included psychostimulants, noradrenergic reuptake inhibitors, antipsychotics, alpha-2 adrenergic agonists, antidepressants, cholinergic and other Alzheimer treatments, and "other" drugs (antiepileptic drug mood stabilizers, N-methyl-D-aspartate (NMDA) receptor antagonists).

Psychostimulants

Because of the volume of research on psychostimulants in patients with intellectual disability (ID) and ADHD symptoms and because of overlap of ID with patients having PDDs, we start with a brief comment on the ID/ADHD research. Arnold and colleagues [3] conducted an exhaustive review of stimulant effects and concluded that they do benefit many people with ID. They noted that most of the sound research was conducted with patients having mild and moderate ID and that efficacy in people with severe or profound ID has not been well demonstrated and may occur at lower rates. Aman and colleagues [4] studied 90 children with ID and ADHD, and reported that 44% of participants showed at least a 30% reduction compared with placebo on teacher ratings when treated once daily with a dose of 0.40 mg/kg methylphenidate. Using the same quantitative definition of response, Pearson and colleagues [5] found that 38% of children with ID receiving 0.30 mg/kg methylphenidate twice a day and 55% of those receiving 0.60 mg/kg methylphenidate twice a day showed a 30% advantage over placebo as rated by teachers on Conners' Abbreviated Symptom Questionnaire (CASQ).

Table 1 presents group studies of psychostimulant treatment in young people with PDDs and ADHD. The earliest studies [6,7] were conducted with preschoolers with autism (but not necessarily with ADHD symptoms) and therapeutic effects on ADHD symptoms were not observed. Furthermore, a variety of adverse events, including irritability, worse stereotypies, and increased hyperactivity, occurred in some children. However, we should not be overly influenced by these reports, as the children were not selected for ADHD symptoms and most of them were preschoolers. We now know that typical preschoolers often show a muted response to stimulants [8]. Five modest studies ran the gamut from totally uncontrolled [9], to confounded with time because of open-label design [10,11], to well controlled [12,13]. All of these reported at least some benefit in ADHD symptoms, and most also reported a variety of adverse events, including irritability, self-injury, social withdrawal, and insomnia. Response rates in these trials ranged from 46% [11] to 62% [13].

Santosh and colleagues [14] reported two comparisons involving children with ADHD plus autism spectrum disorder (ASD). In the first retrospective comparison of 113 children with "pure" ADHD (no ASD) and 61 children with ADHD plus ASD, the percentage of responders (Clinical Global Impression—Improvement [CGI-I] [15] scores of 1 or 2) [15] was 66.3% and 51%, respectively, which did not differ significantly. Remarkably, only 1.6% of the ADHD plus ASD group had bedwetting problems, and only 21.3% had "learning difficulties" (often used in the United Kingdom to refer to ID). In a companion trial that was part of the same publication, Santosh and colleagues [14] compared the progress of 25 "pure" ADHD patients with that of 27 ASD plus ADHD patients. They claimed more-or-less equivalent gains in both groups, although they did not report response rates and used independent t tests where a two-way analysis-of-variance model would have been more appropriate. They reported IQs as 95 for "pure" ADHD and 84 for ADHD plus ASD. These and the low rates of bedwetting (1.6%) and learning difficulties (21.3%) in the first study raise questions about the representativeness of participants with ASDs in these studies since they may have been quite "high-functioning."

The largest and best-controlled trial of stimulant treatment was conducted by the Research Units on Pediatric Psychopharmacology (RUPP) Autism Network [16,17] (see Table 1). Autistic disorder was the predominant diagnosis (74% of sample), but 26% of the sample had PDD-NOS or Asperger's disorder. Placebo and methylphenidate doses approximating 0.125, 0.25, and 0.50 mg/kg were given twice a day with a third dose, which was smaller, given in the late afternoon. As assessed by the Aberrant Behavior Checklist (ABC) [18,19] Hyperactivity subscale, parents rated their children as significantly improved compared with placebo on the low, medium, and high doses (with effect sizes, d, of 0.29, 0.54, and 0.40, respectively). The parent-rated Social Withdrawal subscale on the ABC was significantly worse on the high dose. Thirty-five of the 72 participants (49%) were classified as clinical responders to methylphenidate, whereas 13 participants (18%) exited the study because of intolerable side effects. Irritability,

Table 1
Studies of psychostimulants in young people with PDDs

Investigators	Subjects	Treatment and design	Outcome by variable
Campbell et al, 1972	16 children, ages 3–6 y (mean 4.3 y), with autistic disorder, treated as inpatients; subjects not selected for ADHD symptoms; IQ 28–96	Open-label trial, lasting 3–4 d, comparing baseline with d-amphetamine (mean dose 4.8 mg)	Nonsignificantly worse behavior on CGI (no drug > d-amphetamine); nonsignificantly worse behavior on Fish Symptom Severity Scale (no drug > d-amphetamine); adverse events reported: irritability, hyperactivity, and appetite loss commonly occurring
Campbell et al, 1976	11 children, ages 3–6 y (mean 5.4 y), with autistic disorder, treated as inpatients; IQ 36–90	Levoamphetamine (crossed with levodopa) and with 4-wk washout between active drugs; levoamphetamine dose 3.5–42 mg/d (mean 13.4 mg/d); duration of levoamphetamine 4–12 wk (mean 8.3 wk)	On CGI—Improvement subscale, 7 subjects rated worse, 2 rated as unchanged, and 2 as minimally improved; no change on CGI—Severity scale; hyperactivity declined in 5 of 7 subjects with the symptom; adverse events reported: loss of appetite 7, weight 6, worsening of pre-existing and de novo stereotypies 9, worsening of self-injury 3, worsening of excitability 1
Hoshino et al, 1977	15 children with autism, ages 2–13 y (mean 7.0 y); all but 1 were boys; not clear whether ADHD symptoms problematic at outset	Open-label, variable duration (2 wk–1 y) trial of methylphenidate (0.3–1.0 mg/kg/d); average treatment duration 6.5 mo; no inferential statistics	Werry, Weiss, Peters Activity Scale (parent rated): baseline score 29.9; endpoint 21.9; 6 subjects rated as substantially improved on Werry, Weiss, Peters Activity Scale; 9 cases (60%) considered substantially improved clinically; adverse events: irritability 6 (40%), insomnia 5 (33%), self-injury or aggression 4 (27%), diarrhea 3 (20%)
Birmaher et al, 1988	9 children, ages 4–16 y (mean not reported), with autism and significant ADHD symptoms	Uncontrolled group study comparing 1-week baseline (no drug) with methylphenidate given in doses of 10–50 mg/d (mean dose 25 mg/d) on bid basis for 2 wk	Conners' Parent Rating Scale: methylphenidate > baseline; Conners' Teacher Rating Scale: methylphenidate > baseline; Children's Psychiatric Rating Scale (total score): methylphenidate > baseline. Adverse events reported: mild initial insomnia

Reference	Subjects	Design	Results
Quintana et al, 1995	10 children with autism and symptoms of ADHD; developmental quotient 50–84 (mean 64.3); age 7–11 y (mean 8.5 y)	Double-blind placebo-controlled crossover, with 2 wk on each drug condition; dose was 10 mg methylphenidate bid in first wk and 20 mg in second wk; no drug confounds	Conners' Parent Rating Scale: baseline = methylphenidate; doctor-completed ABC Hyperactivity: methylphenidate > placebo; doctor-completed Connor's Teacher Questionnaire: methylphenidate > placebo; number of clinical responders not reported; investigators characterized findings as significant but modest
Handen et al, 2000	13 children with PDDs and symptoms of ADHD; 9 had autism and 4 had PDD-NOS; 10 boys and 3 girls; age 5.6–11.2 y (mean 7.4 y); 11 of 13 had ID	Double-blind placebo-controlled crossover with treatment trials of 1 wk; placebo compared with methylphenidate 0.3 mg/kg/d and 0.6 mg/kg/d, given 2 or 3 times per d; high dose always followed low dose	Conners' Abbreviated Symptom Questionnaire: high, low > placebo; IOWA Conners' Scale: low > placebo; ABC Hyperactivity: high > placebo; ABC Inappropriate Speech: low, high > placebo; all comparisons based on teacher ratings; adverse events associated with methylphenidate: social withdrawal, dullness, sadness, irritability; 1 child unable to tolerate methylphenidate; 8 (62%) participants subsequently treated clinically with 0.2 to 0.6 mg/kg/d methylphenidate
Di Martino et al, 2004	13 children; 7 with autism, 3 with PDD-NOS, 3 with Asperger's disorder, all with ADHD symptoms; moderate or greater hyperactivity on Hyperactivity subscale of CPRS and t-score ≥ 60 on Conners' Parent and Teacher Revised Scale; age 5–13 y (mean 7.9 y)	Test trial: acute 1-hour open trial with 0.4 mg/kg methylphenidate; efficacy trial: open-label trial, extending from 1 wk (nonresponders) to 3 mo (responders)	Test trial: On CGI—Improvement, 5 children were terminated, 2 had worse hyperactivity, 1 had worse stereotypic behavior, 1 had dysphoria, and 1 had motor tics; 8 children entered remainder of trial. Week 1: 6 of 8 subjects rated 2 or 3 on CGI and followed for 3 mo; 2 subjects unchanged on CGI—Improvement and terminated. 3-Mo comparison: Conners' Parent/Teacher Rating Scales-Revised: Hyperactivity: methylphenidate > placebo; ADHD Index: methylphenidate > placebo; ADHD/DSM total: methylphenidate > placebo (all findings true of parent and teacher ratings). As 5 subjects terminated after test dose and 2 terminated after 1 week, only 6 subjects completed trial; 6 of original 13 subjects (46%) had positive response to methylphenidate

(continued on next page)

Table 1
(*continued*)

Investigators	Subjects	Treatment and design	Outcome by variable
RUPP, 2005	72 children with PDD and ADHD symptoms, ages 5–14 y (mean 7.5 y); 47 (65%) had autism; 14 (19%) had PDD-NOS, 5 (7%) had Asperger's disorder	Methylphenidate: low, medium, high doses (~0.125, 0.250, 0.500 mg/kg) given 3 times daily (last dose about half of morning and midday doses); double-blind crossover placebo-controlled, 1-wk treatment phases	6 subjects (8.3%) did not survive test-dose phase; 1 dropped out before crossover; parent-rated ABC Hyperactivity: low, medium, high > placebo; effect sizes 0.29 (low), 0.54 (medium), and 0.40 (high); parent-rated ABC Social Withdrawal: placebo > high dose (indicates worsening with methylphenidate; effect size 0.37); 35 of 72 subjects (49%) were responders; CGI—Improvement: medium dose > placebo
Santosh et al, 2006 (a)	113 children with "pure" ADHD and 61 children with ASD (by consensus) and ADHD. Mean ages were 13.14 y for children with "pure" ADHD and 12.43 y for children with ADHD and ASD	Open-label, of variable duration; no controls with retrospective ratings from clinical notes; doses did not differ between groups; no data about concomitant treatment or drugs	CGI—Improvement: did not differ statistically between groups; CGI—Improvement 1 or 2 for 63% of ADHD-only group and 51% of ADHD plus ASD group (*P* not reported); efficacy index, taken from CGI: although marginal difference (*P* = .06) favoring ADHD plus ASD, the index did not correspond to the official NIMH form
Santosh et al, 2006 (b)	25 children with "pure" ADHD and 27 children with ADHD and ASD; mean ages were 11.6 y for children with pure ADHD and 10.6 y for children with ADHD and ASD; mean IQs were 95.2 and 84.3, respectively	Open-label trial, of variable duration, with prospective ratings done at baseline and "follow-up" (1–6 mo later; mean 87 d); no control condition or blindness; no data on concomitant treatment or drugs	Internet-based "profile of neuropsychiatric symptoms" used; as assessed by separate *t* tests, both groups improved on hyperactivity, impulsivity, inattention, oppositionality, aggression, and intermittent explosive rage; to properly test for differential effect, 2 × 2 analysis of variance should have been used; CGI, inappropriately analyzed by *t* tests, improved in both groups; response rates not reported

| Posey et al, 2007 | 66 children (of 72 reported in RUPP (2005) with PDD and ADHD symptoms, ages 5–14 y (mean 7.5 y) | Methylphenidate: low-dose (0.125 mg/kg), medium-dose (0.25 mg/kg), and high-dose (0.50 mg/kg) conditions; double-blind placebo-controlled crossover, 1-wk treatment phases | Parent-rated SNAP Hyperactivity: low, medium, high > placebo; teacher-rated SNAP Hyperactivity: medium, high > placebo; low = placebo; parent-rated SNAP ODD: low, medium, high = placebo; teacher-rated SNAP ODD: low, medium, high = placebo; IQ, age, type of PDD did not moderate outcome |

Abbreviations: ABC, Aberrant Behavior Checklist; ASD, Autism spectrum disorder; CGI, Clinical Global Impression; CPRS, Children's Psychiatric Rating Scale; IOWA, Inattention/Overactivity With Aggression; NIMH, National Institute of Mental Health; RUPP, Research Units on Pediatric Psychopharmacology; SNAP, Swanson, Nolan, and Pelham scale; >, better response than; =, no change or equal response compared to.

emotional outbursts, and initial insomnia were the most problematic adverse events.

Posey and colleagues [17] reported additional findings from the RUPP study. On the Swanson, Nolen, and Pelham (SNAP) rating scale (http://www.adhd.net/snap-iv-instructions.pdf) [20], parents rated the children as significantly improved on all three doses. On the teacher-rated SNAP Hyperactivity subscale, the medium and high doses produced significant improvement compared with placebo; the low dose failed to separate from placebo. Posey and colleagues examined age, IQ, and autism versus other PDDs as possible moderators, but none of them influenced outcome.

All in all, the stimulants tend to produce highly variable responses in children with PDDs and ADHD symptoms. Such responses range from substantial improvement with minor side effects through to more problematic behavior and physical or behavioral side effects. Given what we know, stimulants would still be a reasonable first therapeutic choice for previously untreated children with PDDs and uncomplicated ADHD, even though they do not work as well, on average, as they do in typically developing children. Any side effects should be reversible on discontinuing the drug. Clinicians should be candid with parents about the lower likelihood of a positive clinical response and elevated risk of adverse events. Treatment should proceed with low initial doses, small dose increments, and a data-based approach. Both clinicians and parents should be prepared to stop the trial if there is clear evidence of behavioral deterioration or unacceptable adverse events.

Atomoxetine

Atomoxetine (Strattera) is a relatively new noradrenergic reuptake inhibitor frequently used to control symptoms of ADHD in typically developing children. Jou and colleagues [21] were first to report on the effects of atomoxetine on hyperactivity and inattention in children with PDDs. Twenty patients (10 dually diagnosed with mental retardation; 16 with autism, 2 with Asperger's disorder, and 2 with PDD-NOS) were openly treated with atomoxetine for an average of 19.5 weeks. Sixteen (80%) received concomitant medications but no changes in dose or titration in co-therapy were made during the course of the study. Conners' Parent Rating Scale (Conners' PRS) [22] was the main outcome measure. Significant improvement between baseline and endpoint was reported for the Hyperactivity and Inattention subscales. The average baseline Hyperactivity score of 17.1 improved to 13.0 ($t = 3.86$, $P < .001$, $d = 1.77$), while baseline and endpoint Inattention scores were 7.5 and 5.8, respectively ($t = 3.1$, $P = .01$, $d = 1.42$). Twelve (60%) of the participants were responders to atomoxetine based on the CGI-I scores of 1 or 2.

Troost and colleagues [23] did a pilot study of atomoxetine in 12 children with PDD (6 with autism, 5 with PDD-NOS, and 1 with Asperger's disorder). Patients were washed out of psychoactive drugs and treated openly with atomoxetine. Five subjects (42%) discontinued after at least 6 weeks because of side effects, including gastrointestinal complaints. The parent-rated investigator-scored ADHD Rating Scale-IV (ADHD-RS) [24], Conners' PRS, and the ABC were outcome measures. The endpoint total score of the ADHD-RS significantly decreased from a baseline average of 40.33 to 22.42 ($P = .003$, $d = 2.30$). A significant improvement occurred in the Conners' PRS ADHD Index between baseline and endpoint (24.25 and 18.67, respectively; $P = .023$, $d = 0.65$). The Hyperactivity subscale of the Conners' PRS showed a significant reduction from 9.83 to 6.67 ($P = .03$, $d = 0.63$), but the change on the ABC Hyperactivity subscale failed to reach significance (baseline 23.58, endpoint 18.67, $P = .07$). The investigators felt that gastrointestinal symptoms were more severe in their participants than observed in typically developing children, and they speculated that children with PDD may be more susceptible to such effects.

Posey and colleagues [25] conducted an 8-week open-label pilot study that included 16 children with PDDs (7 with autism, 7 with Asperger's disorder, and 2 with PDD-NOS), hyperactivity, and a nonverbal IQ of at least 70. Participants began with a dose of 0.5 mg/kg/d, which was titrated to 1.2 mg/kg/d in the third week. The CGI—Severity (CGI-S) subscale was the primary outcome measure; secondary measures included the ABC, the SNAP-IV, and Conners' Continuous Performance Test (CPT) [26]. After 8 weeks, there was a significant reduction on the CGI-S (5.1 to 3.9; $F_{1,15} = 17.86$, $P = .001$; $d = 1.09$). The ratings of both parents and teachers on the SNAP-IV decreased significantly (44.4 to 22.6, $d = 1.9$; 29.6 to 14.7, $d = 1.4$, respectively; $P < .0001$). Both parents and teachers saw, in addition to decreases on several other subscales of the ABC, improvement on the Hyperactivity subscale (28.4 to 14.2, $P = .0004$, $d = 1.9$; 18.2 to 8.4, $P < .0001$, $d = 1.0$, respectively). No differences were found on the Conners' CPT, which is consistent with a study in typically developing adults with ADHD [27].

Arnold and colleagues [28] completed the first placebo-controlled trial of atomoxetine in children with PDDs. This double-blind pilot study used a crossover design where each condition lasted for 6 weeks (3-week titration), followed by a 1-week washout period. The primary outcome measures were the ABC Hyperactivity subscale, the CGI-I , CGI-S, and SNAP Hyperactivity subscale (each rated on a scale of 0–3). Sixteen children were randomized, and 3 terminated early (2 because of lack of effect with placebo; 1 because of adverse events with atomoxetine). "Responder" status was achieved by a 25% decrease on ABC Hyperactivity subscale and a 1 or 2 on the CGI-I. Nine children (56%) responded to atomoxetine, whereas 4 (25%) responded to placebo. This response rate is lower than that found in studies with typically developing children, although slightly better than the response rate found in the RUPP study using methylphenidate in children with PDD [16]. The slope of response on time was compared for the outcome measures. The slopes for atomoxetine and placebo were significantly different on the ABC Hyperactivity subscale (-5.00 versus 0.56, respectively, $P = .04$; $d = 0.90$) and SNAP Hyperactivity (-5.87 versus -0.82, $P = .005$, $d = 1.27$). The effect sizes of the placebo-controlled impact of atomoxetine on ADHD symptoms were comparable to those found in typically developing children [29–31]. The low incidence of adverse events was impressive; 2 of the 3 individuals who terminated early were in the placebo group. The investigators suggested that future research include a parallel group design to alleviate carryover effects.

Together, these studies suggest that atomoxetine may be useful for controlling ADHD symptoms in children with PDD. Although effect sizes were generally large, this likely was due in part to the open-label design of most studies. In general, the side effects profile appeared to be mild, including mostly tolerable gastrointestinal effects. However, this evidence is preliminary; no large, placebo-controlled, parallel design trials have been published. To our knowledge, no study thus far (either with children having a form of PDD or in typically developing children with ADHD) has demonstrated significant effects of atomoxetine on cognition [25,28,32]. If correct, this stands in contrast to psychostimulants, where enhancement of sustained attention and other performance tests is the norm. This would reflect a true qualitative difference in mode of action between atomoxetine and psychostimulants. It may be tempting to discount atomoxetine because of this, but it is well to remember that no long-term study of the psychostimulants in typically developing children has demonstrated academic gains due to active treatment.

Antipsychotics

Classical antipsychotics

Predictably, most of the work on classical antipsychotics used small sample sizes, and much of it was poorly designed. Waizer and colleagues [33] assessed open-label thiothixene in 18 outpatient "schizophrenic" children diagnosed with Creak's criteria. The children (ages 5–13 years, mean 9.4 years) were rated as significantly improved on ratings of psychomotor activity (36% reduction) and concentration (9%) with a mean dose of 17 mg/d.

Probably the best study of classical antipsychotics came from Magda Campbell's laboratory at New York University [34]. In this investigation, 40 inpatient children, ages 2 to 6 years (mean 4.6 years) with autism were treated over 4 weeks with one of two sequences of medication: haloperidol, placebo, haloperidol; or placebo, haloperidol, placebo. Outcome measures included the Children's Psychiatric Rating Scale (CPRS) [35], CASQ, and the CGI. On the CPRS, the children were rated by clinicians as having significantly less hyperactivity and fidgetiness (both $Ps < .01$)

with haloperidol. The children were rated by their teachers as having significantly lower CASQ scores with haloperidol, and clinicians rated the children as more improved with haloperidol on both the CGI-S and CGI-I. Unfortunately, 11 of the 40 participants (28%) developed dystonic reactions at some stage. In one follow-up study of 118 autistic children treated for 6 to 12 months, Campbell and colleagues [36] found that 34 subjects (29%) showed withdrawal dyskinesias on placebo substitution and 4 subjects (3.4%) showed tardive dyskinesia (total prevalence of dyskinesia of 38 [32.2%]). Despite the positive effects on ADHD symptoms in the acute study, one would want to be very conservative and use haloperidol only where target symptoms are quite extreme in young patients with PDDs.

Atypical antipsychotics

Risperidone

In contrast to conventional antipsychotics, novel agents are reported to activate dopamine neurons in prefrontal cortex and limbic regions (eg, nucleus accumbens) with lower effect in the striatum [37]. Risperidone is such a novel agent. In addition, risperidone has greater $5\text{-}HT_2$ blockade than D_2 blockade. Because risperidone is better researched than the others, we present only controlled studies with risperidone.

Four controlled studies of risperidone in children with PDDs have targeted inattentiveness and hyperactivity (Table 2). The RUPP Autism Network [38] conducted a randomized controlled study of 101 children with autism and disruptive behavior, including hyperactivity. Scores on the ABC Hyperactivity subscale were markedly and significantly lower for risperidone compared with placebo after 8 weeks of treatment ($d = 1.00$). Shea and colleagues [39] also conducted an 8-week, controlled trial and reported significant ABC Hyperactivity subscale reductions. On the parent-rated NCBRF Hyperactive subscale, risperidone produced significant reductions. The effect sizes were smaller in the trial of Shea and colleagues than in the RUPP study, probably because subjects were not selected for extreme behavior in the trial of Shea and colleagues.

Hellings and colleagues [40] randomized subjects first to placebo and then to two risperidone dosing schedules (low and high). In this double-blind placebo-controlled crossover study, the ABC Hyperactivity subscale showed moderate improvements at both a low dose ($d = 0.58$) and a high dose ($d = 0.41$) of risperidone (see Table 2). Finally, Troost and colleagues [41] conducted an open-label study of risperidone with a double-blind placebo-controlled discontinuation phase. The outcome measures were from focused-attention and divided-attention tasks. At endpoint of the open-label (week 24), half of the subjects were tapered off risperidone to placebo over an 8-week period. There were no significant drug group differences on focused attention, but the risperidone group performed better on the divided-attention task in reaction time hits and reaction time for correct

Table 2
Studies of antipsychotics in young people with PDDs

Investigators	Subjects	Treatment and design	Outcome by variable
RUPP, 2002	Children ages 5–17 y (mean 8.8 y); 82 males, 19 females; autistic disorder and serious behavioral problems; N = 101	Double-blind placebo-controlled parallel groups; mean daily dose of risperidone at endpoint was 1.8 mg (range 0.5–3.5 mg); 8-wk acute trial	34 of 49 subjects (69.4%) were risperidone responders; parent-rated ABC Hyperactivity: risperidone > placebo; effect size 1.0; parent-rated ABC Irritability: risperidone > placebo; effect size 1.2; parent-rated ABC Stereotypy: risperidone > placebo; effect size 0.8; clinician-rated CGI-I: risperidone > placebo
Shea et al, 2004	Children, ages 5–12 y (mean 7.45 y); 61 males and 18 females with PDDs; no specific behavioral entry criteria; N = 79	Double-blind placebo-controlled parallel groups; mean daily dose at endpoint 1.48 mg risperidone oral solution; 8-wk acute trial	77 subjects were included in the intent-to-treat efficacy sample; risperidone-treated subjects given lower (better) scores; parent-rated ABC Hyperactivity: risperidone > placebo ($P \leq .001$); parent-rated NCBRF Hyperactive: risperidone > placebo ($P \leq .05$); clinician-rated CGI-I risperidone > placebo
Troost et al, 2005	Children, ages 5–17 y (mean 9.1 y); 22 males and 2 females with PDDs and serious behavioral problems; N = 24	24 wk of open-label risperidone followed by an 8-wk double-blind placebo-controlled discontinuation of risperidone; mean daily dose 1.7 mg	26 subjects met criteria as risperidone responders; 2 subjects terminated early because of weight gain. Parent-rated ABC Hyperactivity subscale: risperidone = placebo ($P = .12$)
Hellings et al, 2006	Children, adolescents, adults, ages 8–56 y (mean 22.0 y), 23 males and 17 females with PDD (n = 36) or ID (n = 4); presence of serious behavioral problems; N = 40	Double-blind placebo-controlled crossover with discontinuation to placebo; low dose = 1 mg bid; high dose = 2 mg/bid; mean daily dose at endpoint for children and adolescents was 1.67 mg and for adults 1.52 mg risperidone oral solution	87.5% of subjects met the criteria as partial or full risperidone responders; parent-rated ABC Hyperactivity: risperidone low dose > placebo 1 and 2 (averaged effect size 0.58; parent-rated ABC Hyperactivity: risperidone high dose > placebo 1 and 2 (averaged effect size 0.41); unable to locate P values for ABC Hyperactivity subscale

Troost et al, 2006	Children, 5–17 y (mean 10.1 y); 22 males and 2 females with PDDs and serious behavioral problems; N = 24	24 wk of open-label risperidone followed by 8-wk double-blind placebo-controlled discontinuation of risperidone; mean dose 1.7 mg/d	12–14 subjects provided valid measures for focused-attention task and divided-attention task following discontinuation phase; significant differences between treatment groups on divided-attention task and reaction time hits under lighter of two memory loads, risperidone > placebo ($\eta^2 = 0.36$); significant difference between groups in reaction time correct rejections during lighter memory load; risperidone > placebo ($\eta^2 = 0.37$); focused attention task: placebo = risperidone
Corson et al, 2004	20 young people with autism, ages 5–28 y (mean 12.1 y), 16 males and 4 females; 12 with autism and 8 with PDD-NOS	Retrospective, nonblinded clinical trials with quetiapine (25–600 mg/d; mean 198 mg/d) over 4–180 wk (mean 60 wk); 5 subjects received other medication	CGI, based on composite of aggression, self-injury, irritability, and hyperactivity: 8 of 20 participants (40%) regarded as responders based on CGI-I score of much improved (n = 6) or very much improved (n = 2)
Hardan et al, 2005	10 young patients, ages 5–19 y (mean 12.0 y) with autism (n = 7) or PDD-NOS (n = 3); 8 males and 4 females	Retrospective nonblind chart review of consecutive patients treated with quetiapine (200–800 mg/d; mean 477 mg/d); 6 subjects received constant doses of other psychotropic drugs; duration of trials from 10–48 wk (mean 22.0 wk)	Parent ratings on Conners' PRS (Goyette et al, 1978): Conduct problem: quetiapine > placebo, (effect size 0.49); Inattention: quetiapine > placebo (effect size 0.93); Hyperactivity, quetiapine > placebo (effect size 0.63); no difference in effects on Psychosomatic, Learning, or Anxiety subscales
Malone et al, 2007	12 adolescents with autism, ages 12–18 y (mean 14.5 y); 2 enrolled as inpatients, 10 as outpatients	Open-label, 6-wk trial of ziprasidone, at 40–160 mg/d (mean 98.3 mg/d); no other medicines permitted; nonblind	ABC Hyperactivity: ziprasidone > baseline (effect size 0.36; CPRS Hyperactivity: ziprasidone = baseline; other: body mass index declined nonsignificantly; Corrected QT interval increased by 14.7 ms ($P = .04$); not clinically significant

(continued on next page)

Table 2
(continued)

Investigators	Subjects	Treatment and design	Outcome by variable
Valicenti-McDermott and Demb, 2006	32 young people, ages 5–19 y (mean 10.9 y); 23 (72%) males, 9 (28%) females; participants chosen for a multitude of "developmental disabilities," including mental retardation (n = 18), autism (n = 15), and PDD (n = 3)	Retrospective chart review of patients who were switched to aripiprazole from multiple other drugs or initiated de novo (n = 4) on aripiprazole; duration of treatment 6–15 months; no standardized behavioral instruments used during treatment	Improvement in hyperactivity occurred in 10 of 21 with the target symptom (48%) and in 5 of 13 children (38%) with a target symptom of impulsivity (disorder not specified); aripiprazole effective in 9 of 24 children (37%) with "autism spectrum disorder," including 4 of 5 children (80%) with "multiple complex developmental disorder"; 6 of 12 children with PDDs with hyperactivity listed as a target symptom were regarded as improved

Abbreviations: >, effect was statistically greater than; =, effect was not statistically different.

rejections. However, the parent-rated ABC Hyperactivity subscale showed no significant group differences [42].

When participants were admitted because of extreme behavior, risperidone had significant and important effects on ADHD symptoms. The effects on attention tests require replication, but they also suggested improvement.

Other atypical antipsychotics

Unfortunately there is no well-controlled research known to us that addresses the effects of other atypical antipsychotics on hyperactivity. We summarize the evidence on quetiapine, ziprasidone, and aripiprazole (see Table 2). The two retrospective reports on quetiapine reported overall gains on the CGI-I, which was based in part on hyperactivity [43], and CPRS parent ratings of inattention and hyperactivity [44]. One very small open-label study of ziprasidone found significant improvement on the ABC Hyperactivity subscale but not on the CPRS Hyperactivity scale [45]. Valicenti-McDermott and Demb [46] described outcomes for a heterogeneous group of young people with "developmental disabilities." Improvement in hyperactivity occurred for 10 of 21 children (48%) with ADHD symptoms as a target of treatment. The investigators felt that children with PDDs responded less well than the other participants.

Alpha-2 adrenergic agonists

Clonidine and guanfacine act on alpha-2 adrenergic presynaptic receptors to inhibit noradrenergic release and synaptic transmission [37]. Guanfacine has a longer action than clonidine has.

Clonidine

Two small studies have investigated clonidine for hyperactivity in autistic disorder. Fankhauser and colleagues [47] conducted a double-blind placebo-controlled crossover study of the clonidine transdermal patch (approximately 0.005 mg/kg/d) in seven autistic males ages 5 to 33 years (mean age 12.9 years) exhibiting "hyperarousal." The parent-rated CASQ did not show a significant difference between groups in hyperactivity and inattentiveness at endpoint. However, CGI-I ratings showed significant gains ($P < .0001$). Jaselskis and colleagues [48] conducted a 12-week double-blind placebo-controlled crossover study of clonidine (0.15–0.20 mg/d) in eight males with autistic disorder and hyperactivity. The results were mixed, showing a significant improvement in ADHD symptoms on the parent-rated CASQ ($P = .03$; $d = .57$) and the teacher-rated ABC Hyperactivity subscale ($P = .03$; $d = .34$), but not on the clinician-rated CPRS Hyperactivity subscale.

Guanfacine

Two studies about guanfacine have been reported. Posey and colleagues [49] conducted a retrospective study of guanfacine in children with target symptoms, including inattentiveness and hyperactivity. Eighty subjects (10 female, 70 males), with a mean age of 7.7 years, met the criteria of a PDD diagnosis and history of guanfacine pharmacotherapy. A determination of global severity and global improvement (based on interfering behaviors, including ADHD symptoms) was made by subjects' treating psychiatrists. Guanfacine was associated with a statistically significant improvement in CGI-S ratings ($P < .001$; $d = 0.58$).

Scahill and colleagues [50] conducted an 8-week open trial of guanfacine in 25 children (23 boys and 2 girls) with a mean age of 9.0 years and a diagnosis of PDD accompanied by hyperactivity. All 25 had failed to respond or could not tolerate methylphenidate. Outcome measures included parent and teacher ratings on the ABC, SNAP-IV, and CGI-I. Dosage ranged from 1.0 to 3.0 mg/d, split into two or three doses. The results showed significant improvement on the parent-rated ABC Hyperactivity subscale ($P < .001$; $d = 1.4$) and the SNAP-IV Hyperactivity subscale ($P < .0001$; $d = 1.5$). Teacher ratings also reflected significant improvement on ABC Hyperactivity ($P < .01$; $d = 0.83$) and on the SNAP-IV ($P = .01$; $d = 0.56$). Forty-eight percent of subjects were rated *much improved* or *very much improved* on the CGI-I. Four subjects terminated early due to irritability and 1 due to agitation.

Antidepressants

Tricyclic antidepressants

Tricyclic antidepressants have a long history of use for ADHD symptoms in typically developing children [51] and in adults. In recent years, however, growing concern about potentially serious cardiovascular effects has curbed the use of this class in children. The literature regarding tricyclic antidepressants in children with developmental disabilities is limited. Gordon and colleagues [52] compared the use of clomipramine and desipramine to treat the associated behaviors of autism in seven children with the disorder. The subjects took part in a 10-week double-blind randomized crossover trial, following 2 weeks of a single-blind placebo period. On the CPRS Hyperactivity subscale, the effects of clomipramine and desipramine after 5 weeks were significantly different from the effects of placebo (115% improvement, 80% improvement, and 2% improvement, respectively; $F = 4.62$, $P = .05$, $d = 1.11$), but not from each other.

Gordon and colleagues [53] followed the 1992 report with a larger double-blind comparison of clomipramine, desipramine, and placebo. Twelve children with autism completed a 10-week double-blind crossover study of clomipramine and placebo, and 12 different subjects with autism participated in an identical study of clomipramine and desipramine. The same pattern of results as in the earlier report was found: Both desipramine and clomipramine had significantly greater effects than placebo on hyperactivity ($F = 14.4$, $P = .0001$, $d = 1.32$), but they were not significantly different from one another. Medication was reduced for 2 patients who experienced cardiac effects with clomipramine (1 experienced tachycardia, another delayed conduction). A third subject had a generalized tonic-clonic seizure. To the best of our knowledge, these promising effects on ADHD symptoms have not been pursued in subsequent research.

Selective serotonin reuptake inhibitors

There are several older reports of fluoxetine (Prozac), an SSRI, for depression in adolescents and adults with autism [54,55], although the only purely adolescent sample was that of Fatemi and colleagues [56]. This open trial included seven patients with autism who had been treated with fluoxetine in the previous 6 years (for an average of 18 months). Mean baseline and endpoint scores on the ABC were compared, and a significant drop was observed in all subscales except Hyperactivity, which increased by 14% (22.21 to 25.80, significance not reported). Although fluoxetine seemed to be beneficial for some autism symptoms, the increase in hyperactivity may be a limiting factor.

There are several reports that venlafaxine, a serotonin-norepinephrine reuptake inhibitor, was useful in young adults with PDD. However, these effects did not seem to appear in children. Hollander and colleagues [57] completed an open-label study of 10 individuals with PDDs. The sample included 8 children (1 with PDD-NOS, 4 with Asperger's disorder, and 3 with autism) and 2 adults. Results were presented qualitatively: Four of the 8 children experienced significant hyperactivity/restlessness as an adverse event of the drug, although 6 of 8 were considered responders (ie, a "much improved" or "very much improved" rating on the CGI-I addressing the core symptoms of autism). The investigators concluded that venlafaxine may bring about some improvement to the core symptoms of autism, although it appeared to exacerbate hyperactivity.

The remaining reports of SSRIs in individuals with autism were specific to symptoms of depression or did not include children. It appears that tricyclic antidepressants may have some role in managing ADHD symptoms in children with PDDs, although potential cardiac effects warrant cautious use. There is little reason to believe that the SSRIs or venlafaxine have utility for managing ADHD symptoms in young people with PDDs and, in fact, they may exacerbate ADHD symptoms.

Anxiolytic agents

The literature on use of anxiolytic agents to control ADHD symptoms in typically developing children is both sparse and weak [58]. Benzodiazepine anxiolytics may produce significant side effects as well as dependence, withdrawal, and rebound symptoms. Not surprisingly, there are no respectable studies of these drugs in children with PDDs.

Two reports of buspirone, which has mixed pharmacologic action on dopamine and serotonin receptors and is marketed as an anxiolytic, were located. Realmuto and colleagues [59] published a case study of four subjects with autism and mild-to-moderate mental retardation. Hyperactivity was a target symptom for three. Each child received 5 mg of buspirone, open-label, three times daily for 4 weeks, followed by methylphenidate or fenfluramine for 4 more weeks. Parents completed the ABC, and teachers completed Conners' Teacher's Rating Scale (Conners' TRS) [60]. Only qualitative data were reported. Two children showed "improvement" in hyperactivity. Another child did not respond to initial treatment. When switched to fenfluramine, he experienced worsening of ADHD symptoms, which improved again when he returned to buspirone.

In a "single-subject study" [61], a child with autism and ADHD symptoms received 3 weeks of placebo, followed by washout and 3 weeks of buspirone (10 mg/d). Improvements on blinded ratings on the CASQ failed to reach significance, although a reliable linear improvement was seen in the number of daily performance tasks completed at school with buspirone.

We were able to find only one other study examining the use of anxiolytic agents in children with PDD, this being with a benzodiazapine. Marrosu and colleagues [62] administered diazepam to seven children with infantile autism (*Diagnostic and Statistical Manual of Mental Disorders, Third Edition*) and disruptive anxiety attacks. Diazepam was given intramuscularly when the children experienced anxiety attacks significant enough to disrupt the class they were attending. Children were rated on the "Children's Diagnostic Scale" in the hour following the administration of the drug. Ratings of hyperactivity worsened for six of the seven participants.

The lack of studies in children with PDD may well be due in part from known effects of anxiolytic agents in typically developing children, where true anxiolytic agents have been shown to cause dysinhibition and sometimes increased activity and impulsiveness [58]. There is little reason to assume that they will be helpful in children with PDDs and ADHD symptoms, and they may have adverse effects.

Cholinesterase inhibitors

Cholinesterase inhibitors increase acetylcholine levels in the brain through the inhibition of the enzyme cholinesterase and have been used for Alzheimer's disease [37]. Postmortem studies have found significant abnormalities of the cholinergic system and its nicotinic receptors in the brains of individuals with autism [63,64].

Donepezil

Very few studies of donepezil have been attempted in ASDs. Hardan and Handen [65] conducted a retrospective study of donepezil and its effects on core symptoms of autism and disruptive behavior in eight young people. Significant improvement was reported for the CGI-S ratings and on the ABC Hyperactivity and Irritability subscales. To date, there is no compelling argument for advocating donepezil for treating either the secondary symptoms or the core features of autism. Rigorous exploratory studies are needed.

Galantamine

Neiderhofer [66] tested the effects of galantamine in a randomized placebo-controlled crossover study of 20 outpatient boys (mean age 7.4 years) with autism diagnosed by *International Statistical Classification of Diseases, 10th Revision* criteria. After combining parent and teacher ratings, the investigators found significant differences favoring galantamine on ABC Irritability, Hyperactivity, and Inappropriate Speech subscales. No side effects were reported. Neiderhofer concluded that galantamine is well tolerated and may be beneficial for treating irritability in children with autism.

Nicolson and colleagues [67] conducted a 12-week open-label study of galantamine in 13 children and adolescents with autism, ages 4 to 17 years. Significant improvement was noted on the ABC for the Irritability and Social Withdrawal subscales, but not for Hyperactivity. Clinician ratings on the CPRS showed significant improvement over time on the Autism and the Anger subscales but not the Hyperactivity subscale. Clinician ratings showed a significant reduction in the autism severity on the CGI-S. This study suggests possible benefit of galantamine for interfering behaviors in children with PDDs, although there was no indication of benefit for ADHD symptoms.

Rivastigmine tartrate

Rivastigmine tartrate has dual actions, inhibiting both acetylcholinesterase and butyrylcholinesterase and enhancing cholinergic function at the synaptic cleft [37]. Chez and colleagues [68] conducted a 12-week open-label study of rivastigmine tartrate in 32 children with PDDs, ages 2 to 12 years. Paired *t* tests indicated significant improvements over time on the Childhood Autism Rating Scale and Conners' PRS-Revised [69]. It was not clear from this report whether the change occurred on the Hyperactivity subscale or on the total score from the Conners' PRS-Revised.

N-methyl-D-aspartate receptor antagonists

Amantadine hydrochloride

Amantadine has been found to have noncompetitive NMDA antagonist activity and has moderate NMDA receptor-blocking properties at doses routinely used for its prescribed indications (ie, influenza, herpes zoster, and Parkinson disease) [70]. It also exerts its activity by increasing dopamine at the receptor [37].

King and colleagues [70] conducted a double-blind placebo-controlled multicenter study of amantadine hydrochloride in 39 subjects with autistic disorder, ages 5 to 19 years. There were no clinically significant differences between treatments on the parent-rated ABC Irritability or Hyperactivity subscales. Investigator-rated ABC scores did reveal a significant treatment difference on the Hyperactivity subscale. There were no significant differences on the CGI-S at the final visit. Amantadine was well tolerated. The investigators concluded that the dose range of 90 to 200 mg (below the recommended 200-mg dose for treatment of influenza) may have been too low to elicit a treatment effect even if amantadine has clinical potential.

Memantine

Memantine is an NMDA antagonist thought to preserve neuronal function. It selectively blocks the excitotoxic effects associated with abnormal glutamate transmission by modulating calcium channels [37]. It has been hypothesized that glutamate is involved in the pathophysiology of PDDs [71,72]. Owley and colleagues [73] conducted an open-label trial of memantine in 14 children with PDDs. There were no significant differences between baseline and endpoint on measures of expressive language, receptive language, nonverbal IQ, or CGI-S. Significant differences were found on a memory test ($P = .02$) and on all subscales of the ABC (especially the Social Withdrawal and Hyperactivity subscales). Conversely, hyperactivity was an adverse event for 5 subjects (36%). The investigators called for double-blind placebo-controlled studies of memantine.

Erickson and colleagues [74] conducted a retrospective chart-review of memantine in 18 children (15 male, 3 female; ages 6–19 years) with PDDs. As part of routine care, the treating physician completed the CGI-S and the CGI-I scales. Six subjects also had ABC baseline and endpoint data available. Eleven of the 18 (61%) were considered responders on the CGI-I and, on the ABC, there was a significant improvement on the Hyperactivity subscale.

There are enough positive data to warrant controlled trials of memantine. Hyperactivity was reported as both a side effect and as an area of therapeutic change. Thus, treatment with memantine is clearly experimental at this time.

Antiepileptic drug mood stabilizers

Many children with ASDs are also diagnosed with epilepsy and receive antiepileptic drugs. Hollander and colleagues [75] reported that 5 of 14 (36%) autistic individuals aged 5 to 40 years became less impulsive after treatment with divalproex sodium, although side effects (fatigue, sedation, behavioral activation) were severe enough for 2 participants to terminate. Uvebrant and Bauziene [76] published an anecdotal report of 50 children treated with lamotrigine. They reported that the children experienced an increase in attention span. However, only 13 of the children (26%) were diagnosed with autism, so it is not clear if these results were true of autism. Belsito and colleagues [77] explored lamotrigine for symptoms of autism in a double-blind placebo-controlled trial. Twenty-eight children with autism were treated with lamotrigine for 8 weeks, followed by a 4-week mainte-nance period. The main outcome measures, the Autism Behavior Checklist [78] and the ABC, showed no differences between placebo and lamotrigine. The investigators concluded that lamotrigine is probably not helpful in treating core symptoms of autism; an effect on ADHD symptoms seems unlikely.

Hardan and colleagues [79] conducted an open-label retrospective chart-review of topiramate in children with PDDs. Fifteen patients were included in the sample (11 with autism, 2 with Asperger's disorder, and 2 with PDD-NOS), and hyperactivity was a target symptom for 8. Eight of the children (53%) were considered responders after achieving a "much improved" or "very much improved" rating on the CGI-I. The children displayed signif-icant reductions on several subscales of Conners' PRS [22]: Inattention declined from 8.5 to 5.3 ($t = 3.11$, $P = .008$, $d = 1.66$), and hyperactivity decreased from 17.9 to 12.5 ($t = 4.30$, $P = .001$, $d = 2.30$). There is a need for double-blind placebo-controlled trials to confirm these impressions.

Overall, few studies and limited evidence supports the use of antiepi-leptic mood stabilizers in improving symptoms of ADHD in children with PDDs, and the positive studies in ASD are all uncontrolled. Despite some positive carbamazepine studies in typically developing children, clin-ical use of these agents for ADHD symptoms in children with PDDs must be considered a personal experiment and should be guided by clin-ical data.

Opiate blockers

Several studies of naltrexone were conducted in children with autism, usually with the hope of reducing core features of autism [80–86]. No effects were consistently found in autism symptoms. What is intriguing is that all of these studies observed reductions in hyperactivity, a finding that was often unanticipated [87].

Summary

Unfortunately, case series, open-label trials, and retrospective reports still dominate the autism field, and blinded placebo-controlled studies make up a small minority of the literature. Although uncontrolled studies *may* reflect true effects, it is equally true that "significant" changes may be due to the passage of time, placebo effects, or the well-known tendency of higher scores to regress to the mean. Such uncontrolled studies may exaggerate effect sizes. Hence, the brunt of the evidence presented here is only suggestive and awaits true assessment in properly controlled studies. At this point, the evidence for a therapeutic effect on hyperactivity and inattention seems best for methylphenidate (although other stimulant preparations probably also work about as well), atomoxetine, certain atypical antipsychotics, and alpha-2 adrenergic agonists. There is not much to commend the SSRIs, venlafaxine, benzodiazepines, or antiepileptic drug mood stabilizers for these symptoms. The case still needs to be made for tricyclic antidepressants, cholinesterase inhibitors, and NMDA receptor blockers, whose use for hyperactivity should be viewed as experimental.

References

[1] Lecavalier L. Behavioral and emotional problems in young people with pervasive developmental disorders: relative prevalence, effects of subject characteristics, and empirical classification. J Autism Dev Disord 2006;36:1101–14.

[2] Aman MG, Tassé MJ, Rojahn J, et al. The Nisonger CBRF: a child behavior rating form for children with developmental disabilities. Res Dev Disabil 1996;17:41–57.

[3] Arnold LE, Gadow KD, Pearson DA, et al. Stimulants. In: Reiss S, Aman MG, editors. Psychotropic medication and developmental disabilities: the international consensus handbook. Columbus (OH): Ohio State University Nisonger Center; 1998. p. 229–57.

[4] Aman MG, Buican B, Arnold LE. Methylphenidate treatment in children with low IQ and ADHD: analysis of three aggregated studies. J Child Adolesc Psychopharmacol 2003;13: 27–38.

[5] Pearson D, Lane D, Santos C, et al. Effects of methylphenidate treatment in children with mental retardation and ADHD: individual variation in medication response. J Am Acad Child Adolesc Psychiatry 2004;43:686–98.

[6] Campbell M, Fish B, David R, et al. Response to tri-iodothyronine and dextroamphetamine: a study of preschool schizophrenic children. J Autism Child Schizophr 1972;2: 343–58.

[7] Campbell M, Small AM, Collins PJ, et al. Levodopa and levoamphetamine:a crossover study in young schizophrenic children. Curr Ther Res Clin Exp 1976;19:70–86.

[8] Connor DF. Psychostimulants in attention deficit hyperactivity attention deficit disorder: theoretical and practical issues for the community practitioner. In: Gozal D, Molfese DL, editors. Attention deficit hyperactivity disorder: from genes to patients. Totowa (NJ): Humana Press; 2007. p. 487–528.

[9] Hoshino Y, Kumashiro H, Kaneko M, et al. Effects of methylphenidate on early infantile autism and its relation to serum serotonin levels. Folia Psychiatrica et Neurologica Japonica 1977;3(4):605–14.

[10] Birmaher B, Quintana H, Greenhill LL. Methylphenidate treatment of hyperactive autistic children. J Am Acad Child Adolesc Psychiatry 1988;27:248–51.

[11] Di Martino A, Melis G, Cianchetti C, et al. Methylphenidate for pervasive developmental disorders: safety and efficacy of acute single dose test and ongoing therapy: an open-pilot study. J Child Adolesc Psychopharmacol 2004;14:207–18.

[12] Quintana H, Birmaher B, Stedge D, et al. Use of methylphenidate in the treatment of children with autistic disorder. J Autism Dev Disord 1995;25:283–94.

[13] Handen BL, Johnson CR, Lubetsky M. Efficacy of methylphenidate among children with autism and symptoms of attention-deficit hyperactivity disorder. J Autism Dev Disord 2000;30:245–55.

[14] Santosh PJ, Baird G, Pityaratstian N, et al. Impact of comorbid autism spectrum disorders on stimulant response in children with attention deficit hyperactivity disorder: a retrospective and prospective effectiveness study. Child Care Hlth Dev 2006;32:575–83.

[15] Guy W. ECDEU assessment manual of psychopharmacology (NIMH Publication 76-338). Washington, DC: Department of Health, Education, and Welfare; NIMH; 1976.

[16] Research Units on Pediatric Psychopharmacology Autism Network. A randomized, double-blind, placebo-controlled, crossover trial of methylphenidate in children with hyperactivity associated with pervasive developmental disorders. Arch Gen Psychiatry 2005;62:1266–74.

[17] Posey DJ, Aman MG, McCracken JT, et al. Positive effects of methylphenidate on inattention and hyperactivity in pervasive developmental disorders: an analysis of secondary measures. Biol Psychiatry 2007;61:538–44.

[18] Aman MG, Singh N, Stewart A, et al. The Aberrant Behavior Checklist: a behavior rating scale for the assessment of treatment effects. Am J Ment Defic 1985;89:485–91.

[19] Aman MG, Singh NN, Stewart AW, et al. Psychometric characteristics of the Aberrant Behavior Checklist. Am J Ment Defic 1985;89:492–502.

[20] Swanson J. School-based assessments and interventions for ADD students. Irvine (CA): KC Publishing; 1992.

[21] Jou R, Handen B, Hardan A. Retrospective assessment of atomoxetine in children and adolescents with pervasive developmental disorders. J Child Adolesc Psychopharmacol 2005;15:325–30.

[22] Goyette C, Conners C, Ulrich R. Normative data on revised Conners Parent And Teacher Rating Scales. J Abnorm Child Psychol 1978;6:221–36.

[23] Troost P, Steenhuis M, Tuynman H, et al. Atomoxetine for attention-deficit/hyperactivity disorder symptoms in children with pervasive developmental disorders: a pilot study. J Child Adolesc Psychopharmacol 2006;16:611–9.

[24] DuPaul G, Power T, Anastopoulos A, et al. ADHD rating scale—IV: checklists, norms, and clinical interpretations. New York: The Guilford Press; 1998.

[25] Posey D, Wiegand R, Wilkerson J, et al. Open-label atomoxetine for attention-deficit/ hyperactivity disorder symptoms associated with high-functioning pervasive developmental disorders. J Child Adolesc Psychopharmacol 2006;16:599–610.

[26] Conners C. Conners' continuous performance test—II. North Tonawanda (NY): Multi Health Systems; 2000.

[27] Spencer T, Biederman J, Wilens T, et al. Effectiveness and tolerability of tomoxetine in adults with attention deficit hyperactivity disorder. Am J Psychiatry 1998;155:693–5.

[28] Arnold L, Aman M, Cook A, et al. Atomoxetine for hyperactivity in autism spectrum disorders: placebo-controlled crossover pilot trial. J Am Acad Child Adolesc Psychiatry 2006;45:1196–205.

[29] Michelson D, Faires D, Wernicke J, et al. Atomoxetine in the treatment of children and adolescents with attention-deficit/hyperactivity disorder: a randomized, placebo-controlled, dose-response study. Pediatrics 2001;108:1–9.

[30] Michelson D, Allen A, Busner J, et al. Once-daily atomoxetine treatment for children and adolescents with attention deficit hyperactivity disorder: a randomized, placebo-controlled study. Am J Psychiatry 2002;159:1896–901.

[31] Sutton V, Milton D, Ruff D, et al. Efficacy of atomoxetine treatment for children and adolescents with attention-deficit/hyperactivity disorder. Paper presented at the 51st Annual

Meeting American Academy of Child and Adolescent Psychiatry. Washington, DC: 2004, October.

[32] Spencer T, Biederman J, Heiligenstein J, et al. An open-label, dose-ranging study of atomoxetine in children with attention deficit hyperactivity disorder. J Child Adolesc Psychopharmacol 2001;11:251–65.

[33] Waizer J, Polizos P, Hoffman SP, et al. A single-blind evaluation of thiothixene with outpatient schizophrenic children. J Autism Child Schizophr 1972;2:378–86.

[34] Anderson LT, Campbell M, Grega DM, et al. Haloperidol in the treatment of infantile autism: effects on learning and behavioral symptoms. Am J Psychiatry 1984;141:1195–202.

[35] Fish B. Children's psychiatric rating scale. Psychopharmacol Bull 1985;21:753–70.

[36] Campbell M, Armenteros JL, Malone RP, et al. Neuroleptic-related dyskinesias in autistic children: a prospective, longitudinal study. J Am Acad Child Adolesc Psychiatry 1997;36: 835–43.

[37] Bezchlibnyk-Butler KZ, Jefferies JJ. Clinical handbook of psychotropic drugs. 15th edition. Ashland (OH): Hogrefe & Huber Publishers; 2005.

[38] Research Units on Pediatric Psychopharmacology Autism Network. Risperidone in children with autism for serious behavioral problems. N Engl J Med 2002;347:314–21.

[39] Shea S, Turgay A, Carroll A, et al. Risperidone in the treatment of disruptive behavioral symptoms in children with autistic and other pervasive developmental disorders. Pediatrics 2004;114:634–41.

[40] Hellings JA, Zarcone JR, Reese RM. A crossover study of risperidone in children, adolescents and adults with mental retardation. J Autism Dev Disord 2006;36:401–11.

[41] Troost PW, Althaus M, Lahius BE. Neuropsychological effects of risperidone in children with pervasive developmental disorders: a blinded discontinuation study. J Child Adolesc Psychopharmacol 2006;16:561–73.

[42] Troost PW, Lahius BE, Steenhuis MP. Long-term effects of risperidone in children with autism spectrum disorders: a placebo discontinuation study. J Am Acad Child Adolesc Psychiatry 2005;44:1137–44.

[43] Corson AH, Barkenbus JE, Posey DJ, et al. A retrospective analysis of quetiapine in the treatment of pervasive developmental disorders. J Clin Psychiatry 2004;65:1531–6.

[44] Hardan AY, Jou RJ, Handen BL. Retrospective study of quetiapine in children and adolescents with pervasive developmental disorders. J Autism Dev Disord 2005;35:387–91.

[45] Malone RP, Delaney MA, Hyman SB, et al. Ziprasidone in adolescents with autism: an open-label pilot study. J Child Adolesc Psychopharmacol 2007;17:779–90.

[46] Valicenti-McDermott MR, Demb H. Clinical effects and adverse reactions of off-label use of aripiprazole in children and adolescents with developmental disabilities. J Child Adolesc Psychopharmacol 2006;16:549–60.

[47] Fankhauser MP, Karumanchi VC, German ML, et al. A double-blind, placebo-controlled study of the efficacy of transdermal clonidine in autism. J Clin Psychiatry 1991;53:77–82.

[48] Jaselskis CA, Cook EH Jr, Fletcher KE, et al. Clonidine treatment of hyperactive and impulsive children with autistic disorder. J Clin Psychopharmacol 1992;12:322–7.

[49] Posey DJ, Puntney JI, Sasher TM, et al. Guanfacine treatment of hyperactivity in pervasive developmental disorders: a retrospective analysis of 80 cases. J Child Adolesc Psychopharmacol 2004;14:233–41.

[50] Scahill L, Aman MG, McDougle CJ, et al. A prospective open-trial of guanfacine in children with pervasive developmental disorders. J Child Adolesc Psychopharmacol 2006;16: 589–98.

[51] Geller B, Reising D, Leonard H, et al. Critical review of tricyclic antidepressant use in children and adolescents. J Am Child Adolesc Psychiatry 1999;38:513–6.

[52] Gordon C, Rapoport J, Hamburger S, et al. Differential response of seven subjects with autistic disorder to clomipramine and desipramine. Am J Psychiatry 1992;149:363–6.

[53] Gordon C, State R, Nelson J, et al. A double-blind comparison of clomipramine, desipramine, and placebo in the treatment of autistic disorder. Arch Gen Psychiatry 1993;50:441–7.

[54] Cook EH, Rowlett R, Jaselskis C, et al. Fluoxetine treatment of children and adults with autistic disorder and mental retardation. J Am Acad Child Adolesc Psychiatry 1992;31: 739–45.

[55] Todd R. Fluoxetine in autism. Am J Psychiatry 1991;148:1089.

[56] Fatemi S, Realmuto G, Khan L, et al. Fluoxetine in treatment of adolescent patients with autism: a longitudinal open trial. J Autism Dev Disord 1998;28:303–7.

[57] Hollander E, Kaplan A, Cartwright C, et al. Venlafaxine in children, adolescents, and young adults with autism spectrum disorders: an open retrospective clinical report. J Child Neurol 2000;15:132–5.

[58] Werry J, Aman MG. Anxiolytics, sedatives, and miscellaneous drugs. In: Werry J, Aman MG, editors. Practitioner's guide to psychoactive drugs for children and adolescents. 2nd edition. New York: Plenum Medical Book Company; 1999. p. 433–69.

[59] Realmuto GM, August GJ, Garfinkel BD. Clinical effect of buspirone in autistic children. J Clin Psychopharmacol 1989;9:122–5.

[60] Conners C. A teacher rating scale for use in drug studies with children. Am J Psychiatry 1969; 126:884–8.

[61] McCormick L. Treatment with buspirone in a child with autism. Arch Fam Med 1997;6(4): 368–70.

[62] Marrosu F, Marrosu G, Rachel M, et al. Paradoxical reactions elicited by diazepam in children with classic autism. Funct Neurol 1987;3:355–61.

[63] Perry EK, Lee ML, Martin-Ruiz CM, et al. Cholinergic activity in autism: abnormalities in the cerebral cortex and basal forebrain. Am J Psychiatry 2001;158:1058–66.

[64] Lee M, Martin-Ruiz C, Graham A, et al. Nicotinic receptor abnormalities in the cerebellar cortex in autism. Brain 2002;125:1483–95.

[65] Hardan AY, Handen BL. A retrospective open trial of adjunctive donepezil in children and adolescents with autistic disorder. J Child Adolesc Psychopharmacol 2002;12:237–41.

[66] Neiderhofer H. Galantamine may be effective in treating autistic disorder. [letters]. BMJ 2002;325:1422–3.

[67] Nicolson R, Craven-Thuss B, Smith J. A prospective, open-label trial of galantamine in autistic disorder. J Child Adolesc Psychopharmacol 2006;16:621–9.

[68] Chez MG, Aimonovich M, Buchanan T, et al. Treating autistic spectrum disorders in children: utility of the cholinesterase inhibitor rivastigmine tartrate. J Child Neurol 2004;19(3): 165–9.

[69] Conners C. Conners' rating scales-revised, technical manual. Toronto: Multi-Health Systems; 1997.

[70] King BH, Wright DM, Handen BL, et al. Double-blind placebo-controlled study of amantadine hydrochloride in the treatment of children with autistic disorder. J Am Acad Child Adolesc Psychiatry 2001;40:658–65.

[71] Carlsson M. Hypothesis: Is infantile autism a hypoglutamatergic disorder? Relevance of glutamate-serotonin interactions for pharmacotherapy. J Neural Transm 1998;105: 525–35.

[72] Lappalainen R, Riikonen R. High levels of cerebrospinal fluid in Rett syndrome. Pediatr Neurol 1996;15:213–6.

[73] Owley T, Salt J, Guter S, et al. A prospective, open-label, trial of memantine in the treatment of cognitive, behavioral, and memory dysfunction in pervasive developmental disorders. J Child Adolesc Psychopharmacol 2006;16:517–24.

[74] Erickson CA, Posey DJ, Stigler KA, et al. A retrospective study of memantine in children and adolescents with pervasive developmental disorders. Psychopharmacology (Berl) 2007;191:141–7.

[75] Hollander E, Dolgoff-Kaspar R, Cartwright C, et al. An open trial of divalproex sodium in autistic disorder spectrum disorders. J Clin Psychiatry 2001;62:530–4.

[76] Uvebrant P, Bauziene R. Intractable epilepsy in children: the efficacy of lamotrigine treatment including nonsiezure-related benefits. Neuropediatrics 1994;25:284–9.

[77] Belsito K, Law P, Kirk K, et al. Lamotrigine therapy for autistic disorder: a randomized dou-ble-blind, placebo-controlled trial. J Autism Dev Disord 2001;31:175–81.

[78] Krug DA, Arick J, Almond P. Autism behavior checklist record form. Austin (TX): PRO-ED; 1993.

[79] Hardan A, Jou R, Handen B. A retrospective assessment of topiramate in children and adolescents with pervasive developmental disorders. J Child Adolesc Psychopharmacol 2004;14:426–32.

[80] Campbell M, Overall JE, Small AM, et al. Naltrexone in autistic children: an acute open dose range tolerance trial. J Am Acad Child Adolesc Psychiatry 1989;28:200–6.

[81] Campbell M, Anderson LT, Small AM, et al. Naltrexone in autistic children: behavioral symptoms and attentional learning. J Am Acad Child Adolesc Psychiatry 1993;32:1283–91.

[82] Kolmen BK, Feldman H, Handen BL, et al. Naltrexone in young autistic children: a double-blind placebo-controlled crossover study. J Am Acad Child Adolesc Psychiatry 1995;34:223–31.

[83] Willemsen-Swinkles SH, Buitelaar JK, Weijnen FG, et al. Placebo-controlled acute dosage naltrexone study in young autistic children. Psychiatry Res 1995;58:203–15.

[84] Willemsen-Swinkles SH, Buitelaar JK, van Engeland H. The effects of chronic naltrexone treatment in young autistic children: a double-blind placebo controlled crossover study. Biol Psychiatry 1996;39:1023–31.

[85] Kolmen BK, Feldman H, Handen BL, et al. Naltrexone in young autistic children: replica-tion study and learning measures. J Am Acad Child Adolesc Psychiatry 1997;36:1570–8.

[86] Willemsen-Swinkles SH, Builtelaar JK, van Berkelaer-Onnes IA, et al. Brief report: six months continuation treatment in naltrexone-responsive children with autism: a double blind placebo-controlled crossover study. J Autism Dev Disord 1999;29:167–9.

[87] Aman MG, Langworthy KS. Pharmacotherapy for hyperactivity in children with autism and other pervasive developmental disorders. J Autism Dev Disord 2000;30:451–9.

ELSEVIER
SAUNDERS

Child Adolesc Psychiatric Clin N Am
17 (2008) 739–752

CHILD AND
ADOLESCENT
PSYCHIATRIC CLINICS
OF NORTH AMERICA

Pharmacotherapy of Irritability in Pervasive Developmental Disorders

Kimberly A. Stigler, MD[a],*, Christopher J. McDougle, MD[b]

[a]Department of Psychiatry, Indiana University School of Medicine, Riley Hospital for Children, Room 4300, 702 Barnhill Drive, Indianapolis, IN 46202-5200, USA
[b]Department of Psychiatry, PB 2nd Floor, 1111 W. 10th Street, Indiana University School of Medicine, Indianapolis, IN 46202-4800, USA

Autistic disorder (autism) and related pervasive developmental disorders (PDDs) are lifelong neuropsychiatric disorders characterized by impairments in social interaction and communication, as well as restricted interests and activities [1]. Children and adolescents diagnosed with a PDD often suffer from severe irritability, including aggression, self-injurious behavior (SIB), and tantrums. In addition to its inherent potential dangerousness, irritability is frequently of sufficient severity to negatively impact educational and therapeutic interventions [2]; therefore, the importance of effectively targeting this symptom domain is clear. The treatment of irritability in PDDs is multimodal and includes the use of behavioral and pharmacologic approaches.

The pharmacotherapy of irritability (aggression, SIB, tantrums) in children and adolescents with PDDs primarily encompasses the atypical antipsychotics, which are emerging as the first-line pharmacologic treatment for this target symptom domain. Other pharmacologic agents that have been investigated for the treatment of irritability include the α-2 adrenergic agonists, as well as the anticonvulsants and mood stabilizers.

This work was supported in part by a Research Unit on Pediatric Psychopharmacology-Psychosocial Intervention grant (U10 MH066766) from the National Institute of Mental Health (NIMH) to Indiana University (Drs. McDougle and Stigler), research grant (R01 MH072964) from the NIMH (Drs. McDougle and Stigler), a General Clinical Research Center grant (M01 RR00750) from the National Institutes of Health to Indiana University (Drs. McDougle and Stigler), and a Daniel X. and Mary Freedman Psychiatric Research Fellowship Award (Dr. Stigler).

* Corresponding author. Christian Sarkine Autism Treatment Center, James Whitcomb Riley Hospital for Children, Room 4300, 702 Barnhill Drive, Indianapolis, IN 46202-5200.
E-mail address: kstigler@iupui.edu (K.A. Stigler).

Antipsychotics

Typical antipsychotics

Research into the pharmacotherapy of autism and related disorders began in the 1960s. The development of the typical antipsychotic chlorpromazine for schizophrenia led to the dawn of a new era in psychiatry based on the pharmacologic treatment of psychiatric disorders. Over time as more compounds were developed investigators actively sought to determine their potential use in targeting the severe and often debilitating symptoms of aggression and SIB in autism; however, these studies were methodologically flawed, and concerns were raised regarding diagnostic accuracy [3]. At the same time efforts were being made to develop well-designed studies, attention was shifting away from the low-potency antipsychotics due to their propensity for sedation and cognitive adverse effects. Researchers were increasingly drawn toward antipsychotics with potent dopamine (DA) D_2 receptor antagonism, such as haloperidol, in their search for an effective treatment.

Systematic research into the pharmacotherapy of autism and related disorders began with the work of Campbell and colleagues [4] who conducted several well-designed studies of haloperidol in individuals with autism. In their first study, haloperidol (mean dosage, 1.7 mg/d) was compared with placebo in combination with one of two language training groups in children with autism aged 2.6 to 7.2 years. Significant improvement was recorded in symptoms of withdrawal and stereotypy in youth aged 4.5 years and older who were randomized to haloperidol as measured by the Children's Psychiatric Rating Scale [5]. Adverse effects included dose-related sedation in 12 of 20 (60%) subjects and acute dystonia in 2 of 20 (10%) subjects.

Several subsequent studies demonstrated that haloperidol was effective in targeting a range of maladaptive behavioral symptoms in youth with autism [6–8]; however, the drug was found to frequently be associated with acute dystonic reactions and dyskinesias (particularly withdrawal). Investigators sought to better understand the frequency of dyskinesias associated with haloperidol treatment in this population. One study enrolled 60 children (age range, 2.3–7.9 years) with autism who were responders to haloperidol [9]. The subjects were randomized to continuous or discontinuous (5 days on and 2 days off) treatment with haloperidol for 6 months, after which they all received 4 weeks of placebo. Although all were reversible, three youth developed dyskinesias during haloperidol treatment and nine developed withdrawal dyskinesias during the placebo period. Another study prospectively monitored the emergence of tardive dyskinesia and withdrawal dyskinesia in 118 children with autism aged 2.3 to 8.2 years [10]. The youth received 6 months of haloperidol followed by 1 month of placebo, after which the need for another cycle of haloperidol treatment followed by placebo was assessed. In this study, 40 of 118 (33.9%) subjects developed dyskinesias, primarily reversible withdrawal dyskinesias. Of the individuals on a higher mean dosage (3.4 mg/d) of haloperidol during the study, 9 of 10 (90%) developed dyskinesias. Taken together, although potentially beneficial, the current role of haloperidol is limited to treatment-refractory patients due to concerns regarding its associated adverse effects.

Atypical antipsychotics

In contrast to the typical antipsychotics, the atypical antipsychotics exhibit a profile of potent antagonism at serotonin (5-hydroxytryptamine) and DA receptors, which purportedly results in decreased propensity for tardive dyskinesia and extrapyramidal symptoms (EPS) [11]. The following atypical antipsychotics are discussed in this article: clozapine, risperidone, olanzapine, quetiapine, ziprasidone, and aripiprazole. Selected placebo-controlled studies of atypical antipsychotics for the treatment of irritability in children and adolescents with autism and related PDDs are shown in Table 1.

Clozapine

Three known reports have been published on the use of clozapine in the treatment of individuals with autism. Zuddas and colleagues [12] treated three children with autism aged 8 to 12 years with clozapine (dose range, 200–450 mg/d) who had not responded to haloperidol for up to 8 months. Clozapine treatment resulted in decreased aggression, marked hyperactivity, and negativism. Although two children demonstrated sustained improvement, one child relapsed after 5 months. All three youth experienced transient sedation and enuresis. Another report found that clozapine treatment at 275 mg/d significantly reduced "overt tension," hyperactivity, and stereotypies in a 17-year-old male inpatient with autism and severe mental retardation over a duration of 15 days [13]. Mild constipation and sialorrhea were among the adverse effects reported. The use of clozapine at a dosage of 300 mg/d in a 32-year-old male patient with autism and profound mental

Table 1

Selected placebo-controlled studies of antipsychotics for irritability in pervasive developmental disorders

Drug and reference	Sample	Design	Mean dosage	Responders
Haloperidol [4]	n = 40; 2–7 years; autism	8-week crossover	1.7 mg/d	Haloperidol > placebo
Risperidone [15]	n = 101; 5–17 years; autism	8-week parallel groups	1.8 mg/d	Risperidone > placebo; 69%
Risperidone [22]	n = 79; 5–12 years; PDD	8-week parallel groups	1.2 mg/d	Risperidone > placebo; 87%
Olanzapine [30]	n = 11; 6–14 years; PDD	8-week parallel groups	10 mg/d	Olanzapine > placebo; 50%

Abbreviation: n, number of subjects.

retardation was described [14]. Marked improvement in treatment-refractory aggressive behavior and social interaction was noted after 2 months, with progressive improvement recorded over 5 years of treatment. No EPS or agranulocytosis was reported.

The dearth of reports on the use of clozapine in PDDs is most likely due to its potential to cause life-threatening agranulocytosis as well as its propensity to lower the seizure threshold. Moreover, patients with an impaired ability to communicate and cognitive impairment would likely encounter difficulty tolerating weekly to biweekly venipuncture to monitor white blood cell counts.

Risperidone

Several case series and open-label trials as well as double-blind, placebo-controlled studies have found risperidone effective in targeting symptoms of irritability in children and adolescents with autism and related disorders. The Research Units on Pediatric Psychopharmacology (RUPP) Autism Network [15] conducted the first double-blind, placebo-controlled study of risperidone in children and adolescents with autism. In this 8-week study, 101 youth (mean age, 8.8 years) were randomly assigned to receive risperidone or placebo. At baseline, all subjects had significant irritability defined as aggression, SIB, and tantrums as determined by an Aberrant Behavior Checklist (ABC) Irritability subscale score of 18 or greater [16]. Risperidone treatment at a mean dosage of 1.8 mg/d resulted in a 57% reduction on the ABC Irritability subscale score compared with a 14% decrease in the placebo group. Based on a ≥25% improvement on the ABC Irritability subscale score and a rating of "much improved" or "very much improved" on the Clinical Global Impressions-Improvement (CGI-I) scale, 69% of the risperidone-treated subjects were considered responders compared with 12% of those who received placebo. Risperidone was associated with a mean weight gain of 5.9 lbs compared with 1.8 lbs with placebo. Although drooling was more frequently reported in subjects receiving risperidone, clinician-administered standardized measures of acute EPS and tardive dyskinesia were not significantly different between groups.

Four other subscales of the ABC, including social withdrawal, stereotypy, hyperactivity, and inappropriate speech, were also examined by the RUPP Autism Network [15]. Although risperidone was associated with greater improvement on all of the ABC subscales, reductions in social withdrawal and inappropriate speech were not statistically significant following Bonferroni correction for multiple comparisons. In an effort to better understand the efficacy of risperidone for core symptoms of autism, McDougle and colleagues [17–19] further explored secondary outcome measures that included the modified Ritvo-Freeman Real Life Rating Scale (R-F RLRS) and modified Children's Yale-Brown Obsessive Compulsive Scale (CY-BOCS). Significant improvement was observed on the following subscales of the R-F RLRS: sensory motor behaviors, affectual reactions, and sensory responses; however, no significant change on the social relationship to people or language subscales was found. Measures on the CY-BOCS revealed that risperidone was more efficacious than placebo for decreasing interfering repetitive behavior.

In a companion study to the initial 8-week acute risperidone trial by the RUPP Autism Network [20], 63 responders continued on open-label risperidone for an additional 16 weeks. During this phase, the mean dosage remained stable, and there was no clinically significant worsening of target symptoms. Risperidone was discontinued in two subjects due to loss of effectiveness and in one subject due to an adverse event. Over the entire 6 months of risperidone treatment, the children and adolescents gained an average of 11.2 lbs. After the 16-week open-label continuation phase, the 32 subjects who continued to be classified as responders were randomized to either continued risperidone treatment or gradual placebo substitution over the course of 3 weeks. Ten of 16 (62.5%) subjects randomized to placebo showed significant worsening of symptoms, whereas 2 of 16 (12.5%) subjects who continued on risperidone worsened. This finding suggests that risperidone treatment beyond 6 months is necessary to prevent relapse. It has been confirmed in another placebo-controlled discontinuation study of risperidone in autism and other PDDs [21].

Investigators in Canada conducted a second 8-week multicenter, placebo-controlled study of risperidone in children and adolescents with PDDs [22]. In that study, 79 youth (mean age, 7.5 years) were randomly assigned to risperidone (mean dose, 1.2 mg/d) or placebo. Entry criteria included a diagnosis of a PDD and a Childhood Autism Rating Scale (CARS) score greater than 30 [23]; however, the mean baseline ABC Irritability subscale score was 20, indicating that the subjects were highly symptomatic. Risperidone treatment resulted in a 64% reduction in the ABC Irritability subscale score in comparison with 31% with placebo. Furthermore, 53% of the subjects given risperidone were considered responders compared with 18% of those given placebo. Significant improvement was recorded on all five subscales of the ABC, with the greatest magnitude of improvement observed for irritability and hyperactivity. In the risperidone group, social withdrawal decreased by 63% versus 40% in the placebo group. The mean weight gain was 5.9 lbs in the risperidone group and 2.2 lbs in the placebo group. No differences in EPS were measured by standardized rating scales.

The results of these two randomized controlled trials demonstrating the efficacy and tolerability of risperidone led to its approval by the US Food and Drug Administration (FDA) for the treatment of irritability in children and adolescents with autism aged 5 to 16 years. To date, risperidone is the only FDA-approved drug for the treatment of symptoms in children and adolescents with autism or any other PDD.

Recently, a 12-week double-blind trial of risperidone versus haloperidol was completed in 30 children and adolescents (age range, 8–18 years) with autism [24]. The subjects received 0.01 to 0.08 mg/kg/d of either drug.

Risperidone was associated with significantly greater reductions in total ABC scores combined with clinically significant improvement in general behavior among other symptoms in comparison with the results in the haloperidol group. Subjects randomized to risperidone exhibited significant increases in serum prolactin, whereas the haloperidol group had increased alanine amino transferase levels. Overall, both risperidone and haloperidol were considered safe and well tolerated by the investigators.

Risperidone has also been investigated in samples that included even younger children with PDDs. Nagaraj and colleagues [25] published a placebo-controlled study of 40 children with autism aged 2 to 9 years. Youth as young as 2 years of age were given a risperidone dosage of 1 mg daily. Risperidone was highly efficacious as determined by ratings on the CARS and Children's Global Assessment Scale. Another recent 6-month, placebo-controlled trial of 24 children less than 6 years of age diagnosed with PDDs found risperidone (dose range, 0.5–1.5 mg/d) to be minimally efficacious versus placebo [26]; however, high degrees of irritability were not required for study entry, which may have contributed to the limited improvement observed in this trial.

Olanzapine

The ability of olanzapine to effectively target behavioral symptoms in autism and other PDDs has been shown in three open-label trials and one small placebo-controlled study. Potenza and colleagues [27] conducted a 12-week open-label study evaluating olanzapine (mean dose, 7.8 mg/d) in eight children, adolescents, and adults with autism and other PDDs (mean age, 20.9 years; age range, 5–42 years). Six of seven (86%) subjects who completed the trial were considered responders, with significant improvement recorded in overall symptoms of autism, hyperactivity, social relatedness, affectual reactions, sensory responses, language usage, irritability, anxiety, and depressive symptoms. No change in repetitive behavior was observed. Prominent adverse events included increased appetite and weight gain in six subjects (mean weight gain, 18.4 lbs at week 12), as well as sedation in three subjects. Significant EPS were not recorded.

A 6-week open-label study employing a parallel groups design was conducted of olanzapine (mean dose, 7.9 mg/d) versus haloperidol (mean dose, 1.4 mg/d) in 12 children with autism (mean age, 7.8 years) [28]. In the olanzapine group, five of six (83%) subjects were judged responders, whereas in the haloperidol group, three of six (50%) subjects were responders. Weight gain was significantly higher in the olanzapine group (mean, 9 lbs; range, 5.9–15.8 lbs) when compared with the haloperidol group (mean 3.2 lbs; range, −5.5 to +8.8 lbs).

A 3-month open-label trial of olanzapine (mean dose, 10.7 mg/d) in 25 children (mean age, 11.2 years) with a PDD found the drug effective in only 3 (12%) subjects [29]. The low response rate in this trial may have been due to the low level of irritability recorded on the ABC Irritability subscale at baseline. The mean baseline ABC Irritability subscale score in this study was 11, which is significantly less than in the previously described two large placebo-controlled studies of risperidone in youth with PDDs. Furthermore, the other two olanzapine studies described previously had specific entry criteria based on the degree of irritability.

To date, one small 8-week, placebo-controlled study of olanzapine has been published in children and adolescents with a PDD [30]. The 11 study participants aged 6 to 14 years were randomly assigned to olanzapine (mean dose, 10 mg/d) or placebo. Three of six (50%) subjects receiving olanzapine versus one of five (20%) receiving placebo were deemed treatment responders. The mean weight gain recorded in the olanzapine group was 7.5 lbs versus 1.5 lbs with placebo.

Quetiapine

To date, four reports of quetiapine in the treatment of individuals with autism and other PDDs have been published. A 16-week open-label study of quetiapine (mean dose, 225 mg/d) was conducted in six youth (age range, 6–15 years) with autism [31]. Only two of six (33%) subjects were considered responders. The remaining four subjects discontinued treatment prematurely, with three withdrawing due to sedation or lack of response and one withdrawing after a possible seizure. In addition, increased appetite and weight gain (range, 2–18 lbs) were recorded. Overall, it was concluded that quetiapine was generally ineffective and poorly tolerated.

Findling and colleagues [32] completed a 12-week open-label trial of quetiapine (mean dose, 292 mg/d; range, 100–450 mg/d) in 9 youth (mean age, 14.6 years; range, 12–17 years) with autism. Although six of nine (67%) subjects completed the trial, only two of nine (22%) were determined to be responders. Two subjects discontinued prematurely, one subject due to sedation and one due to agitation and aggression. Adverse events included sedation, weight gain, agitation, and aggression.

A retrospective case series of 20 subjects (mean age, 12.1 years; range, 5–28 years) with a PDD who had received quetiapine (mean dose, 249 mg/d; range, 25–600 mg/d) for at least 4 weeks (mean duration, 59.8 weeks; range, 4–180 weeks) was conducted [33]. In that study, no subject was being treated concurrently with another antipsychotic or mood stabilizing agent. The investigators found that 8 of 20 (40%) subjects responded to quetiapine. Fifty percent (50%) of the subjects experienced adverse events, 15% of which led to drug discontinuation. In another retrospective case series, 10 subjects aged 5 to 19 years with PDD and mental retardation were prescribed quetiapine (mean dose, 477 mg/d) [34]. Subjects taking concomitant medications were included if the drug dosages were held constant during the study. Significant improvement occurred in symptoms of hyperactivity and inattention. Six of 10 (60%) subjects were considered treatment responders. Overall, quetiapine was well tolerated, with mild sedation, sialorrhea, and weight gain reported.

Ziprasidone

McDougle and colleagues [35] conducted a study of the effectiveness and safety of ziprasidone in 12 individuals (mean age, 11.6 years; range, 8–20 years) with autism or PDD not otherwise specified. Six of 12 (50%) subjects receiving open-label treatment with ziprasidone (mean dose, 59.2 mg/d; range, 20–120 mg/d) for a minimum of 6 weeks (mean duration, 14.2 weeks; range, 6–30 weeks) were deemed responders. Improvement in aggression, agitation, and irritability was reported. The most common adverse effect was transient sedation. No cardiovascular adverse effects were observed or reported. The mean change in weight was −5.8 lbs (range, −35 to +6 lbs). The weight loss was likely due to subjects being switched from other medications that had caused significant weight gain. In a second study, 10 adults with autism and mental retardation were switched to ziprasidone from other atypical antipsychotics (clozapine, risperidone, quetiapine), most often because of excessive weight gain [36]. After 6 months of ziprasidone treatment, the subjects had lost significant weight (mean, −9.5 lbs). In regards to symptom improvement, six subjects had an improvement in maladaptive behavior, one was unchanged, and three worsened.

Recently, Malone and colleagues [37] published a 6-week prospective, open-label pilot study of ziprasidone (mean dosage, 98.3 mg/d; range, 20–160 mg/d) in 12 adolescents (mean age, 14.5 years; range, 12–18 years) with autism. Nine of 12 (75%) subjects were considered responders. Ziprasidone treatment resulted in a reduction in disruptive behaviors, including irritability, aggression, and hyperactivity. Ziprasidone was found to be weight neutral. Measures of total cholesterol decreased, whereas levels of prolactin remained the same. Two subjects experienced acute dystonic reactions. A mean increase in QTc of 14.7 ms was recorded at study endpoint.

The potential for QTc interval prolongation with ziprasidone on electrocardiography led to an FDA warning regarding its use. Ziprasidone should not be given to individuals with known cardiac disease such as cardiac arrhythmias or a long QT syndrome or who are taking other drugs that can prolong the QTc interval without careful monitoring and consultation with a cardiologist.

Aripiprazole

Preliminary results of aripiprazole treatment for irritability in children and adolescents with PDDs have been published. In a prospective, open-label case series, five subjects (mean age, 12.2 years; range, 5–18 years) with autism were treated with aripiprazole (mean dose, 12 mg/d; range 10–15 mg/d) for an average of 12.8 weeks (range, 8–16 weeks) [38]. All five subjects were considered responders, with significant improvement observed in aggression, SIB, and tantrums. Aripiprazole was well tolerated, with no acute EPS or clinically significant changes in heart rate or blood pressure recorded. Two subjects experienced mild transient somnolence. The mean change in weight was −8.2 lbs (range, −30 to +1 lb), most likely due to discontinuation of prior atypical antipsychotics that had led to significant weight gain.

A retrospective chart review of the first 32 individuals aged 5 to 19 years (mean age, 10.9 years) with a PDD, mental retardation, or both who were prescribed aripiprazole (mean dose, 10.6 mg/d; range, 1.25–30 mg/d) for 6 to 15 months was undertaken [39]. Aripiprazole was reported to be effective in 18 of 32 (56%) subjects, including 9 (37%) of the 24 youth with a PDD. Adverse effects were recorded in 50% of the subjects, which led to drug discontinuation in seven children. The mean body mass index (BMI) increased from 22.5 (n = 27) to 24.1 (n = 23), with greater weight gain noted in youth less than 12 years of age.

Most recently, preliminary results of a 14-week prospective, open-label study of aripiprazole (mean dose, 7.8 mg/d; range, 2.5–15 mg/d) in 25 children and adolescents (mean age, 8.6 years; range, 5–17 years) with PDD not otherwise specified or Asperger's disorder were presented [40]. In that study, 22 of 25 (88%) subjects were determined responders with target symptoms of aggression, SIB, and severe tantrums. The ABC Irritability subscale score decreased from a mean score of 29 at baseline to a mean score of 8.1 at study endpoint. Sixteen subjects had mild tiredness, and one subject had moderate tiredness. Mild EPS were recorded in nine subjects. Nineteen subjects gained weight during the study (mean, +2.3 lbs; range, −3.3 to + 7.7 lbs).

Other psychotropic agents

α-2 Adrenergic agonists

Clonidine

A 6-week double-blind, placebo-controlled crossover study of clonidine was conducted in eight children and adolescents aged 5 to 13 years (mean, 8.1 years) with autism [41]. Treatment at doses ranging from 4 to 10 μg/kg/d led to significant improvement of irritability, hyperactivity, stereotypies, inappropriate speech, and oppositional behavior according to parent and teacher ratings on the ABC and Connors scales; however, the investigators did not record any significant changes. Adverse effects included hypotension, sedation, and decreased activity. Transdermal clonidine (mean dosage, 3.6 μg/kg/d; range, 0.16–0.48 mg/d) was investigated in a 4-week double-blind, placebo-controlled crossover study in nine individuals with autism aged 5 to 33 years (mean age, 12.9 years). Clonidine was determined to be beneficial for impulsivity, hyperarousal, and self-stimulation [42]. Adverse effects, most prominent during the first 2 weeks of treatment, included fatigue and sedation.

Guanfacine

A retrospective analysis of guanfacine (mean dosage, 2.6 mg/d; range, 0.25–9.0 mg/d) was completed in 80 subjects aged 3 to 18 years (mean age, 7.7 years) with a PDD [43]. Nineteen of 80 (23.8%) patients were deemed responders as determined by ratings of "much improved" or "very much improved" on the CGI-I. Individuals diagnosed with Asperger's disorder or PDD not otherwise specified demonstrated greater response than those diagnosed with autism. Guanfacine was effective in 10 of 69 (14%) patients with significant aggression. The most common reported adverse effect was transient sedation.

Mood stabilizers and anticonvulsants

Lithium

To date, one known case report has been published on lithium for symptoms of irritability in autism not associated with mania or bipolar disorder. This report described the augmentation of fluvoxamine with lithium (900 mg/d) [44]. After 2 weeks of treatment, a marked decrease in aggression and impulsivity was reported.

Divalproex sodium

An open-label study of divalproex sodium (mean dosage, 768 mg/d; range 125–2500 mg/d; mean blood level, 75.8 µg/mL) was conducted in 14 subjects aged 5 to 40 years (mean age, 17.9 years) with a PDD [45]. Ten of 14 (71%) subjects were judged responders as determined by ratings of "much improved" or "very much improved" on the CGI-I. Improvement was observed in several symptoms, including impulsivity, aggression, and affective instability. Adverse effects were mild-to-moderate and included sedation, weight gain, behavioral activation, hair loss, and elevated liver enzymes.

An 8-week double-blind, placebo-controlled study of divalproex sodium was conducted in 30 subjects aged 6 to 20 years with a PDD and associated significant aggression [46]. At study endpoint, the mean trough blood level was 77.8 µg/mL. No significant treatment difference was reported between the divalproex sodium and placebo groups based on their primary outcome measure, the ABC Irritability subscale. Adverse effects included increased appetite, skin rash resulting in study discontinuation, and hyperammonemia.

Lamotrigine

In 13 youth with autism initially prescribed lamotrigine for intractable epilepsy, 8 of 13 (62%) patients exhibited subsequent improvement in interfering behavioral symptoms [47]. Nevertheless, a double-blind, placebo-controlled trial of lamotrigine in 14 subjects aged 3 to 11 years (mean age, 5.8 years) with autism did not find a significant difference between drug and placebo on behavioral scores of the Autism Behavior Checklist and ABC [48]. The children received lamotrigine (5 mg/kg/d) over a maintenance period of 4 weeks. Insomnia and hyperactivity were the most common adverse effects.

Topiramate

Mazzone and Ruta [49] reported on the use of topiramate in five youth aged 9 to 13 years (mean age, 11.4 years) with autism and treatment-refractory severe behavioral problems. The drug was started at 0.5 mg/kg/d and titrated up to a maximum of 2.5 mg/kg/d. The duration of treatment ranged from 10 to 33 weeks (mean duration, 22 weeks). Two patients received add-on sertraline at 6 months for obsessive behavior. One patient was on long-term treatment with risperidone. Two patients were judged responders as defined by ratings of "much improved" or "very much improved" on the CGI-I for symptoms of irritability, anger, and hyperactivity, among others. Three other patients showed no improvement, with one patient discontinuing treatment at 10 weeks. Adverse effects were mild, with one patient exhibiting mild sedation. The BMI was significantly reduced in one patient (-2.1) over 12 weeks and slightly reduced (-0.9) in another patient. The investigators concluded that topiramate response was variable and that most children tolerated the medication well but did not show notable improvement.

Levetiracetam

Levetiracetam was investigated for the treatment of aggression, hyperactivity, mood lability, and impulsivity in 10 children aged 4 to 10 years with autism [50]. Subjects were treated for a mean duration of 4.1 weeks. Although the investigators recorded improvement in all of the symptoms, only subjects who were not recently weaned from drugs targeting aggression (eg, risperidone) showed significant improvement in aggression. A 10-week double-blind, placebo-controlled study of levetiracetam (mean dosage, 862.5 mg/d) was conducted in 20 children and adolescents (age range, 5–17 years) with autism [51]. The investigators assessed aggression and affective instability with the ABC parent and teacher rating, finding no significant difference between levetiracetam and placebo. Adverse effects included agitation and aggression.

Summary

Research to date supports use of the atypical antipsychotics as a first-line pharmacologic treatment for children and adolescents with PDDs and associated irritability (aggression, SIB, tantrums). Indeed, the only medication treatment currently approved for irritability in youth with autism is risperidone. Other atypical antipsychotics, including olanzapine and aripiprazole, are currently being investigated via double-blind, placebo-controlled trials. In addition to ongoing research on the atypical antipsychotics in PDDs, large-scale placebo-controlled studies of other medications such as guanfacine are clearly needed to better determine their efficacy in this diagnostic group. The use of anticonvulsants and mood stabilizers has been evaluated in studies in which aggression was a primary target of pharmacotherapy in youth with PDDs, however, controlled studies supporting their use have not been reported. Although additional research regarding their use can be expected in the future, the available research suggests that mood stabilizers and anticonvulsants will not be as effective as atypical antipsychotics for the treatment of irritability in this population. Taken together, the evidence to date most robustly supports the efficacy and tolerability of the atypical antipsychotics for the treatment of irritability in children and adolescents with autism and other PDDs.

References

[1] American Psychiatric Association. Diagnostic and statistical manual of mental disorders. 4th edition, text revision (DSM-IV-TR). Washington, DC: American Psychiatric Publishing; 2000.

[2] McDougle CJ, Posey DJ, Stigler KA. Pharmacological treatments. In: Moldin SO, Rubenstein JLR, editors. Understanding autism: from basic neuroscience to treatment. Boca Raton (FL): CRC Press; 2006. p. 417–42.

[3] Campbell M, Geller B, Cohen IL. Current status of drug research and treatment with autistic children. J Pediatr Psychol 1977;2:153–61.

[4] Campbell M, Anderson LT, Meier M, et al. A comparison of haloperidol and behavior therapy and their interaction in autistic children. J Am Acad Child Psychiatry 1978;17:640–55.

[5] Fish B. Children's Psychiatric Rating Scale (scoring). Psychopharmacol Bull 1985;21: 753–64.

[6] Cohen IL, Campbell M, Posner D, et al. Behavioral effects of haloperidol in young autistic children. J Am Acad Child Adolesc Psychiatry 1980;19:665–77.

[7] Anderson LT, Campbell M, Grega DM, et al. Haloperidol in the treatment of infantile autism: effects on learning and behavioral symptoms. Am J Psychiatry 1984;141:1195–202.

[8] Anderson LT, Campbell M, Adams P, et al. The effects of haloperidol on discrimination learning and behavioral symptoms in autistic children. J Autism Dev Disord 1989;19:227–39.

[9] Perry R, Campbell M, Adams P, et al. Long-term efficacy of haloperidol in autistic children: continuous versus discontinuous drug administration. J Am Acad Child Adolesc Psychiatry 1989;28:87–92.

[10] Campbell M, Armenteros JL, Malone RP, et al. Neuroleptic-related dyskinesias in autistic children: a prospective, longitudinal study. J Am Acad Child Adolesc Psychiatry 1997;36: 835–43.

[11] Pierre JM. Extrapyramidal symptoms with atypical antipsychotics: incidence, prevention and management. Drug Saf 2005;28:191–208.

[12] Zuddas A, Ledda MG, Fratta A, et al. Clinical effects of clozapine on autistic disorder. Am J Psychiatry 1996;153(5):738.

[13] Chen NC, Bedair HS, McKay B, et al. Clozapine in the treatment of aggression in an adolescent with autistic disorder. J Clin Psychiatry 2001;62(6):479–80.

[14] Gobbi G, Pulvirenti L. Long-term treatment with clozapine in an adult with autistic disorder accompanied by aggressive behavior. J Psychiatry Neurosci 2001;26:340–1.

[15] Research Units on Pediatric Psychopharmacology Autism Network. Risperidone in children with autism and serious behavioral problems. N Engl J Med 2002;347:314–21.

[16] Aman MG, Singh NN, Stewart AW, et al. The aberrant behavior checklist: a behavior rating scale for the assessment of treatment effects. Am J Ment Defic 1985;5:485–91.

[17] McDougle CJ, Scahill L, Aman MG, et al. Risperidone for the core symptom domains of autism: results from the study by the autism network of the Research Units on Pediatric Psychopharmacology. Am J Psychiatry 2005;162:1142–8.

[18] Freeman BJ, Ritvo ER, Yakota A, et al. A scale for rating symptoms of patients with the syndrome of autism in real life settings. J Am Acad Child Adolesc Psychiatry 1986;25:130–6.

[19] Scahill L, Riddle MA, McSwiggin-Hardin M, et al. Children's Yale-Brown Obsessive Compulsive Scale: reliability and validity. J Am Acad Child Adolesc Psychiatry 1997;36:844–52.

[20] Research Units on Pediatric Psychopharmacology Autism Network. Risperidone treatment of autistic disorder: longer-term benefits and blinded discontinuation after 6 months. Am J Psychiatry 2005;162:1361–9.

[21] Troost PW, Lahuis BE, Steenhuis MP, et al. Long term effects of risperidone in children with autism spectrum disorders: a placebo discontinuation study. J Am Acad Child Adolesc Psychiatry 2005;44:1137–44.

[22] Shea S, Turgay A, Carrol A, et al. Risperidone in the treatment of disruptive behavioral symptoms in children with autistic and other pervasive developmental disorders. Pediatrics 2004;114:e634–641.

[23] Schopler E, Reichler RJ, DeVellis RF, et al. Toward objective classification of childhood autism: childhood autism rating scale (CARS). J Autism Dev Disord 1980;10:91–103.

[24] Miral S, Gencer O, Inal-Emiroglu FN, et al. Risperidone versus haloperidol in children and adolescents with AD: a randomized, controlled, double-blind trial. Eur Child Adolesc Psychiatry 2008;17:1–8.

[25] Nagaraj R, Singhi P, Malhi P. Risperidone in children with autism: randomized, placebo-controlled, double-blind study. J Child Neurol 2006;21:450–5.

[26] Luby J, Mrakotsky C, Stalets MM, et al. Risperidone in preschool children with autistic spectrum disorders: an investigation of safety and efficacy. J Child Adolesc Psychopharmacol 2006;16:575–87.

[27] Potenza MN, Holmes JP, Kanes SJ, et al. Olanzapine treatment of children, adolescents, and adults with pervasive developmental disorders: an open-label pilot study. J Clin Psychopharmacol 1999;19:37–44.

[28] Malone RP, Cate J, Sheikh RM, et al. Olanzapine versus haloperidol in children with autistic disorder: an open pilot study. J Am Acad Child Adolesc Psychiatry 2001;40:887–94.

[29] Kemner C, Willemsen-Swinkels SH, de Jonge M, et al. Open-label study of olanzapine in children with pervasive developmental disorder. J Clin Psychopharmacol 2002;22:455–60.

[30] Hollander E, Wasserman S, Swanson EN, et al. A double-blind placebo-controlled pilot study of olanzapine in childhood/adolescent pervasive developmental disorder. J Child Adolesc Psychopharmacol 2006;16:541–8.

[31] Martin A, Koenig K, Scahill L, et al. Open-label quetiapine in the treatment of children and adolescents with autistic disorder. J Child Adolesc Psychopharmacol 1999;9:99–107.

[32] Findling RL, McNamara NK, Gracious BL, et al. Quetiapine in nine youths with autistic disorder. J Child Adolesc Psychopharmacol 2004;14:287–94.

[33] Corson AH, Barkenbus JE, Posey DJ, et al. A retrospective analysis of quetiapine in the treatment of pervasive developmental disorders. J Clin Psychiatry 2004;65:1531–6.

[34] Hardan AY, Jou RJ, Handen BL. Retrospective study of quetiapine in children and adolescents with pervasive developmental disorders. J Autism Dev Disord 2005;35:387–91.

[35] McDougle CJ, Kem DL, Posey DJ. Case series: use of ziprasidone for maladaptive symptoms in youths with autism. J Am Acad Child Adolesc Psychiatry 2002;41:921–7.

[36] Cohen SA, Fitzgerald BJ, Khan SR, et al. The effect of a switch to ziprasidone in an adult population with autistic disorder: chart review of naturalistic, open-label treatment. J Clin Psychiatry 2004;65:110–3.

[37] Malone RP, Delaney MA, Hyman SB, et al. Ziprasidone in adolescents with autism: an open-label pilot study. J Am Acad Child Adolesc Psychiatry 2007;17(6):779–90.

[38] Stigler KA, Posey DJ, McDougle CJ. Case report: aripiprazole for maladaptive behavior in pervasive developmental disorder. J Child Adolesc Psychopharmacol 2004;14:455–63.

[39] Valicenti-McDermott MR, Demb H. Clinical effects and adverse reactions of off-label use of aripiprazole in children and adolescents with developmental disabilities. J Child Adolesc Psychopharmacol 2006;16:549–60.

[40] Stigler KA, Diener JT, Kohn AE, et al. Aripiprazole in Asperger's disorder and pervasive developmental disorder not otherwise specified: a 14-week prospective, open-label study. Program No. 35, Abstract Viewer. Boca Raton (FL): American College of Neuropsychopharmacology; 2007.

[41] Jaselskis CA, Cook EH, Fletcher KE, et al. Clonidine treatment of hyperactive and impulsive children with autistic disorder. J Clin Psychopharmacol 1992;12:322–7.

[42] Fankhauser MP, Karumanchi VC, German ML, et al. A double-blind, placebo-controlled study of the efficacy of transdermal clonidine in autism. J Clin Psychiatry 1992;53(3):77–82.

[43] Posey DJ, Decker J, Sasher TM, et al. Guanfacine treatment of hyperactivity and inattention in autism: a retrospective analysis of 80 cases. J Child Adolesc Psychopharmacol 2004;14: 233–41.

[44] Epperson CN, McDougle CJ, Anand A, et al. Lithium augmentation of fluvoxamine in autistic disorder: a case report. J Child Adolesc Psychopharmacol 1994;4:201–7.

[45] Hollander E, Dolgoff-Kaspar R, Cartwright C, et al. An open trial of divalproex sodium in autism spectrum disorders. J Clin Psychiatry 2001;62(7):530–4.

[46] Hellings JA, Weckbaugh M, Nickel EJ, et al. A double-blind, placebo-controlled study of valproate for aggression in youth with pervasive developmental disorders. J Child Adolesc Psychopharmacol 2005;15(4):682–92.

[47] Uvebrant P, Bauzine R. Intractable epilepsy in children: the efficacy of lamotrigine treatment, including non–seizure-related benefits. Neuropediatrics 1994;25:284–9.

[48] Belsito KM, Law PA, Kirk KS, et al. Lamotrigine therapy for autistic disorder: a randomized, double-blind, placebo-controlled trial. J Autism Dev Disord 2001;31(2):175–81.

[49] Mazzone L, Ruta L. Topiramate in children with autistic spectrum disorders. Brain Dev 2006;28(10):668.

[50] Rugino TA, Samsock TC. Levetiracetam in autistic children: an open-label study. J Dev Behav Pediatr. 2002;23(4):225–30.

[51] Wasserman S, Iyengar R, Chaplin WF, et al. Levetiracetam versus placebo in childhood and adolescent autism: a double-blind placebo-controlled study. Int Clin Psychopharmacol 2006;21(6):363–7.

ELSEVIER
SAUNDERS

Child Adolesc Psychiatric Clin N Am
17 (2008) 753–771

CHILD AND
ADOLESCENT
PSYCHIATRIC CLINICS
OF NORTH AMERICA

Psychopharmacologic Interventions for Repetitive Behaviors in Autism Spectrum Disorders

Latha Soorya, PhD*,
Jessica Kiarashi, Eric Hollander, MD

Department of Psychiatry, Seaver & New York Autism Center of Excellence, Mount Sinai School of Medicine, One Gustave L. Levy Place, Box 1230, New York, NY 10029, USA

The core symptom domain of restrictive, repetitive, and stereotyped patterns of behavior historically has been understudied relative to other core symptom domains in autism spectrum disorder (ASD). Several factors may contribute to the relative inattention given to the restricted, repetitive behaviors and interests (RRBIs) domain, including uncertainties about the specificity of RRBIs to ASD [1]. Namely, the presence of RRBIs in normal infant development and the high prevalence in other developmental disabilities [1,2] may have reduced the relevance of this domain to ASD researchers in the past.

Recent research, however, has provided greater insight into the nature of the RRBI domain and its importance in the conceptualization of ASD. Studies suggest RRBIs in ASD are differentiated in the severity, frequency, and topography from repetitive behaviors observed in developmentally disabled (DD) and typically developing (TD) populations, with individuals who have ASDs showing increased symptom severity and behaviors associated with maintaining routines and order [3,4]. Furthermore, RRBIs have shown strong heritability, particularly for compulsive behaviors [5] and may be the most enduring diagnostic marker of ASD in children [6]. Research also suggests the broad category of RRBIs may be conceptualized with greater specificity, with potentially differing etiologies and treatments associated with specific RRBI categories.

Importantly, repetitive and compulsive behaviors are an important intervention target in improving overall outcomes for individuals who have

---

* Corresponding author.
E-mail address: latha.soorya@mssm.edu (L. Soorya).

ASD. RRBIs can create considerable disturbance in daily family activities and often interfere with progress in educational and psychosocial interventions. Moreover, medical and behavioral intervention research in the area of repetitive behaviors in ASD is relatively scarce. Table 1 presents the handful of placebo-controlled trials evaluating pharmacologic interventions for repetitive behaviors in ASDs. Pharmacologic approaches receiving the most attention include selective serotonin reuptake inhibitor (SSRI) interventions, which have shown promise in three controlled clinical trials. Nevertheless, SSRIs rapidly have become the most prescribed medication in pediatric ASD populations, a likely reflection of the demand for interventions providing respite from the distress and disruption caused by this core symptom domain [7]. This article provides an in-depth overview of the empiric research on SSRI and other pharmacologic interventions, preceded by a brief introduction of the literature on the phenomenology and potential etiologies of the repetitive behavior domain in ASD.

Defining the repetitive and compulsive behavior domain in autism spectrum disorder

The repetitive behavior domain in ASD is comprised of diverse behaviors characterized by repetition, rigid behavioral or thought patterns, insistence on preserving the status-quo, and intense interests that are distinguished by their all-encompassing nature or unusual content. The *Diagnostic and Statistical Manual of Mental Disorders, Fourth Edition* (DSM-IV) [8] description of RRBIs includes:

A preoccupation with stereotyped and restricted patterns of interest
Inflexibility in adhering to routines and rituals
Stereotyped and repetitive motor mannerisms
Persistent preoccupation with parts of objects

Although descriptive of the range of common repetitive behavior topographies observed in ASDs, DSM-IV descriptions of RRBIs in ASDs fail to account for several factors, including repetitive self-injury, hoarding, and obsessive thought patterns often observed in individuals who have ASDs.

Several investigations have provided alternative conceptual and quantitative categorizations of repetitive behaviors. A series of investigations aimed at characterizing the RRBI domain in ASD relative to other populations, including clinical and neurotypical samples, has been completed. As mentioned, RRBIs in individuals who have ASD display more severe RRBIs than DD or TD individuals, across many parameters (eg, frequency, duration, and interference on family life) [9,10]. Compared with adults who had obsessive–compulsive disorder (OCD), McDougle and colleagues [11] found differences in the severity and pattern of OCD behaviors in autistic adults on the Yale-Brown Obsessive Compulsive Scale (YBOCS). Adults who had autism exhibited more compulsive than obsessive behaviors and a more limited range of obsessions, with significantly fewer obsessions surrounding sex, religion, symmetry, contamination, and aggression than adults who had OCD. Fewer compulsive-type behaviors often seen in OCD (eg, cleaning, counting, checking) were reported for the autism population. The presence of behaviors such as touching, tapping, rubbing, hoarding, and self-damaging and the absence of repetitive thoughts about aggression, symmetry, checking, and counting seemed to characterize the autism group in this study.

A general conceptual categorization of RRBIs includes two categories of RRBIs: lower-order repetitive motor and sensory behaviors and higher-order ritualistic and compulsive behaviors [1,4]. Lower-order behaviors include stereotyped motor mannerisms (eg, hand flapping); repetitive use of objects;=, repetitive self-injury, spontaneous dyskinesias, and unusual sensory interests (eg, sniffing and/or mouthing objects). Higher-order repetitive behaviors include OCD-like behaviors such as compulsions, a desire to maintain sameness, ritualistic behaviors, and circumscribed interests or preoccupations.

Other recent studies chose quantitative approaches to defining subdomains of RRBIs through factor analytic approaches [4,12]. Richler and colleagues [4] evaluated RRBIs as reported on the repetitive behavior domain of the Autism Diagnostic Interview-Revised (ADI-R) in young children who had autism (ie, under 3 years old). Results of the factor analysis confirmed previous research on the factor structure of the ADI-R and conceptual models of lower/higher-order repetitive behaviors [12,13], with findings suggesting the ADI-R repetitive behavior domain consists of two factors: repetitive sensorimotor behaviors and insistence on sameness. Recent factor analyses, using instruments designed to provide detailed assessment of the repetitive behavior domain, such as the Repetitive Behavior Scale-Revised (RBS-R) and YBOCS suggest greater distinction in the behaviors comprising the RRBI categories in ASDs [14,15]. Lam and Aman [14] identified six factors on the RBS-R, a parent report measure of RRBIs modified for autism, including ritualistic behavior, sameness behavior, stereotypic behavior, self-injurious behavior, compulsive behavior, and restricted interests. In contrast, Anagnostou and colleagues [15] analyzed Y-BOCS data in ASD populations and identified a four-factor solution describing RRBIs in ASDs, including obsessions, higher-order repetitive behaviors, lower-order repetitive behaviors, and hoarding.

Although research in these categorizations of RRBIs is in its early stages, investigations suggest utility in this conceptualization in aiding genetics research, which indicates a familial pattern in first-degree relatives of individuals who have ASD for higher-order compulsive behaviors, but not for lower-order repetitive behaviors [5].

Table 1
Double-blind, placebo-controlled psychopharmacological intervention for repetitive behaviors in autism spectrum disorders

Author	Design	Sample	Medication	Measures	Outcome	Adverse effects across all groups	Dosing start/mean final dose
Gordon et al, 1993 [32]	Double-blind, placebo-controlled crossover	12 children	Clomipramine versus desipramine and placebo	Children's Psychiatric Rating Scale, CGI, obsessive compulsive subscale of Comprehensive Psychopathological Rating Scale	Significant improvements in clomipramine group in reducing hyperactivity, stereotypies, compulsive behaviors, and anger	Reported adverse effects included fatigue, tremors, tachycardia, insomnia, nausea, diaphoresis, and behavioral problems	25 mg/152 mg/d
McDougle et al, 1996 [37]	Double-blind, placebo-controlled	30 adults	Fluvoxamine	YBOCS, CGI, Vineland, Brown, Ritvo-Freeman	Significant improvements in repetitive behavior and aggression	Reported adverse effects included nausea and sedation	50 mg/d/276−7 ± 41.7 mg daily
Hollander et al, 2004 [70]	Placebo controlled crossover	45 children and adolescents	Fluoxetine	CGI-AD, C-YBOCS	Significant decrease in repetitive behavior	No overall difference between groups, but patients on fluoxetine reported less anxiety than placebo group	2.5 mg/d/9.90 ± 4.35 mg daily

Study	Design	n	Drug	Measures	Results	Adverse effects	Dose
Buchsbaum et al, 2001 [40]	Placebo-controlled crossover	6 adults	Fluoxetine	YBOCS, HAM-A	Significant improvement in obsessions, repetitive behaviors, and anxiety	Headaches (in 1 patient the day of fluoxetine treatment)	10 mg/d/target end dose = 40 mg/d
McDougle et al, 2005 [62]	Double-blind, placebo-controlled	101 children and adolescents	Risperidone	ABC, CGI, C-YBOCS, Ritvo-Freeman, Vineland	Significant improvement in restricted, repetitive, and stereotyped behaviors, interests, and activities	Weight gain was the most significant adverse effect and increased appetite, fatigue, and drowsiness were more common in risperidone group than placebo group	0.5–3.5 mg/d/1.8 ± 0.7 mg/d 16-week open label: 2.0 mg/d /2.1 mg/d
Hollander et al, 2006 [69]	Double-blind, placebo-controlled	12 children and adolescents and 1 adult	Divalproex sodium	C-YBOCS	Significant improvements in repetitive behaviors	Reported adverse effects included irritability, weight gain, anxiety, and aggression	125 mg/d/822.92 ± 326.2 mg/d

(continued on next page)

Table 1
(*continued*)

Author	Design	Sample	Medication	Measures	Outcome	Adverse effects across all groups	Dosing start/mean final dose
Hollander et al, 2003 [68]	Double-blind, placebo-controlled	15 adults	Oxytocin	YBOCS	Significant decrease in frequency and severity of repetitive behaviors and frequency	Reported adverse effects included anxiety, depression, drowsiness, stomach cramps, and headache	Intravenous infusion: 10 mL/h increased every 15 minutes the first hour, 50 mL the second hour, 100 mL the third hour, and held constant at 700 mL the fourth hour

Abbreviations: ABC, Aberrant Behavior Checklist; Brown, Brown Aggression Scale; CARS, Child Autism Rating Scale; CGI, Clinical Global Impressions scale; CGI-AD, CGI adapted for global autism; CGI, Clinical Global Impressions scale; CY-BOCS, Children's Yale-Brown Obsessive Compulsive Scale; HAM-A, Hamilton Rating Scale for Anxiety; Ritvo-Freeman, Ritvo-Freeman Real Life Rating Scale; Vineland, Vineland maladaptive behavior subscales; YBOCS, Yale-Brown Obsessive Compulsive Scale.

Data from Kolevzon, A, Mathewson, KA, Hollander, E. Selective serotonin reuptake inhibitors in autism: a review of efficacy and tolerability. J Clin Psychiatry 2006;67(3):407–14.

Etiologic hypotheses of repetitive behaviors and interests in autism spectrum disorders

The underlying cause of repetitive behaviors, whether as a cohesive category or within particular classes of RRBIs, is not known. Several theories from across disciplines—biological, behavioral, neuropsychological and translational neuroscience—have been proposed to describe the underlying pathology of RRBIs in ASDs. Neuropsychological theories include the role of executive function deficits and weak central coherence in the presence of RRBIs [1]. Major biological theories include hypotheses about the role of repetitive behavior in regulating dysfunctional arousal regulation systems in ASDs [16], sensitivity to dopamine and endogenous opioids, and serotonin dysregulation [17]. Research investigating animal models of ASD may provide insight into potential etiologies for repetitive behaviors including reports of an inbred mouse strain, BTBR T + tf/J [18], which expresses an endophenotype with social recognition deficits and rigid behavioral/cognitive patterns (exemplified by failure of this strain on reversal learning tasks). Although several theories have been posited for the underlying causes of repetitive behaviors in ASD, interdisciplinary research aimed at integrating endophenotyping, genetics, and pharmacologic findings is needed to refine theories and address potentially different etiologies for specific classes of repetitive behaviors.

Serotonin dysregulation in autism spectrum disorders: implications for intervention research

Several investigations support the role of serotonin in the underlying pathophysiology of autism, with converging support from genetics, pharmacologic, biological, and neuroimaging research [15–18]. The role of the serotonin system in autism has received considerable attention since a study by Schain and colleagues [19], which found elevated blood serotonin levels (ie, hyperserotonemia) in patients who had autism. Since the Schain and Freedman study, several studies have confirmed hyperserotonemia as a common biological deficit in ASD, with approximately one third of individuals in studies expressing elevated platelet serotonin levels [17,20]. Further support has been found in pharmacologic studies, including a study by McDougle and colleagues [21], in which medication-naïve adults who had ASD underwent a tryptophan depletion trial to reduce 5-hydroxytyptamine (5HT) synthesis, release, and neurotransmission. Results indicated adults who had autism exhibited more repetitive behaviors such as whirling, flapping, pacing, banging, rocking, and self-injury. In a similar investigation of sumatriptan, the authors found that sensitivity of the 5HT1d receptor, as measured by growth hormone response, positively correlated with severity of the repetitive behavior domain, but not other core domains or global autistic symptoms [22].

Hypotheses regarding serotonin dysregulation as a potential underlying cause of ASD and specifically repetitive behaviors are also appealing because of the broad effects of the serotonin system with other neurotransmitter systems and on a range of human behaviors. Serotonin has been implicated in many behaviors observed in individuals who have ASD, including aggression, anxiety, repetitive behaviors, mood, impulsivity, sleep, ingestion, reward systems, and psychosis [17]. The serotonin system is also of interest in autism research given its essential role in brain development and impact on critical areas of the brain, including the cerebellum, thalamus, and frontal cortex, which may be dysfunctional in individuals who have autism [23].

In addition to evidence for serotonin dysfunction from biological and pharmacologic challenge studies, similarities between RRBIs in ASD and the repetitive and obsessive behaviors observed in OCD, where pharmacologic treatments with SSRIs are considered a first-line treatment, led to research on the effects of SSRI interventions in ASDs [24] SSRIs are a class of agents that inhibit central nervous system neuronal uptake of serotonin [25] through blocking the reuptake of (5HT) and increasing 5HT levels in the synapse by preventing reuptake of 5HT by the presynaptic nerve terminal [26]. SSRIs also may alter the 5HT receptors to bring about long-term changes, but because each specific SSRI has other pharmacologic characteristics, they produce different adverse effects and vary in effectiveness.

Treatment with serotonin reuptake inhibitors and selective serotonin reuptake inhibitors

Several recent articles provide overviews of research on the efficacy of SRIs in treating core and associated symptoms of ASD [27–29]. The SRI/SSRI treatment literature, however, is small, consisting of three randomized trials and several open-label studies. Pharmacologic agents reviewed in this class include the SRI clomipramine, and SSRIs, including citalopram, escitalopram, fluoxetine, fluvoxamine, and sertraline. The limited pool of controlled and open-label research points to benefits of SSRI treatments in improving the core symptom domain of repetitive behaviors; potentially in associated symptoms, such as anxiety and aggression; and overall global functioning. The effects on other core and associated symptoms have been less striking, although the existing research has not been designed well to study the effects on social and communication deficits in ASD. Existing data suggest differential efficacy and tolerability profiles, with overall greater efficacy and tolerability profile for SSRIs compared with SRIs, and potentially more generalized efficacy for fluoxetine across the spectrum of individuals with ASDs. In addition, commonly reported adverse effects, particularly in pediatric populations, include what has come to be known as activation symptoms, describing the potential increased hyperactivity, sleep disturbance, and general overall increase in agitation and irritability that may result from some SSRIs and ultimately result in termination of SSRI interventions. Greater details on the effects of each pharmacologic agent will be summarized.

Clomipramine

Much of the SRI research in ASDs has drawn from the success of SRIs in treating repetitive motor behaviors, compulsions, and obsessions in pediatric and adult OCD populations. The success of clomipramine hydrochloride, a tricyclic antidepressant, in treating repetitive and stereotyped obsessive–compulsive motor behaviors in OCD populations in both placebo-controlled [30] and comparison randomized controlled trials (RCTs) with desipramine hydrochloride [31] presented the possibility of similar efficacy in ASDs. An RCT of clomipramine in children who had autism compared clomipramine, desipramine, and placebo in a cross-over design [32]. The design involved a 2-week single-blind placebo phase, followed by a 10-week cross-over phase with two arms: clomipramine/placebo (n = 12) and clomipramine/desipramine (n = 12). Results indicated clomipramine was more effective than placebo and desipramine in decreasing abnormal behaviors on the autism subscale of the Children's Psychiatric Rating Scale, and in improving OCD symptoms as measured by several outcomes. Adverse events reflected those seen in the OCD literature and included lowering of the seizure threshold, with one brief seizure reported in a patient in this trial, who subsequently was removed from the study.

Subsequent open-label [33,34] and placebo-controlled studies [35], however, suggest limited efficacy for clomipramine, and considerable safety and tolerability concerns. In the open-label pediatric research, one study [33] reported five of five young children had initially positive responses to clomipramine but developed serious adverse effects, including serotonin syndrome, resulting in withdrawal of treatment. Another open-label study reported increased irritability, self-injury, aggression toward others, and urinary retention requiring catheterization as common adverse events [34]. Remington and colleagues [35] conducted a double-blind, placebo-controlled cross-over trial of clomipramine, haloperidol, and placebo in children and adults, evaluating effects on the core domains and associated features of ASD. The Aberrant Behavior Checklist (ABC) was used to measure problem behaviors, including stereotypy. Results indicated comparable efficacy for clomipramine and placebo on stereotypy. Twenty of 32 participants, however, prematurely terminated Clomipramine, compared with only 10 of 33 participants receiving haloperidol. Investigators reported high rates of adverse effects with clomipramine, including fatigue, tremors, tachycardia, diaphoresis, and significant behavior problems.

Fluvoxamine

The ASD literature includes two double-blind, placebo-controlled trials, one adult and one pediatric, of fluvoxamine. In addition to its primary effects on the serotonin transporter, fluvoxamine also may have effects on σ_1 receptors, involved in dopamine regulation and modulation of N-methyl-D-asparate receptors [36]. McDougle and colleagues [37] conducted a placebo-controlled study of fluvoxamine versus placebo in 30 adults who had autism. Participants enrolled in the 12-week trial were rated on the Clinical Global Impressions scale (CGI), with results indicating 8 of 15 patients who received fluvoxamine (276.7 mg/d) were responders compared with 0 of 15 in the placebo group. Significant improvements in repetitive thoughts and behaviors, aggression, social relatedness, and repetitive language were noted. Minor adverse efforts were reported and included nausea and sedation.

In a subsequent unpublished pediatric study by the same laboratory [38], children and adolescents (mean age 9.5 years) who had ASDs were reported to have a poor response to fluvoxamine, with notable adverse effects in 14 of 18 children on the active medication. Reported adverse effects suggest limited tolerability that potentially is related to activation, despite a starting dose of 25 mg every other day which is less than that recommended by the US Food and Drug Administration (FDA) for treating pediatric OCD. In addition, it is important to note that plasma levels of fluvoxamine are substantially higher in child populations than in adolescent and adult populations. The pharmacokinetic properties suggest C_{max} of fluvoxamine plasma levels, and the area under the curve is tripled in children versus adolescents. Interestingly, C_{max} is also higher in girls compared with boys [39]. Only 1 out of 18 children randomized to fluvoxamine showed clinically significant improvement in the target symptoms. The pharmacokinetic findings and discrepant results from adult and pediatric fluvoxamine studies suggest treatment with SSRIs in developmental conditions such as ASD require sensitivity to developmental processes, particularly given the role of serotonin in early brain development.

Fluoxetine

Fluoxetine is an SSRI known to be a potent inhibitor of 5HT uptake. In addition, it may have effects on the $5HT_{2c}$ receptor and indirectly influence noradrenergic and dopaminergic systems. Fluoxetine has been studied in separate controlled investigations in pediatric and adult populations [40,41]. These suggest that fluoxetine is tolerated well and efficacious in reducing repetitive, stereotyped behaviors and restricted interest patterns in individuals who have ASD. In addition, several open-label studies have shown improvement of autistic symptoms with fluoxetine in adults and children [42,43]. A large open-label fluoxetine study found a 69% improvement in 129 autistic children, aged 2 to 8 [44].

Hollander and colleagues [39] conducted a 20-week double-blind, placebo-controlled cross-over trial of low-dose liquid fluoxetine treatment in 45 children and adolescents with autism (ages 5 to 16 years). The study design included three phases, starting with an 8-week phase of fluoxetine versus placebo, followed by a 4-week washout phase and an 8-week double-blind cross-over trial. Dosing started at a fixed dose of 2.5 mg/d and followed-with a flexible titration based on weight and tolerability to a maximum target dose at week 4 of 0.8 mg/kg/d (actual mean final dose = .4 mg/kg/d). Measurements included the children's form of the YBOCS (CY-BOCS) [45] and the Clinical Global Improvement Scale Adapted to Global Autism (CGI-AD), a CGI-Severity (CGI-S) score focused on core autism symptoms independent of associated symptom domains. Fluoxetine treatment resulted in significant reductions in repetitive behaviors as measured by the CY-BOCS, with results suggesting a moderate-to-large effect size (.76). Global autism severity as measured by the CGI-AD did not improve in this trial, although results from a global composite measure weighted for repetitive behaviors were suggestive of improvements in global autism symptoms. Adverse effects as measured by the Fluoxetine Side Effects Checklist indicated minor adverse effects such as diarrhea, weight gain, insomnia, and anxiety in the fluoxetine group. The adverse effects were not statistically significant compared with the placebo group [29]. Thus, these results suggest fluoxetine was tolerated well and effective in reducing repetitive behaviors in children who had autism. The study was limited by the short duration (8 weeks) for fluoxetine treatment in the cross-over design and the limited evaluation of effects on other core and associated symptom domains (eg, socialization and anxiety).

In adults, a single pilot, double-blind, placebo controlled cross-over study in a small sample (n = 6) was conducted to evaluate the effects of fluoxetine treatment on repetitive behaviors and global autism severity. In addition, investigators aimed to develop hypotheses regarding predictors of treatment responsiveness through measuring baseline and post-treatment serotonin metabolism through positron emission tomography (PET) imaging [40]. Participants significantly improved during the fluoxetine arm of the cross-over study on the obsession subscale of the Y-BOCS, with three of six participants also demonstrating improvement on global measures of autism severity. Of interest, results from the PET imaging suggested that higher baseline metabolism rates in medial frontal and anterior cingulate cortices were associated with treatment response, supporting similar findings by this research group in individuals who had depression [40]. The authors' group also conducted a larger, double-blind, placebo-controlled trial of fluoxetine in adults who had ASDs. Results from this study will represent the first double-blind, placebo-controlled trial of fluoxetine in adults who have ASDs.

Sertraline

Two open-label studies have been published of sertraline an SSRI, which also has dopamine uptake-blocking properties. The studies suggest sertraline may be an effective treatment for repetitive behaviors, anxiety, and irritability/aggression [46,47]. McDougle [46] conducted a 12-week open-label trial of sertraline in 42 adults who had pervasive developmental disorders (PDDs) using the YBOCS, Ritvo-Freeman Real-Life Rating Scale to measure autism symptomatology, and the Self-Injurious Behavior Questionnaire. Authors reported 24 of 42 patients improved on measures of repetitive and aggressive behaviors, but not social relatedness. On the CGI, 15 of 22 patients who had autism and 9 of 14 with PDD-not otherwise specified were much improved or very much improved on CGI-Improvement (CGI-I) ratings, while none of the six patients who had Asperger's disorder improved with sertraline treatment. The authors suggest that lower baseline repetitive behavior and ASD symptom scores in the Asperger's group may have contributed to the limited efficacy observed for Asperger's participants. Three of the 42 patients experienced agitation and anxiety resulting in termination. Sertraline showed no serious cardiovascular effects or seizures and was tolerated well.

Sertraline's effectiveness also was assessed in children in an open-label trial [47]. Nine children with autism between the ages of 6 and 12 were administered sertraline for the treatment of transition-associated anxiety and agitation. It was found that 89% of the subjects had a positive response. Results suggest the importance of future controlled investigation of sertraline in pediatric and adult ASD populations.

Citalopram

Citalopram is one of the most highly selective SSRIs [48]. A published open-label, chart-review of citalopram in 15 children and adolescents who had PDDs suggested improvements in repetitive behaviors and anxiety based on CGI-S and CGI-I ratings [49]. The study reported a mean dose of citalopram was 16.9 mg plus or minus 12.1 mg daily (range 5 to 40 mg), with children treated over an average period of 218.8 plus or minus 167.2 days. Of the 15 cases, 11 were much improved or very much improved. The longer the subject was on the treatment, the more positive the response. As noted, anxiety and repetitive behaviors or stereotypies were most responsive to citalopram, with 10 of the 15 subjects showing improvement in anxiety, presumably related to reduced rigidity in adherence to routines and rituals. Although length of treatment time correlated positively with response, higher dosages did not.

A National Institutes of Health (NIH)-sponsored STAART (Studies to Advance Autism Research and Treatment) network study has been funded to study the effects of liquid citalopram on global improvement and repetitive behaviors in a large, multisite randomized controlled trial enrolling participants ages 5 to 17 meeting criteria for an ASD by DSM-IV-Text Revision criteria. Results from this trial will represent the largest evaluation of an psychopharmacological intervention, and an SSRI, in the ASD literature to date.

Escitalopram

A 10-week open-label trial also was conducted to evaluate the safety and efficacy of escitalopram [50], the S-enantiomer of citalopram, which like citalopram, is highly selective for the serotonin reuptake site and has no affinity for norepinephrine or dopamine reuptake sites [51]. The study focused on escitalopram's impact on global severity and irritability in individuals who had PDD. There were 28 individuals between the ages of 6 and 17 included in the study. The dose began at 2.5 mg/d and increased every week until a maximum of 20 mg/d. The investigators reported improvement was observed in global functioning as measured by the CGI-I. Additionally, 17 out of 28 children were reported as less irritable on the ABC-Community Version (ABC-CV) irritability subscale. Adverse events included reports of hyperactivity and irritability in 18 participants, none in five participants and no reports of more severe adverse events (eg, self-injury, suicidal ideation, sleep disturbance). These reports suggest a promising safety, tolerability, and efficacy profile for escitalopram to evaluate in larger-scale controlled studies.

Early intervention with selective serotonin reuptake inhibitors

SSRIs have been presented as a model pharmacologic treatment, because serotonin is known to enhance synapse refinement in the brains of autistic children [52]. In the developing cortex, serotonin is concerned with maturation of thalamic afferents, cortical dendrites, and axons, with alterations in the levels of serotonin potentially resulting in negative effects. High levels of serotonin may reduce pruning of the dendritic branches [53,54], with too little serotonin causing a smaller number of dendritic spines than usual, miniscule dendritic arbors and somatosensory barrels, and a decrease in synaptic density [55–57]. Thus, interventions targeting normalization of serotonin regulation in the developing brain of young children who have autism has been proposed as a novel, early intervention strategy [52]. A pilot, randomized, placebo-controlled trial is being funded by the NIH STAART network in toddlers and preschoolers who have autism to evaluate the effects of liquid fluoxetine on global improvements and alterations in developmental progressions in young children who have ASDs.

Other treatments for repetitive behaviors and interests in autism spectrum disorder

Atypical antipsychotics

Following two large-scale, randomized controlled trials of the atypical antipsychotic risperidone [58,59], atypical antipsychotics increasingly have been prescribed to children who have ASDs [60]. Traditional and atypical antipsychotics are prescribed conventionally for managing severe maladaptive behaviors associated with ASD, including irritability, aggression, and self-injury. In addition to improving associated symptoms of irritability and aggression, results from a few controlled studies [58] suggest utility for the atypical risperidone in improving the core symptom of repetitive behaviors and restricted interests. Risperidone's action on postsynaptic serotonin receptors, in addition to dopamine and reports of its effectiveness in treating refractory OCD when combined with SSRIs [61], suggests its utility for treating RRBIs in ASDs. McDougle and colleagues [61] conducted the first double-blind, placebo-controlled trial of risperidone in 31 adults who had ASDs and found risperidone treatment (mean dose = 2.9 mg/d) significantly improved repetitive behaviors on the Y-BOCS compulsion subscale items. Additionally, improvements were noted in the associated symptoms of aggression, irritability, and anxiety. Overall, risperidone was tolerated well in the adult sample, with adverse events including mild, transient sedation, particularly during initial dosing period, with no reports of serious adverse effects. McDougle and colleagues [62] reported on the efficacy of risperidone on core symptom domains of ASD in a follow-up article to the multisite RUPP (Research Units on Pediatric Psychopharmacology) Autism Network study, which had a primary aim of evaluating short- and long-term effects of risperidone treatment in children and adolescents who had high levels of disruptive behaviors. Results suggested risperidone significantly improved repetitive behaviors as measured by the C-YBOCS [44] and the Ritvo-Freeman Real-Life Rating Scale subscales of sensory–motor behaviors, but did not influence social or communication skills as measured by the Ritvo-Freeman scale. These studies suggest efficacy for use of atypical antipsychotics in treating interfering repetitive behaviors in ASD. Risks associated with long-term use of atypical antipsychotics such as the development of metabolic syndrome, however, warrant further research, including research evaluating long-term adverse effects, effects on particular classes of repetitive behaviors in ASD, and use of risperidone as an adjunctive therapy in nonresponders to other interventions.

Divalproex sodium

Although SSRIs are a potentially potent treatment for repetitive behaviors in ASD, a common adverse effect of SSRIs, irritability and hyperactivity, reduces the tolerability of these medications, particularly in pediatric populations. For some patients, these negative adverse effects may inhibit them from continuing medication even if there are positive results. Efforts aimed at improving the tolerability of SSRIs in pediatric populations include initiating treatment with low, minimally therapeutic doses, and slowly titrating to clinically effective levels. In addition, it has been hypothesized that treatment with medications such as divalproex sodium, which has shown effectiveness in ameliorating irritability in some disorders [63], may hold potential as an alternative treatment or lead-in to SSRI interventions.

Hollander and colleagues [39] evaluated the use of divalproex sodium in directly targeting the core symptom domain of repetitive behaviors in ASDs. This study was the first randomized, double-blind, placebo-controlled trial using divalproex sodium, and the authors hypothesized that repetitive behaviors would be reduced with divalproex sodium based on reports from the treatment of refractory OCD with SSRIs augmented by anticon-vulsants such as divalproex sodium [64]. Thirteen subjects were randomized (12 children, 1 adult). There was a 2:1 ratio in place for subjects in the drug group versus placebo group, with dosing starting at 125 mg/d, increasing to 125 mg every 4 days during the 2 weeks of the treatment. Significant group differences were seen on the C-YBOCS, with improvements in repetitive be-haviors for the treatment group and a worsening of symptoms observed in the placebo group. Reported adverse events included weight gain, irritabil-ity, anxiety, and aggression in both the divalproex sodium and placebo groups. The authors postulated that divalproex sodium's efficacy in treating repetitive behaviors in ASD may result from the reduced irritability and dis-tress associated with repetitive behaviors. Analysis of individual items from the C-YBOCS, however, suggested divalproex sodium decreased the actual number of hours spent on repetitive behaviors, suggesting future research is needed to replicate these findings and evaluate the direct or indirect influ-ence of divalproex sodium on repetitive behaviors in ASD.

Oxytocin

The role of oxytocin in the pathophysiology of ASD is based on several intriguing lines of investigation, which collectively suggest a role for oxyto-cin in improving core symptoms of ASD. Oxytocin is a nine-amino acid pep-tide hormone that has peripheral and centrally mediated actions, acts as a neuromodulator in the brain, and is of interest in autism research because of findings from animal studies highlighting oxytocin's role in two core domains of ASD: socialization (eg, affiliative behaviors) and repetitive behaviors (eg, grooming, stretching) [65]. Recent studies also have investi-gated the role of centrally mediated oxytocin on human social behavior, including trust [66] and emotional perception [67].

Few studies of oxytocin exist in individuals who have autism, with exist-ing research suggesting children who have ASD may have deficits in endo-crine oxytocin system [68] and have lower plasma levels of oxytocin compared with typically developing children [68].

Evidence for the role of oxytocin in social and repetitive behaviors in individuals who had ASD was evaluated by members of the authors' research group in a double-blind, placebo-controlled cross-over trial evalu-ating the effects of oxytocin on repetitive behaviors in an intravenous infu-sion study of oxytocin versus placebo [68]. Fifteen adults who had autism received an intravenous infusion of oxytocin versus placebo over a 4-hour period, with oxytocin dosing slowly titrated to 700 mL/h at the beginning of the fourth hour. The infusion was repeated approximately 2 to 3 weeks after the initial infusion. Ratings were made on clinician-rated scale evalu-ating the specific repetitive behaviors, including need to know, repeating, ordering, telling/asking, self-injury, and touching. Results suggested decreases in the severity, frequency, and number of repetitive behaviors observed in participants during the oxytocin infusion compared with placebo. An ongoing trial by the authors' research group is investigating the safety, tolerability, and efficacy of intranasal oxytocin infusion in adults who have ASD in a 6-week trial using standardized and clinician-rated measures of socialization and repetitive behaviors.

Summary

The available, although somewhat limited, treatment literature on repetitive behaviors in ASD shows benefits from SSRIs, the most commonly prescribed medication in children who have ASDs [7] in some studies and in some patients. The review of SRI/SSRI interventions highlights the variability often observed in intervention research in ASD. Some trials suggest certain SSRIs such as fluoxetine may improve repetitive behaviors in children and adults [39,40], with the potential for others (eg, fluvoxamine in adults) to influence aggression and social relatedness [36]. Future research with SSRIs may benefit from systematic assessment of other relevant domains such as anxiety, communication, and sociability. Trials of some SRIs/SSRIs (eg, fluvoxamine), however, reveal inconsistent results. The variability may result from methodological differences among trials (eg, dosing) and individual variability that may influence treatment response. One level of individual variability may be age-related differences in serotonin metabolism [20], which should be investigated further as potential reasons for differences observed in pediatric and adult trials. In addition, future work defining and evaluating activation, a commonly reported adverse effect of SRI treatment, is needed, with some efforts in this area underway in collaborative treatment networks.

Research on other potential medication treatments for repetitive behaviors include atypical antipsychotics, anticonvulsants, and the neuropeptide oxytocin. Research on the atypical antipsychotic risperidone suggests risperidone is effective in reducing repetitive behaviors in children who have high levels of irritability and aggression [61]. Similar findings were reported for the anticonvulsant divalproex sodium, which reduced repetitive behaviors in one report of individuals who had ASD [69]. Preliminary results with divalproex sodium suggest that combination therapy may be a way to deal with activation. As increased attention is paid to repetitive behaviors in ASD, and new molecular targets arise from animals models, future research may provide new treatment data on short- versus long-term benefits, direct versus indirect treatment effects, and specificity of treatment effects within subclasses of RRBIs to best facilitate informed clinical decision making.

References

[1] Turner M. Annotation: repetitive behaviour in autism: a review of psychological research. J Child Psychol Psychiatry 1999;40(6):839–49.
[2] Baumeister AA, Forehand R. Effects of contingent shock and verbal command on body rocking of retardates. J Clin Psychol 1972;28(4):586–90.

[3] Bodfish JW, Symons FJ, Parker DE, et al. Varieties of repetitive behavior in autism: comparisons to mental retardation. J Autism Dev Disord 2000;30(3):237–43.

[4] Richler J, Bishop SL, Kleinke JR, et al. Restricted and repetitive behaviors in young children with autism spectrum disorders. J Autism Dev Disord 2007;37(1):73–85.

[5] Silverman JM, Smith CJ, Schmeidler J, et al. Symptom domains in autism and related conditions: evidence for familiality. Am J Med Genet 2002;114(1):64–73.

[6] Lord C, Risi S, DiLavore PS, et al. Autism from 2 to 9 years of age. Arch Gen Psychiatry 2006;63(6):694–701.

[7] Aman MG, Lam KS, Van Bourgondien ME. Medication patterns in patients with autism: temporal, regional, and demographic influences. J Child Adolesc Psychopharmacol 2005; 15(1):116–26.

[8] DSM-IV, Diagnostic and Statistical Manual of Mental Disorders (Fourth ed.), American Psychiatric Association, Washington, DC (1994).

[9] Lord C, Pickles A. Language level and nonverbal social–communicative behaviors in autistic and language-delayed children. J Am Acad Child Adolesc Psychiatry 1996;35(11): 1542–50.

[10] Szatmari P, Bartolucci G, Bremner R. Asperger's syndrome and autism: comparison of early history and outcome. Dev Med Child Neurol 1989;31(6):709–20.

[11] McDougle CJ, Kresch LE, Goodman WK, et al. A case-controlled study of repetitive thoughts and behavior in adults with autistic disorder and obsessive–compulsive disorder. Am J Psychiatry 1995;152(5):772–7.

[12] Cuccaro ML, Shao Y, Grubber J, et al. Factor analysis of restricted and repetitive behaviors in autism using the Autism Diagnostic Interview-R. Child Psychiatry Hum Dev 2003;34(1):3–17.

[13] Bishop SL, Richler J, Lord C. Association between restricted and repetitive behaviors and nonverbal IQ in children with autism spectrum disorders. Child Neuropsychol 2006; 12(4–5):247–67.

[14] Lam KS, Aman MG. The repetitive behavior scale-revised: independent validation in individuals with autism spectrum disorders. J Autism Dev Disord 2007;37(5):855–66.

[15] Anagnostou E, Chaplin W, Dryden W, et al. Factor analysis of the Y-BOCS in autistic disorder. Neuropsychopharmacology 2005;30(1):S153.

[16] Hutt C, Hutt SJ, Ounsted C. The behaviour of children with and without upper CNS lesions. Behaviour 1965;24(3):246–68.

[17] Cook EH, Leventhal BL. The serotonin system in autism. Curr Opin Pediatr 1996;8(4): 348–54.

[18] McFarlane HG, Kusek GK, Yang M, et al. Autism-like behavioral phenotypes in BTBR T+tf/J mice. Genes Brain Behav 2008;7(2):152–63.

[19] Schain RJ, Freedman DX. Studies on 5-hydroxyindole metabolism in autistic and other mentally retarded children. J Pediatr 1961;58:315–20.

[20] Owley T. The pharmacological treatment of autistic spectrum disorders. CNS Spectr 2002; 7(9):663–9.

[21] McDougle CJ, Naylor ST, Cohen DJ, et al. Effects of tryptophan depletion in drug-free adults with autistic disorder. Arch Gen Psychiatry 1996;53(11):993–1000.

[22] Novotny S, Hollander E, Allen A, et al. Increased growth hormone response to sumatriptan challenge in adult autistic disorders. Psychiatry Res 2000;94(2):173–7.

[23] Chugani DC, Muzik O, Behen M, et al. Developmental changes in brain serotonin synthesis capacity in autistic and nonautistic children. Ann Neurol 1999;45(3):287–95.

[24] Kaplan A, Hollander E. A review of pharmacologic treatments for obsessive–compulsive disorder. Psychiatr Serv 2003;54(8):1111–8.

[25] Moore ML, Eichner SF, Jones JR. Treating functional impairment of autism with selective serotonin reuptake inhibitors. Ann Pharmacother 2004;38(9):1515–9.

[26] Stahl SM. Mechanism of action of serotonin selective reuptake inhibitors. Serotonin receptors and pathways mediate therapeutic effects and side effects. J Affect Disord 1998;51(3): 215–35.

[27] Posey DJ, Erikson CA, Stigler KA, et al. The use of selective serotonin reuptake inhibitors in autism and related disorders. J Child Adolesc Psychopharmacol 2006;16(1–2):181–6.

[28] Kolevzon A, Mathewson KA, Hollander E. Selective serotonin reuptake inhibitors in autism: a review of efficacy and tolerability. J Clin Psychiatry 2006;67(3):407–14.

[29] Hollander, E, Anagnostou, E, editors. Clinical manual for the treatment of autism. Treatment of autism with selective serotonin reuptake inhibitors and other antidepressants. Washington, D.C.: American Psychiatric Publishing; 2007; 81–97.

[30] Flament MF, Rapaport JL, Berg CJ, et al. Clomipramine treatment of childhood obsessive–compulsive disorder. A double-blind controlled study. Arch Gen Psychiatry 1985;42(10): 977–83.

[31] Leonard HL, Swedo SE, Rapaport JL, et al. Treatment of obsessive–compulsive disorder with clomipramine and desipramine in children and adolescents. A double-blind crossover comparison. Arch Gen Psychiatry 1989;46(12):1088–92.

[32] Gordon CT, State RC, Nelson JE, et al. A double-blind comparison of clomipramine, desipramine, and placebo in the treatment of autistic disorder. Arch Gen Psychiatry 1993;50(6): 441–7.

[33] Brasic JR, Barnett JY, Sheitman BB, et al. Adverse effects of clomipramine. J Am Acad Child Adolesc Psychiatry 1997;36(9):1165–6.

[34] Sanchez LE, Campbell M, Small AM, et al. A pilot study of clomipramine in young autistic children. J Am Acad Child Adolesc Psychiatry 1996;35(4):537–44.

[35] Remington G, Sloman L, Konstantareas M, et al. Clomipramine versus haloperidol in the treatment of autistic disorder: a double-blind, placebo-controlled, crossover study. J Clin Psychopharmacol 2001;21(4):440–4.

[36] Narita N, Hashimoto K, Tomitaka S, et al. Interactions of selective serotonin reuptake inhibitors with subtypes of sigma receptors in rat brain. Eur J Pharmacol 1996;307(1):117–9.

[37] McDougle CJ, Naylor ST, Cohen DJ, et al. A double-blind, placebo-controlled study of fluvoxamine in adults with autistic disorder. Arch Gen Psychiatry 1996;53(11):1001–8.

[38] McDougle CJ, Kresch LE, Posey DJ. Repetitive thoughts and behavior in pervasive developmental disorders: treatment with serotonin reuptake inhibitors. J Autism Dev Disord 2000;30(5):427–35.

[39] Fluvoxamine [package insert]. Switzerland: Solvay Pharmaceuticals; 1984.

[40] Hollander E, Phillips, A, Chaplin W, et al. A placebo-controlled crossover trial of liquid fluoxetine on repetitive behaviors in childhood and adolescent autism. Neuropsychopharmacology 2005;30(3):582–9.

[41] Buchsbaum MS, Hollander E, Haznedar MM, et al. Effect of fluoxetine on regional cerebral metabolism in autistic spectrum disorders: a pilot study. Int J Neuropsychopharmacol 2001; 4(2):119–25.

[42] Fatemi SH, Realmuto JM, Khan L, et al. Fluoxetine in treatment of adolescent patients with autism: a longitudinal open trial. J Autism Dev Disord 1998;28(4):303–7.

[43] Markowitz PI. Effect of fluoxetine on self-injurious behavior in the developmentally disabled: a preliminary study. J Clin Psychopharmacol 1992;12(1):27–31.

[44] DeLong GR, Ritch CR, Burch S. Fluoxetine response in children with autistic spectrum disorders: correlation with familial major affective disorder and intellectual achievement. Dev Med Child Neurol 2002;44(10):652–9.

[45] Scahill L, Riddle MA, McSwiggen-Hardin M, et al. Children-s Yale-Brown Obsessive Compulsive Scale: reliability and validity. J Am Acad Child Adolesc Psychiatry 1997;36(6): 844–52.

[46] McDougle CJ, Brodkin ES, Naylor ST, et al. Sertraline in adults with pervasive developmental disorders: a prospective open-label investigation. J Clin Psychopharmacol 1998;18(1): 62–6.

[47] Steingard RJ, Zimnitzky B, DeMaso DR, et al. Sertraline treatment of transition-associated anxiety and agitation in children with autistic disorder. J Child Adolesc Psychopharmacol 1997;7(1):9–15.

[48] Willetts J, Lippa A, Beer B. Clinical development of citalopram. J Clin Psychopharmacol 1999;19(5 Suppl 1):36S–46S.

[49] Namerow LB, Thomas P, Bostic JQ, et al. Use of citalopram in pervasive developmental disorders. J Dev Behav Pediatr 2003;24(2):104–8.

[50] Owley T, Walton L, Salt J, et al. An open-label trial of escitalopram in pervasive developmental disorders. J Am Acad Child Adolesc Psychiatry 2005;44(4):343–8.

[51] Carrasco JL, Sandner C. Clinical effects of pharmacological variations in selective serotonin reuptake inhibitors: an overview. Int J Clin Pract 2005;59(12):1428–34.

[52] Sikich L, Hickok JM, Todd RD. 5-HT1A receptors control neurite branching during development. Brain Res Dev Brain Res 1990;56(2):269–74.

[53] Mooney RD, Shi MY, Rhoades RW. Modulation of retinotectal transmission by presynaptic 5-HT1B receptors in the superior colliculus of the adult hamster. J Neurophysiol 1994; 72(1):3–13.

[54] Salichon N, Gaspar P, Upton AL, et al. Excessive activation of serotonin (5-HT) 1B receptors disrupts the formation of sensory maps in monoamine oxidase a and 5-ht transporter knock-out mice. J Neurosci 2001;21(3):884–96.

[55] Mazer C, Muneyyirci J, Taheny K, et al. Serotonin depletion during synaptogenesis leads to decreased synaptic density and learning deficits in the adult rat: a possible model of neurodevelopmental disorders with cognitive deficits. Brain Res 1997;760(1–2):68–73.

[56] Osterheld-Haas MC, Hornung JP. Laminar development of the mouse barrel cortex: effects of neurotoxins against monoamines. Exp Brain Res 1996;110(2):183–95.

[57] Yan W, Wilson CC, Haring JH. 5-HT1a receptors mediate the neurotrophic effect of serotonin on developing dentate granule cells. Brain Res Dev Brain Res 1997;98(2):185–90.

[58] McDougle CJ, Homes JP, Carlson DC, et al. A double-blind, placebo-controlled study of risperidone in adults with autistic disorder and other pervasive developmental disorders. Arch Gen Psychiatry 1998;55(7):633–41.

[59] McDougle CJ, Fleishmann RL, Epperson CN, et al. Risperidone addition in fluvoxamine-refractory obsessive–compulsive disorder: three cases. J Clin Psychiatry 1995;56(11):526–8.

[60] Witwer A, Lecavalier L. Treatment incidence and patterns in children and adolescents with autism spectrum disorders. J Child Adolesc Psychopharmacol 2005;15(4):671–81.

[61] McDougle CJ, Epperson CN, Pelton GH, et al. A double-blind, placebo-controlled study of risperidone addition in serotonin reuptake inhibitor-refractory obsessive–compulsive disorder. Arch Gen Psychiatry 2000;57(8):794–801.

[62] McDougle CJ, Scahil L, Aman MG, et al. Risperidone for the core symptom domains of autism: results from the study by the autism network of the research units on pediatric psychopharmacology. Am J Psychiatry 2005;162(6):1142–8.

[63] Hollander E, Tracey KA, Swann AC, et al. Divalproex in the treatment of impulsive aggression: efficacy in cluster B personality disorders. Neuropsychopharmacology 2003;28(6):1186–97.

[64] Hollander E. Managing aggressive behavior in patients with obsessive–compulsive disorder and borderline personality disorder. J Clin Psychiatry 1999;60(Suppl 15):38–44.

[65] Insel TR, O'Brien DJ, Leckman JF. Oxytocin, vasopressin, and autism: is there a connection? Biol Psychiatry 1999;45(2):145–57.

[66] Kosfeld M, Heinrichs M, Zak PJ, et al. Oxytocin increases trust in humans. Nature 2005; 435(7042):673–6.

[67] Domes G, et al. Oxytocin improves mind-reading in humans. Biol Psychiatry 2007;61(6): 731–3.

[68] Hollander E, Novotny S, Hanratty M, et al. Oxytocin infusion reduces repetitive behaviors in adults with autistic and Asperger's disorders. Neuropsychopharmacology 2003;28(1):193–8.

[69] Hollander E, Soorya S, Wasseman S, et al. Divalproex sodium vs. placebo in the treatment of repetitive behaviours in autism spectrum disorder. Int J Neuropsychopharmacol 2006;9(2): 209–13.

[70] Hollander E, Soorya L, Chaplin W, et al. Placebo-controlled trial of fluoxetine for repetitive behaviors and global severity in adult autistic disorder. In preparation.

ELSEVIER
SAUNDERS

Child Adolesc Psychiatric Clin N Am
17 (2008) 773–785

CHILD AND
ADOLESCENT
PSYCHIATRIC CLINICS
OF NORTH AMERICA

Assessment and Pharmacologic Treatment of Sleep Disturbance in Autism

Kyle P. Johnson, MD[a],*, Beth A. Malow, MD, MS[b]

[a]*Department of Psychiatry, Oregon Health & Science University,
DC-7P, 3181 SW Sam Jackson Park Road, Portland, OR 97239, USA*
[b]*Department of Neurology, Vanderbilt University,
A-0118 Medical Center North, 1161 21st Avenue South, Nashville, TN 37232-2551, USA*

According to estimates, 20% to 30% of children experience significant sleep disturbances [1–3]. Children with sleep problems suffer daytime consequences, including behavior difficulties and mood instability [4–6]. Additionally, insufficient sleep can adversely impact neurocognitive functioning, including memory, attention, verbal creativity, cognitive flexibility, and abstract reasoning [6–8]. Research in children with obstructive sleep apnea (OSA) clearly shows this relationship between disrupted sleep and daytime impairments because OSA is a natural model for fragmenting sleep via repetitive arousals [9–13]. Moreover, adenotonsillectomy, the typical treatment for pediatric OSA, can lead to improvement in the neurocognitive and behavioral problems associated with OSA [14,15].

The recognition that interventions that improve sleep often result in improved daytime functioning has fueled interest in identifying and treating the sleep problems experienced by children with developmental disabilities, including those with autism spectrum disorders (ASD). Furthermore, parents see this as a significant problem, as numerous surveys attest [16–18]. In fact, a recent study showed that sleep problems rank as one of the most common concurrent clinical disorders [19]. Additionally, there is overlap of neurobiologic factors impacting the regulation of the sleep-wake cycle and those implicated in ASD. Several neurotransmitter systems implicated in promoting sleep and establishing a regular sleep-wake cycle are also affected by autism.

Johnson received support for this article from the Autism Treatment Network. Malow received support for this article from the Autism Speaks Foundation.

* Corresponding author.
E-mail address: johnsoky@ohsu.edu (K.P. Johnson).

Their aberrations in autism may be responsible for a component of the sleep disturbances experienced by children with ASD. These neurotransmitter systems include gamma-aminobutyric acid (GABA), serotonin, and melatonin.

The preoptic area of the hypothalamus is a major sleep-promoting system that uses GABA as a neurotransmitter. Sleep-active neurons in the preoptic area project to brainstem regions that contain neurons involved in arousal from sleep.Inhibiting these regions, in turn, promotes sleep. These regions include the pedunculopontine and laterodorsal tegmental nuclei, the locus coeruleus, and the dorsal raphe [20]. In autism, GABAergic interneurons appear disrupted [21] and a genetic susceptibility region has been identified on chromosome 15q,which contains GABA-related genes [22]. The expression of these autism-susceptibility genes may affect sleep by interfering with the normal inhibitory function of GABA via the preoptic area neurons.

Additionally, several studies have demonstrated abnormal melatonin regulation in individuals with ASD, including elevated daytime melatonin and significantly lower nocturnal melatonin [23–25]. A recent study shows significantly lower excretion rates of urinary 6-sulphatoxymelatonin, the major metabolite of melatonin, in children and adolescents with autism compared with age-and-gender matched controls, with more marked differences in pre-pubertal subjects [26].

The abnormalities in GABA, serotonin, and melatonin production in ASD, along with accumulating evidence of clinical sleep and circadian disturbances, provide evidence for involvement of the neurobiological networks regulating sleep in autism. Studies linking these neurotransmitter abnormalities to the severity of sleep disturbances in ASD have yet to be investigated. Whether subsets of children with ASD who have clinical abnormalities in their sleep-wake cycle are more likely to exhibit abnormalities in sleep-related neurotransmitters remains to be determined.

Sleep disorders likely to occur in children with autism spectrum disorders

Insomnia

Insomnia is the most common sleep disorder experienced by children with ASD. Pediatric insomnia has been defined by recent consensus as "repeated difficulty with sleep initiation, duration, consolidation, or quality that occurs despite age-appropriate time and opportunity for sleep and results in daytime functional impairment for the child and/or family" [27]. Between 44% and 86% of children with ASD have sleep problems, particularly insomnia [19,28–30]. Additionally, children with ASD suffer from irregular sleep-wake patterns, early morning awakenings, and poor sleep routines [31,32]. Because the majority of studies have examined children with classic autism, and because most of these children also have intellectual deficits (ID), these prevalence rates need to be evaluated in the context of the prevalence of sleep problems in patients with ID. Attempts have been made to control for the confounding variable of ID, and it appears that ASD is an independent risk factor for sleep problems [30,33,34].

Insomnia is a symptom and thus can have various causes (Box 1). Behavioral and environmental factors are the main culprits in typically developing children, and they play an important role in the insomnia experienced by children with ASD as well. According to the classification system of the American Academy of Sleep Medicine, there are two types of behavioral insomnia of childhood: (1) behavioral insomnia associated with sleeponset and (2) limit-setting behavioral insomnia [35]. Children with ASD are at high risk for behavioral insomnia either in its pure form or in conjunction with other more biologically determined insomnia. To aid in a child's sleep onset, parents often institute maladaptive sleep associations, which, in the long run, contribute to more sleep disturbances. For example, a parent will hold a child at bedtime to help the child fall asleep, and then put the child, once asleep, in bed. Although this practice facilitates sleep at bedtime, this sleep-onset association has to be repeated when the child has a natural awakening later in the night.

Much like typically developing children, there is a subset of children with ASD who have insomnia not complicated by behavioral or environmental factors. In fact, children with ASD may be more prone to this form of

---

Box 1. Causes of insomnia in children with ASD

Neurobiological (eg, synaptic transmission, deficiency, metabolism)
  GABA
  Melatonin
Behavioral
  Inadequate sleep hygiene
  Behavioral insomnia of childhood
    Sleep-onset association
    Limit-setting
Coexisting neurologicdisorder (eg, epilepsy)
Coexisting medical disorder (eg, gastrointestinal reflux disease)
Coexisting psychiatric disorder (eg, anxiety)
Medications (eg, corticosteroids, bronchodilators)
Other sleep disorders
  Obstructive sleep apnea
  Restless legs syndrome
  Periodic limb movements of sleep
  Delayed sleep-phase disorder
  Irregular sleep-wake rhythm

insomnia because of the neurobiologic overlap mentioned earlier and other concurrent medical and psychiatric problems. An association between sleep problems and gastrointestinal dysfunction has been described in children with ASD [19]. Because gastrointestinal dysfunction is known to be associated with increased night awakenings and pain, it is possible that insomnia in some children with ASD is due to gastrointestinal disorders, such as gastroesophageal reflux [36]. Epilepsy, which occurs in a significant minority of patients with ASD, may negatively impact sleep [37]. Moreover, sleep deprivation from whatever cause likely has a seizure-promoting effect. Therefore, children with ASD and epilepsy should particularly be evaluated for sleep disturbances.

Psychiatric symptoms may interfere with sleep initiation and maintenance. Children with ASD often have difficulties regulating emotions. Insomnia commonly results from anxiety manifesting in the evening as bedtime preparations are being made. Children with ASD are at increased risk for developing major depressive disorder, a condition associated with insomnia, particularly sleep-onset insomnia. Insomnia may also result from a variety of medications used to treat coexisting conditions. Examples include corticosteroids and asthma medications, stimulants for attention-deficit/hyperactivity disorder, activating serotonin uptake inhibitors for depression, and stimulating antiepileptic drugs for epilepsy or mood stabilization.

Circadian rhythm dysfunction may contribute to the insomnia observed in patients with ASD. As mentioned above, several studies have demonstrated abnormal melatonin regulation in individuals with ASD compared with controls, including elevated daytime melatonin and significantly lower nocturnal melatonin [23–26]. Melatonin, the "darkness hormone," is involved in signaling the appropriate timing of the sleep and wake cycle. If there are abnormalities in nocturnal production relative to daytime production or if the timing (phase) of melatonin production is abnormal, insomnia in various forms could result, including the circadian rhythm sleep disorders of delayed sleep-phase syndrome, advanced sleep-phase syndrome, or irregular sleep-wake rhythm.

Obstructive sleep apnea

OSA, which may affect up to 3% of children in the general population, is characterized by loud snoring or noisy breathing (usually worse in the supine position) in association with restless sleep, frequent awakenings, and sweating in sleep. While daytime sleepiness is common in adults with OSA, children may not appear sleepy but instead exhibit symptoms of hyperactivity and other problematic behaviors. Children with craniofacial abnormalities or neuromuscular compromise are at an increased risk for OSA. Diagnosis is made by overnight polysomnography (PSG), with monitoring of respiratory airflow and effort, as well as oxygenation. In children diagnosed with OSA, tonsillectomy and adenoidectomy is the first line of therapy. If symptoms persist or surgery is not an option, the child may be a candidate for continuous positive airway pressure, which overcomes the upper airway obstruction with pressurized air delivered through a mask. Desensitization of patients to continuous positive airway pressure is often required and can be achieved, often in conjunction with a sleep technologist.

While children with ASD do not appear to be at an increased risk for OSA, it is important to recognize the risk factors for this condition and seek appropriate evaluation since treatment can lead to significant improvement in sleep and daytime behavior [38]. A case report of a girl with ASD and OSA documented improvement in a variety of domains measured by pre- and posttreatment questionnaires, including social interaction and ability to focus, repetitive behavior, and auditory sensitivity, after treatment of sleep apnea with adenotonsillectomy.

Other sleep disorders

There are a few case series reports suggesting other sleep pathology in patients with ASD, including nocturnal events. Sleep-related events need to be distinguished from epileptic seizures in this population, given the increased prevalence of epilepsy in autism [39]. Such events include the non-rapid eye movement (REM) arousal disorders, REM sleep behavior disorder, and rhythmic movement disorder. Nocturnal events can usually be distinguished by history, although video-electroencephalogram-PSG in a sleep center is occasionally warranted. One of the cardinal distinguishing features of epileptic seizures in their stereotyped appearance, as well as the presence of tonic or dystonic limb posturing.

The non-REM arousal disorders consist of a spectrum of events of aberrant arousal arising from non-REM sleep stages 3 and 4 (deep) sleep, ranging from confusional arousals, to sleepwalking, to night terrors. There is often a family history of similar spells in parents or siblings, supporting a genetic predisposition. Precipitants include sleep deprivation, emotional stress, medical illness, and other conditions that contribute to disruption of normal sleeping patterns [40]. Research regarding the prevalence of non-REM arousal disorders in the ASD population is mixed with some studies suggesting an increased prevalence and others demonstrating no increase [29,30,32,41,42].

In REM sleep behavior disorder, individuals "act out their dreams" because of an interruption of physiologic muscle atonia during REM sleep. This disorder has been reported in one case series of children with ASD disrupted sleep who were studied with PSG [43]. However, a larger study of PSG in children with ASD who were medication-free did not identify REM sleep without atonia [38]. REM sleep behavior disorder is usually associated with older age and has been related to degeneration of dopaminergic neurons in the substantia nigra, a subcortical region involved in motor control. REM sleep behavior disorder can also occur in association with psychotropic medications that affect REM sleep, such as the selective serotonin reuptake inhibitors [44]. Related abnormalities, such as increased phasic muscle activity in REM sleep in mentally retarded individuals with autism [45], raise the possibility that neurostructural or neurochemical abnormalities involving the brainstem or subcortical regions may be associated with autism. If borne out in future investigations, the presence of REM sleep behavior disorder in autism may provide valuable clues to the etiology of ASD.

Rhythmic movement disorder is characterized by repetitive motion of the head (including head banging), trunk, or limbs, usually during the transition from wakefulness to sleep [46]. It may also arise during sustained sleep. Although the condition most often affects infants and toddlers in a transient and self-limited fashion, it may persist in children with autism and other developmental disabilities.

Assessment

Given the high prevalence of sleep problems, all children with ASD should be screened for sleep disturbances. Sleep questionnaires can facilitate the assessment of sleep problems. The Pediatric Sleep Questionnaire [47] and the Children's Sleep Habits Questionnaire [48] are two published sleep questionnaires often used in clinical practice. Each of these questionnaires asks screening questions for sleep-disordered breathing, a clinical condition not to be missed. If symptoms or signs of sleep-disordered breathing are discovered, the individual should be referred to a sleep specialist as overnight PSG may be indicated. In some cases, children with suspected OSA can be referred directly to an otolaryngologist. Although ASD in and of itself does not appear to be an independent risk factor for OSA, some children with ASD have other risk factors, including adenotonsillar hypertrophy, obesity, and craniofacial abnormalities, such as micrognathia. If restless legs syndrome or excessive movements while asleep are suspected, a referral to a sleep specialist is warranted. Unusual behaviors at night suggestive of parasomnias, such as sleep terrors or sleep walking, may warrant a referral to a sleep specialist, especially if the behavior poses a risk to safety or disturbs the sleep of family members. In the ASD population with their increased risk for epilepsy, consideration must be given to nocturnal seizures being the etiology of unusual behaviors in sleep.

The most common sleep problem in this population is insomnia. If insomnia is the primary sleep complaint, the clinician should obtain a careful history regarding the sleep environment and behaviors related to sleep onset or middle-of-the-night awakenings because improved sleep hygiene and behavioral interventions can be helpful in many cases and might potentially all that is needed to cure the insomnia. See later article by Kodak and Piazza, elsewhere in this issue for further exploration of this topic. PSG is not indicated in the assessment of insomnia unless one is concerned about potential sleep apnea; nocturnal events, such as seizures; or periodic limb movements as the cause. Otherwise, PSG should be reserved for treatment of refractory insomnia. Sleep diaries and actigraphy are useful in the assessment of insomnia. In actigraphy, the child wears an activity meter on the wrist that quantifies movement and rest, which serve as surrogates of activity and sleep. Actigraphy is more convenient and less intrusive and expensive than PSG, and data can be collected for multiple nights [49]. Although characterized as an objective measure of the rest-activity (sleep-wake) cycle, actigraphy has its limitations in that the device may interpret periods of quiet wakefulness as sleep, and periods of restless sleep as wakefulness. Therefore, data from actigraphy is best interpreted in the context of sleep diaries [50]. Behavioral interventions should be offered to all children with ASD and insomnia, but they may not be adequate to address the problem in some children. In those children, pharmacotherapy may be indicated. If the clinician assessing the child with ASD and severe insomnia is not comfortable implementing behavioral measures or prescribing medications for insomnia, a referral to a sleep specialist should be made. The next section focuses on pharmacologic treatments of sleep problems, especially insomnia. Nonpharmacologic treatments for insomnia are discussed by Kodak and Piazza, elsewhere in this issue.

Pharmacologic treatment of sleep disorders in children with autism spectrum disorders

Insomnia

Before engaging in a discussion of the pharmacologic treatment of insomnia in children with ASD, it is important to note that there are no Food and Drug Administration (FDA)–approved medications for pediatric insomnia. With this said, there is some research to support the use of pharmacologic agents, particularly melatonin, in the ASD population.

Melatonin, a neurohormone that promotes sleep, is produced from serotonin in the pineal gland [51]. Exogenous melatonin has shown promise in promoting sleep, although controlled studies of its efficacy and tolerability are limited. Its low cost, relative availability (does not require a prescription), and favorable safety profile make it an attractive choice for treating insomnia in children with ASD. Melatonin is considered a nutritional supplement and is not regulated by the FDA. Although melatonin has not been rigorously tested for safety, efficacy, or purity of preparation, no serious long-term adverse effects have been seen in this widelyused supplement.

The mechanisms by which melatonin may promote sleep in people with ASD are not known. Melatonin may be acting to entrain a circadian clock that is out of alignment with desired sleep-wake schedule. An alternative explanation is that children with ASD may produce deficient amounts of melatonin that exogenous melatonin supplements. As referenced earlier, initial evidence supports this theory [23–26]. Furthermore, melatonin may act nonspecifically as a hypnotic to promote sleep, or may promote sleep by decreasing core body temperature or through anxiolytic mechanisms [52].

Several small studies of melatonin in neurodevelopmental disabilities and ASD have been conducted. These have demonstrated favorable results. Children with neurodevelopmental disorders given supplemental melatonin experience reductions in sleep latency (time to fall asleep) and improvements in total sleep time and sleep efficiency (time-asleep/time-in-bed), with no or minimal adverse effects [53–56]. In these studies, seizures did not occur in children who had been seizure-free and did not increase in those with epilepsy. Only one study, that of five children with refractory epilepsy, reported increased seizures during melatonin treatment [57]. A large retrospective study of over 100 children with ASD treated with melatonin documented minimal adverse effects, with improved sleep in 85% of children treated [58].

Two trials have used melatonin exclusively in children with ASD. In an open-label trial, investigators administered 3 mg of immediate-release melatonin 30 minutes before bedtime for 2 weeks in 15 children with Asperger's syndrome [59]. All children had severe sleep problems and none were taking psychotropic medications. Sleep latency, as measured by actigraphy, decreased significantly from 40 to 21 minutes during treatment. Improvement in behavior also occurred, as measured by several domains on the Child Behavior Checklist. Adverse events were limited to 2 children experiencing mild tiredness and difficulty awakening, and 1 child suffering headaches. An additional child dropped out because of extensive tiredness, difficulty staying awake, dizziness, and diarrhea, with symptoms resolving immediately after melatonin discontinuation. A second open-label study of combined fast- and controlled-release melatonin (3–6 mg) in autism showed improvement in sleep diaries and questionnaires in all children [60]. One month after melatonin was discontinued, 16 children returned to pretreatment sleep scores.

Given its relatively short half-life, melatonin should be given approximately 30 minutes before the desired bedtime. In addition to acting as a hypnotic, melatonin also has a chronobiotic (phase-shifting) effect and therefore may be more effective in individuals with delayed sleep phase when given several hours before bedtime. Physiologic doses ($<$500 μg) are effective in causing phase shifts, but doses of 1 to 3 mg are more commonly used because of sedative effects. Dosage is usually started at 1 mg and titrated up to 3 mg if needed, by 1 mg every 1 to 2 weeks. Doses of 6 mg or higher are needed on occasion. When using melatonin, it is important to continue to use the same formulation, as the bioavailability of melatonin may vary widely among manufacturers. Because it is not regulated by the FDA and is available over-the-counter, it is important to instruct parents to read the label carefully and avoid choosing a brand with other active ingredients (eg, diphenhydramine). Extended-release melatonin may be helpful for the child with sleep-maintenance difficulties, although studies have been limited [61]. Liquid formulations are available and useful in children who will not swallow tablets. Attempts should be made to discontinue melatonin once a sleep cycle is established for 6 weeks or more, although long-term use appears safe and may be necessary.

Although little data supports the use of other medications in the treatment of insomnia in children with ASD, clinicians may need to consider prescribing sedating medications when safety is an issue. Pharmacologic treatment should be tailored to the cause of the individual child's sleep problem and used in conjunction with behavioral interventions. It is important to be conservative when using sedating medications to address insomnia, starting with low doses and increasing gradually. The child should be monitored closely for adverse effects because children with autism may be unable to verbally describe side effects.

Whenever possible, medicines should be prescribed that also assist with other conditions. In children with coexisting epilepsy, antiepileptic drugs with sedating properties can be used. Often, antiepileptic medications can be administered in a way that promotes nocturnal sleep. For example, carbamazepine, gabapentin, and topiramate are usually dosed two or three times a day but can be adjusted to give the higher dose at bedtime. Valproic acid comes in an extended-release form, which can be given once a day at bedtime.

Children with insomnia associated with aggression, extreme irritability, or self-injurious behavior may benefit from treatment with atypical neuroleptics. Risperidone has FDA approval for treating severe irritability and aggression in children with autism. In a child with insomnia coupled with these difficulties, risperidone could be initiated at bedtime or, if multiple doses are needed, the total daily dosage could be adjusted to give the higher dose at bedtime.

In the anxious or depressed child, specific antidepressants that promote sleep may be considered. These include the highly sedating drugs mirtazapine and trazodone. However, trazodone should be avoided in males who cannot communicate reliably because of the risk of priapism. The mildly sedating serotonin reuptake inhibitor fluvoxamine and the tricyclic antidepressants are useful, especially in children with obsessional thoughts that interfere with sleep onset. In the child experiencing sleep-onset insomnia in part due to hyperarousal, clonidine may be beneficial, as would a benzodiazepine, such as clonazepam.

Other sleep disorders

Clonazapam is often effective for treatment of non-REM arousal disorders; the tricyclic antidepressants given at night can also be useful. In rhythmic movement disorder, children exhibit repetitive, stereotyped, and rhythmic motor behaviors that occur predominantly during drowsiness and transition to sleep. Treatment should be initiated when the potential for injury is present. Clonazapam is the recommended choice, although not universally effective. Individuals suffering with REM sleep behavior disorder "act out their dreams" due to an interruption of physiologic muscle atonia during REM sleep. REM sleep behavior disorder often responds to clonazapam, although dopaminergic agents and melatonin have also been tried [45]. In all of these parasomnias, attention to safety issues is paramount. Children with these conditions are at risk to leave the bed or bedroom, placing themselves at risk for injury. Bedside monitors, as well as alarms or bells placed on a door that indicate to parents when a child has left the room, may be necessary.

Summary

Children with ASD frequently have significant sleep problems, most commonly insomnia. Fortunately, there are a variety of treatments available, including behavioral interventions and pharmacotherapy. When establishing a treatment plan, it is imperative to understand the underlying etiology of the sleep problem, which in many cases is multifactorial. Identifying and treating sleep disorders may result not only in improved sleep, but also impact favorably on daytime behavior and family functioning.

References

[1] Lozoff B, Wolf AW, Davis NS. Sleep problems seen in pediatric practice. Pediatrics 1985;75: 477–83.

[2] Armstrong KL, Quinn RA, Dadds MR. The sleep patterns of normal children. Med J Aust 1994;161:202–6.

[3] Owens JA, Spirito A, McGuinn M, et al. Sleep habits and sleep disturbance in elementary school–aged children. J Dev Behav Pediatr 2000;21:27–36.

[4] Zuckerman B, Stevenson J, Bailey V. Sleep problems in early childhood: continuities, predictive factors, and behavioral correlates. Pediatrics 1987;80(5):664–71.

[5] Smedje H, Broman JE, Hetta J. Associations between disturbed sleep and behavioral difficulties in 635 children aged six to eight years: a study based on parents perceptions. Eur Child Adolesc Psychiatry 2001;10:1–9.

[6] O'Brien LM, Gozal D. Neurocognitive dysfunction and sleep in children: from human to rodent. Pediatr Clin North Am 2004;51:187–202.

[7] Dahl RE. The impact of inadequate sleep on children's daytime cognitive function. Semin Pediatr Neurol 1996;3:44–50.

[8] Fallone G, Acebo C, Arnedt JT, et al. Effects of acute sleep restriction on behavior, sustained attention, and response inhibition in children. Percept Mot Skills 2001;93:213–29.

[9] Hansen DE, Vandenberg B. Neuropsychological features and differential diagnosis of sleep apnea syndrome in children. J Clin Child Psychol 1997;26(3):304–10.

[10] Owens J, Opipari L, Nobile C, et al. Sleep and daytime behavior in children with obstructive sleep apnea and behavioral sleep disorders. Pediatrics 1998;102(5):1178–84.

[11] Beebe DW, Wells CT, Jeffries J, et al. Neuropsychological effects of pediatric obstructive sleep apnea. J Int Neuropsychol Soc 2004;10:962–75.

[12] Kennedy JD, Blunden S, Hirte C, et al. Reduced neurocognition in children who snore-Pediatr Pulmonol 2004;37:330–7.

[13] Halbower AC, Mahone EM. Neuropsychological morbidity linked to childhood sleep disordered breathing. Sleep Med Rev 2006;10(2):97–107.

[14] Friedman BC, Hendeles-Amitai A, Kozminsky E, et al. Adenotonsillectomy improves neurocognitive function in children with obstructive sleep apnea syndrome. Sleep 2003;26: 999–1005.

[15] Chervin RD, Ruzicka DL, Giordani BJ, et al. Sleep-disordered breathing, behavior, and cognition in children before and after adenotonsillectomy. Pediatrics 2006;117:e769–778.

[16] Quine L. Sleep problems in children with mental handicap. J Ment Defic Res 1991;35(4): 269–90.

[17] Richdale A, Francis A, Gavidia-Payne S, et al. Stress, behaviour, and sleep problems in children with an intellectual disability. J Intellect Dev Disabil 2000;25(2):147–61.

[18] Polimeni MA, Richdale AL, Francis AJP. A survey of sleep problems in autism, Asperger's disorder and typically developing children. J Intellect Disabil Res 2005;49(4):260–8.

[19] Ming X, Brimacombe M, Chaaban J, et al. Autism spectrum disorders: concurrent clinical disorders. J Child Neurol 2008;23(1):6–13.

[20] Saper CB, Chou T, Scammell TE. The sleep switch: hypothalamic control of sleep and wakefulness. Trends Neurosci 2001;24:726–31.

[21] Levitt P, Eagleson KL, Powell EM. Regulation of neocortical interneuron development and the implications for neurodevelopmental disorders. Trends Neurosci 2004;27:400–6.

[22] McCauley JL, Olson M, Delahanty R, et al. A linkage disequilibrium map of the 1-Mb 15q12 GABAA receptor subunit cluster and association to autism. Am J Med Genet 2004;131: 51–9.

[23] Ritvo ER, Ritvo R, Yuwiler A, et al. Elevated daytime melatonin concentrations in autism: a pilot study. Eur Child Adolesc Psychiatry 1993;2(2):75–8.

[24] Nir I, Meir D, Zilber N, et al. Brief report: circadian melatonin, thyroid-stimulating hormone, prolactin, and cortisol levels in serum of young adults with autism. J Autism Dev Disord 1995;25:641–54.

[25] Kulman G, Lissoni P, Rovelli F, et al. Evidence of pineal endocrine hypofunction in autistic children. Neuro endocrinol Lett 2000;20:31–4.

[26] Tordjman S, Anderson GM, Pichard N, et al. Nocturnal excretion of 6-sulphatoxymelatonin in children and adolescents with autistic disorder. Biol Psychiatry 2005;57:134–8.

[27] Mindell JA, Emslie G, Blumer J, et al. Pharmacologic management of insomnia in children and adolescents:consensus statement. Pediatrics 2006;117:e1223–32.

[28] Wiggs L, Stores G. Severe sleep disturbance and daytime challenging behaviour in children with severe learning disabilities. J Intellect Disabil Res 1996;40(6):518–28.

[29] Patzold LM, Richdale AL, Tonge BJ. An investigation into sleep characteristics of children with autism and Asperger's disorder. J Paediatr Child Health 1998;34:528–33.

[30] Richdale AL, Prior MR. The sleep/wake rhythm in children with autism. Eur Child Adolesc Psychiatry 1995;4(3):175–86.

[31] Honomichl RD, Goodlin-Jones BL, Burnham M, et al. Sleep patterns of children with pervasive developmental disorders. J Autism Dev Disord 2002;32(6):553–61.

[32] Schreck KA, Mulick JA. Parental report of sleep problems in children with autism. J Autism Dev Disord 2000;30(2):127–35.

[33] Bradley EA, Summers JA, Wood HL, et al. Comparing rates of psychiatric and behavior disorders in adolescents and young adults with severe intellectual disability with and without autism. J Autism Dev Disord 2004;34(2):151–61.

[34] Couturier JL, Speechley KN, Steele M, et al. Parental perception of sleep problems in children of normal intelligence with pervasive developmental disorders: prevalence, severity, and pattern. J Am Acad Child Adolesc Psychiatry 2005;44(8):815–22.

[35] American Academy of Sleep Medicine. International classification of sleep disorders. Westchester (IL): American Academy of Sleep Medicine; 2005.

[36] Johnson DA. Gastroesophageal reflux disease and sleep disorders: a wake-up call for physicians and their patients. Rev Gastroenterol Disord 2005;5(Suppl 2):S3–11.

[37] Malow BA. Sleep disorders, epilepsy, and autism. Ment Retard Dev Disabil Res Rev 2004; 10(2):122–5.

[38] Malow BA, McGrew SG, Harvey M, et al. Impact of treating sleep apnea in a child with autism spectrum disorder. Pediatr Neurol 2006;34(4):325–8.

[39] Tuchman R, Rapin I. Epilepsy in autism. Lancet Neurol 2002;1:352–8.

[40] Mahowald M, Bornemann MAC. NREM sleep-arousal parasomnias. In: Kryger MH, Roth T, Dement WC, editors. Principles and practice of sleep medicine. 4th edition. Philadelphia: Elsevier/Saunders; 2005. p. 889–96.

[41] Liu X, Hubbard JA, Fabes RA, et al. Sleep disturbances and correlates of children with autism spectrum disorders. Child Psychiatry Hum Dev 2006;37:179–91.

[42] Wiggs L, Stores G. Sleep patterns and sleep disorders in children with autistic spectrum disorders: insights using parent report and actigraphy. Dev Med Child Neurol 2004;46:372–80.

[43] Thirumalai SS, Shubin RA, Robinson R. Rapid eye movement sleep behavior disorder in children with autism. J Child Neurol 2002;17:173–8.

[44] Mahowald M, Schenck C. REM sleep parasomnias. In: Kryger MH, Roth T, Dement WC, editors. Principles and practice of sleep medicine. 4th edition. Philadelphia: Elsevier/Saunders; 2005. p. 897–916.

[45] Diomedi M, Curatolo P, Scalise A, et al. Sleep abnormalities in mentally retarded autistic subjects: Down's syndrome with mental retardation and normal subjects. Brain Dev 1999; 21:548–53.

[46] Hoban T. Rhythmic movement disorder in children. CNS Spectr 2003;8:135–8.

[47] Chervin RD, Hedger K, Dillon JE, et al. Pediatric sleep questionnaire (PSQ): validity and reliability of scales for sleep-disordered breathing, snoring, sleepiness, and behavioral problems. Sleep Med 2000;1(1):21–31.

[48] Owens JA, Spirito A, McGuinn M. The children's sleep habits questionnaire (CSHQ): psychometric properties of a survey instrument for school-aged children. Sleep 2000;23(8): 1043–51.

[49] Ancoli-Israel S, Cole R, Alessi C, et al. The role of actigraphy in the study of sleep and circadian rhythms. Sleep 2003;26:342–92.

[50] Sadeh A, Acebo C. The role of actigraphy in sleep medicine. Sleep Med Rev 2002;6:113–24.

[51] Claustrat B, Brun J, Chazot G. The basic physiology and pathophysiology of melatonin. Sleep Med Rev 2005;9:11–24.

[52] Heuvel CJVD, Ferguson SA, Macchi MM, et al. Melatonin as a hypnotic: con. Sleep Med Rev 2005;9:71–80.

[53] Jan JE, Esperzedl H, Appleton RE. The treatment of sleep disorders with melatonin. Dev Med Child Neurol 1994;36:97–107.

[54] Ross C, Davies P, Whitehouse W. Melatonin treatment for sleep disorders in children with neurodevelopmental disorders: an observational study. Dev Med Child Neurol 2002;44: 339–44.

[55] Phillips L, Appleton R. Systematic review of melatonin treatment in children with neurodevelopmental disabilities and sleep impairment. Dev Med Child Neurol 2004;46:771–5.

[56] Dodge NN, Wilson GA. Melatonin for treatment of sleep disorders in children with developmental disabilities. J Child Neurol 2001;16:581–4.

[57] Sheldon S. Pro-convulsant effects of oral melatonin in neurologically disabled children. Lancet 1998;351:1254.

[58] Andersen I, Kaczmarska J, McGrew SG, et al. Melatonin for insomnia in children with autism spectrum disorders. J Child Neurol 2008;23:482–5.

[59] Paavonen E, von Wendt T, Vanhala N, et al. Effectiveness of melatonin in the treatment of sleep disturbances in children with Asperger disorder. J Child AdolescPsychopharmacol 2003;13:83–95.

[60] Giannotti F, Cortesi F, Cerquiglini A, et al. An open-label study of controlled release melatonin in treatment of sleep disorders in children with autism. J Autism Dev Disord 2006; 36(6):741–52.
[61] Jan JE, Hamilton D, Seward N, et al. Clinical trials of controlled-release melatonin in children with sleep-wake cycle disorders. J Pineal Res 2000;29(1):34–9.

ELSEVIER
SAUNDERS

Child Adolesc Psychiatric Clin N Am
17 (2008) 787–801

Developing Drugs for Core Social and Communication Impairment in Autism

David J. Posey, MD, MS[a,b,*], Craig A. Erickson, MD[a,b], Christopher J. McDougle, MD[a,b]

[a]Department of Psychiatry, Indiana University School of Medicine,
1111 West 10th Street, Indianapolis, IN 46202-4800, USA
[b]Christian Sarkine Autism Treatment Center, Department of Psychiatry,
Indiana University School of Medicine, Riley Hospital for Children, Room 4300,
702 Barnhill Drive, Indianapolis, IN 46202-5200, USA

Autistic disorder (autism) is defined by specific impairments affecting socialization, communication, and stereotyped behavior which together are called the "core symptoms" of autism. The article by Soorya and colleagues in this issue addresses stereotyped and repetitive behavior. This article focuses on the development of drugs for core social and communication impairment in autism and other pervasive developmental disorders (PDDs).

The impairment in reciprocal social interaction and communication in autism is severe and persistent and usually includes problems with eye-to-eye gaze, facial expression, body posture, and gestures. Some individuals may have little or no interest in establishing friendships. Others may have an interest in developing relationships, but lack understanding of how to go about it. Individuals with autism often exhibit a significant delay in language acquisition and have difficulty communicating even if language is obtained. Echolalia is also common. Persons with Asperger's Disorder and PDD not otherwise specified (NOS) may have relatively intact language, but have difficulty with conversational or pragmatic language.

Finding drugs to effectively target socialization and communication has been challenging to say the least. Many of the drugs showing efficacy in autism are most helpful for symptoms distinct from the core symptoms. Risperidone, the only FDA approved treatment for autism, is specifically indicated for

---

This work was supported in part by a grant from the National Institute of Mental Health (K23 MH68627).

* Corresponding author. Riley Hospital for Children, Room 4300, 702 Barnhill Drive, Indianapolis, IN 46202.

E-mail address: dposey@iupui.edu (D.J. Posey).

1056-4993/08/$ - see front matter © 2008 Elsevier Inc. All rights reserved.
doi:10.1016/j.chc.2008.06.010
childpsych.theclinics.com

irritability associated with autism. Other associated symptoms that often cause clinically significant problems include inattention, hyperactivity, anxiety, and sleep disturbance [1]. Psychiatric drugs are frequently used to address these symptoms in children with autism [2], although the evidence base supporting this clinical practice is still evolving. In contrast, there are no drugs that are commonly used or proven effective in treating the core social and communication impairments that are the hallmarks of PDDs.

A number of challenges to developing drugs that effectively treat social and communication impairment in autism are discussed in this article. We will also summarize past and recent research involving drugs to treat these core symptoms of autism.

Challenges to drug development

Researchers are just beginning to understand the neurobiology of autism and other PDDs. Early research focused on neurochemical abnormalities such as elevated whole-blood serotonin (5-hydroxytryptamine [5-HT]), found in a large minority of children with autism. Twin studies have clearly indicated a high degree of heritability with one study finding a monozygotic concordance rate of 92% compared with a dizygotic concordance rate of 10% [3]. Structural neuroimaging has found that brain growth trajectory is altered in young children with autism [4]. Functional neuroimaging has begun to unravel some aspects of the social brain [5]. Despite these emerging findings, the lack of reproducible neurobiological findings has hampered translational research efforts.

Part of the difficulty in understanding the basic pathophysiology may be due to the heterogeneity of those classified as having a PDD. The consistent use of standardized semistructured diagnostic measures such as the Autism Diagnostic Interview–Revised [6] in research studies has led to consistency across academic centers. However, within this group there continues to be significant differences between patients. Patients may differ widely in terms of the degree of impairment in various core symptoms, as well as intellectual and adaptive functioning. In addition, the number of patients diagnosed as having PDDs is rapidly increasing, owing partly to better recognition and the identification of milder cases which may further lead to this phenotypic heterogeneity.

Despite the increased prevalence of PDDs, these disorders are still relatively uncommon, which leads to further challenges in conducting clinical trials of promising drugs. Recent epidemiologic research suggests that PDDs are present in 1 out of 166 preschool children [7]. However, the rate of narrowly-defined autism may still be only 1 in 500. Timely recruitment of subject volunteers into clinical research protocols is difficult, but has been improved by the establishment of multisite research networks such as the Research Units on Pediatric Psychopharmacology (RUPP) Autism Network [8] and industry-sponsored multisite studies. Identifying patients who are not taking concomitant psychotropic medications is challenging in a disorder where as many as 50% of patients are taking medications for associated symptoms like irritability or hyperactivity [2].

The study of core social and communication difficulties brings additional challenges. In the majority of children with autism these symptoms improve naturally over time. For example, some children who are not talking at age three years may begin talking by age five years. They continue to demonstrate impairment relative to unaffected peers, but the symptoms improve nevertheless. Assessing the efficacy of drugs on this moving developmental target can be difficult. Placebo-controlled studies are essential given improvement which occurs simply with the passage of time, education, and regular speech and language therapy.

Finally, there is a lack of agreement on which outcome measures are best at assessing the core symptoms of autism and whether any of them will ultimately prove useful in clinical trials. Designing an ideal outcome measure is also challenging because of the heterogeneity of presentation discussed above.

Drugs not effective for social and communication impairment

Fenfluramine

Fenfluramine is an indirect 5-HT receptor agonist with structural similarities to amphetamine that was a Food and Drug Administration (FDA)-approved treatment for obesity. In 1997, it was voluntarily withdrawn from the market because of concern that it contributed to the development of cardiac valvular disease [9]. In the 1980s, however, fenfluramine was the target of much interest as a potential treatment for autism because of preliminary reports of efficacy combined with its potential to decrease 5-HT blood levels [10]. Although a subsequent double-blind crossover study was positive [11], more definitive studies failed to find consistent benefit and suggested that fenfluramine may adversely affect learning [12].

Naltrexone

Naltrexone is an opioid receptor antagonist that is FDA-approved for the treatment of alcoholism and opioid dependence. It has also been studied as a potential treatment for self-injury and core autistic symptoms based on possible links between autism and opioid dysregulation [13].

Several double-blind, placebo-controlled studies of naltrexone in autism have been published. One of the larger of these was completed by Campbell and colleagues [14] who randomly assigned 41 hospitalized young children (ages 2.9–7.8 years) with autism to either three weeks of naltrexone (1 mg/kg/d) or placebo treatment. Naltrexone-treated patients showed significant improvement in hyperactivity, but no improvement in learning or core autistic symptoms. Adverse effects were minimal. Another naltrexone (1.48–2.35 mg/kg/d) trial of similar design by Willemsen-Swinkels and colleagues [15] replicated this in 23 children (ages 3–7 years) with autism. Willemsen-Swinkels and colleagues [16] also conducted a 4-week, double-blind, placebo-controlled crossover study in adults with mental retardation, 23 of whom had autism. In this study, naltrexone (50 mg) was no better than placebo, and was actually worse on a staff-rated Clinical Global Impressions (CGI) scale [17].

Double-blind, placebo-controlled studies have failed to support the initial hypothesis that naltrexone alters the core symptoms of autism, including social behavior. Although the drug may improve certain symptoms in some individuals with autism, its effectiveness in the majority of patients is questionable. The most consistent findings coming from these controlled studies are that naltrexone is well tolerated and may be effective in reducing motor hyperactivity.

Secretin

Secretin is the most recent agent to receive attention as a possible pharmacologic treatment for core symptoms of autism. Secretin is a gastrointestinal polypeptide hormone that is FDA-approved for use in the diagnosis of certain gastrointestinal diseases. It also has the distinction of being one of the best studied treatments for autism owing to widespread use following a well-publicized case report of three patients with PDD who showed marked improvement when given it as part of a diagnostic evaluation for gastrointestinal problems [18]. As discussed in the article on complementary and alternative treatments by Levy and Hyman in this issue, none of the randomized placebo-controlled studies of secretin have confirmed any positive effect.

Drugs where more research is needed

Selective serotonin reuptake inhibitors

Selective serotonin reuptake inhibitors (SSRIs) are increasingly being prescribed to children with PDDs. Aman and colleagues [2] recently compared two North Carolina community surveys of psychotropic medication use in autism and found a use of 21.4% for all antidepressants, the majority of which were SSRIs. In the article by Soorya and colleagues in this issue, several potential reasons behind this widespread use of SSRIs in autism are discussed including documented abnormalities in 5-HT function in autism and the shared features with obsessive-compulsive disorder (OCD).

McDougle and colleagues [19] treated 30 adults with autism with either fluvoxamine (276.7 mg/d) or placebo over the course of a 12-week, double-blind study. Eight of 15 (53%) fluvoxamine-treated subjects were rated as responders compared with 0 of 15 placebo-treated subjects. Improvement was seen in repetitive thoughts and behavior, maladaptive behavior, and repetitive language usage. A subsequent unpublished 12-week, double-blind, placebo-controlled study in 34 children and adolescents (ages 5–18 years; mean age 9.5 years) with PDDs found that only 1 of 18 subjects treated with fluvoxamine (106.9 mg/d) responded [20]. There was also a high rate of adverse events including insomnia, hyperactivity, agitation, and aggression despite using doses that are usually well tolerated in children with OCD. Thus, fluvoxamine may improve repetitive language or echolalia secondary to autism in adults, but should be used cautiously in children.

Hollander and colleagues [21] administered fluoxetine to 39 children (ages 5–16 years; mean age 8.2 years) during a 20-week (8 weeks on drug) placebo-controlled crossover study. Liquid fluoxetine was dosed starting at 2.5 mg/d and increased on a weekly basis to reach a maximal target dose of 0.8 mg/kg/d by week 4, if needed. The mean final dose was 0.4 mg/kg/d (mean dose 9.9 mg/d, range 2.4–20 mg/d). Fluoxetine was significantly better than placebo for reducing repetitive behaviors on the Children's Yale-Brown Obsessive Compulsive Scale (CY-BOCS) [22]. There was no improvement on measures of speech or social interaction. Side effects were not significantly different between fluoxetine and placebo. Thus, fluoxetine may lead to a reduction in repetitive behavior or stereotypy in children with PDD.

Placebo-controlled trials support the use of fluvoxamine in adults with autism and fluoxetine in children with PDD for select symptoms, but to date these drugs have not been shown to significantly improve core social and language impairment in controlled studies. Additional uncontrolled reports have reported benefits from other SSRIs including sertraline, paroxetine, citalopram, and escitalopram [23]. Overall, improvements have been most commonly reported in symptoms of anxiety, mood disturbance, aggression, and repetitive behavior. A more optimistic view of the effectiveness of SSRIs has been put forth by DeLong and colleagues [24]. In their clinical treatment of 129 young children (ages 2–8 years) with autism, fluoxetine treatment (4–40 mg/d over 5–76 months) was associated with a positive response in 89 of 129 (69%) children. Their report is intriguing in that improvements in a number of core autistic symptoms were reported. However, the data is difficult to interpret in comparison to controlled studies given the lack of standardized outcome measures and placebo control.

Atypical antipsychotics

Risperidone, an atypical antipsychotic, is the only FDA-approved treatment for autism. Specifically, it is approved for children, ages 5 to 16 years, with autism accompanied by irritability including aggression, self-injury, tantrums, and mood swings. Much of the research supporting its use has focused on children with high degrees of irritability (see article by Stigler and McDougle in this issue). However, some families report improvement in other symptoms including social interaction. Thus, it is informative to examine social and communication outcomes in these studies.

Risperidone

The first placebo-controlled trial of risperidone conducted in autism involved 31 adults (mean age 28.1 years) with autism or PDD NOS [25]. Risperidone (mean dose 2.9 mg/d) was significantly more efficacious than placebo, with 8 of 14 (57%) subjects categorized as responders on the CGI-Improvement scale versus 0 of 16 in the placebo group. Risperidone was beneficial for reducing interfering repetitive behavior as well as aggression, but did not lead to improvement in social relatedness or language.

The logical next step was to study risperidone in children with autism. The RUPP Autism Network randomized 101 children (mean age 8.8 years) to 8 weeks of risperidone or placebo [26]. At baseline, all patients had significant irritability, aggression, or self-injury as rated by the Aberrant Behavior Checklist (ABC) [27]. Risperidone led to significant reduction on all of the ABC subscales compared with placebo, but the reductions in social withdrawal and inappropriate speech were only significant at the $P = .03$ level (insignificant following Bonferroni correction for multiple analyses). To further analyze the efficacy of risperidone on the core symptoms of autism in this group of highly irritable patients, McDougle and colleagues [28] examined secondary outcome measures that included a modified Ritvo-Freeman Real Life Rating Scale (R-F RLRS) [29] and modified CY-BOCS [30]. On the R-F RLRS, significant improvement was seen on the following subscales: sensory motor behaviors, affectual reactions, and sensory responses. However, there was no significant change on the social relationship to people or language subscales.

A second multicenter, placebo-controlled study of risperidone in children with PDD was conducted in Canada [31]. Seventy-nine children (mean age 7.5 years) were randomized to either risperidone (mean dose 1.2 mg/d) or placebo for 8 weeks. Significant improvement ($P < .05$) was seen on all subscales of the ABC, but was of greatest magnitude for irritability and hyperactivity. Social withdrawal decreased by 63% in the risperidone group compared with 40% for the placebo group ($P < .01$).

Studies have also examined risperidone in even younger children. Risperidone is occasionally needed in very young children due to the severity of the irritability and agitation, which can be extreme [32]. Nagaraj and colleagues [33] randomized 39 children (ages 2–9 years; mean age 5 years) to risperidone 1 mg/d or placebo and examined ratings on the Childhood Autism Rating Scale (CARS) [34]. The children had variable presenting symptoms, but 36 of 39 (92%) were considered to have problems with irritability. At 6 months, 12 of 19 (63%) children treated with risperidone showed a 20% improvement in CARS score compared with 0 of 20 (0%) treated with placebo. In a study by Luby and colleagues [35], 23 children (ages 2–6 years;

mean age 4 years) also received risperidone (0.5–1.5 mg/d) or placebo for 6 months. However, these investigators found risperidone only minimally efficacious compared with placebo at 6 months possibly owing to group differences at baseline or small sample size. In contrast to the study by Nagaraj and colleagues [33], high degrees of irritability were not required for study entry.

These studies suggest that risperidone may have modest benefit for reducing social withdrawal, repetitive language, or core symptoms of autism (as rated by CARS) in children with PDD exhibiting high levels of baseline irritability. It is unclear whether risperidone improves these symptoms in the absence of irritability.

Other atypical antipsychotics

Three prospective open-label trials [36–38] and one small placebo-controlled trial [39] of olanzapine in PDD have been published. All of these studies with the exception of the one from Kemner and colleagues [38] were positive in terms of olanzapine efficacy. In the latter study, only 3 of 25 (12%) children (mean age 11 years) with PDD receiving olanzapine (mean dose 10.7 mg/d) responded at 3 months. In contrast to the other studies, disruptive behavior or irritability was not an entry criterion. Potenza and colleagues [36] found improvement in core social and language impairment in addition to other disruptive behavior and irritability. Excessive weight gain was prominent in all four studies.

Quetiapine, ziprasidone, and aripiprazole have also been examined in pediatric and adult populations with PDD. All of these studies have been open-label in design and are described by Stigler and McDougle in another article in this issue. None of them reported significant improvements in core social and language impairment in PDD. This is not surprising given the preliminary nature of the research, as well as its focus on the use of these drugs to treat irritability and disruptive behavior. Larger placebo-controlled trials of olanzapine and aripiprazole are underway [40] and will lead to more information on the effects of these medications on core social and language impairment in PDD, at least in the subset of patient with irritability and disruptive behavior.

Cholinesterase inhibitors

Recently, several investigators have explored the use of four acetylcholinesterase inhibitors: tacrine, donepezil, rivastigmine, and galantamine. All of these drugs are FDA-approved to treat Alzheimer's disease. Tacrine was the first of these drugs to be marketed, but is less frequently prescribed given problems with dosing, tolerability, and safety. A brief case report found only modest benefit of tacrine in three patients with autism [41].

Hardan and Handen [42] reviewed the charts of eight patients with autism (ages 7–19 years; mean age 11 years) treated with donepezil (modal dose 10 mg/d) and found that 4 of 8 (50%) showed significant improvement.

Improvement was seen on ABC ratings of irritability and hyperactivity, but not social withdrawal, inappropriate speech, or stereotypy. Doyle and colleagues [43] also found open-label donepezil beneficial for attention-deficit/hyperactivity disorder symptoms in another eight youth (ages 10–17 years) with PDDs.

Results from a double-blind, placebo-controlled trial of donepezil have also been published [44]. In this study, 43 children (ages 2–10 years; mean age 7 years) with PDDs received either donepezil (2.5 mg/d) or placebo for 6 weeks in double-blind fashion. At least 28 (65%) of the subjects had nocturnal epileptiform activity on EEG, and the majority were taking concomitant psychotropic medications. During the first6 weeks of the trial, donepezil treatment, but not placebo, was associated with a statistically significant improvement in standardized ratings of receptive and expressive language compared with baseline. However, an opposite effect was seen on other core symptoms of autism; placebo treatment, but not donepezil, led to significant improvement on the CARS compared with baseline. Irritability occurred in 5 of 23 (22%) of subjects initially receiving donepezil compared with 0 of 20 (0%) subjects receiving placebo.

The efficacy of 12 weeks of open-label rivastigmine (0.4–0.8 mg given twice daily) has also been examined in 32 children (ages 3–12 years; mean age 7 years) with PDDs [45]. The sample included 13 (41%) subjects who had nocturnal epileptiform activity and 23 (72%) who were taking concomitant medications with psychotropic activity. At weeks 6 and 12 of treatment, subjects showed improvement on the CARS compared with baseline. Measures of expressive language, but not receptive language, improved over time as well. However, caution in the interpretation of this is needed given the lack of a control group.

Finally, Nicolson and colleagues [46] recently published an open-label trial of galantamine in 13 drug-free children (ages 4–17 years; mean age 9 years) with autism. Galantamine was started at 2 mg/d and titrated up to a maximum dose of 24 mg/d. Three subjects withdrew due to either worsening target symptoms (n = 2) or headache (n = 1). Eight (62%) subjects were rated as responders by CGI. Treatment led to improvements in CGI global severity, ABC Irritability and Social Withdrawal subscales, and Children's Psychiatric Ratings Scale [47] Autism and Anger factors.

These preliminary studies of cholinesterase inhibitors are noteworthy. More rigorously controlled trials of donepezil and galantamine have been completed and will likely be published shortly [40]. Until then, it is uncertain whether these drugs have any role in treating the core social and language impairment of autism.

Glutamatergic drugs

A role for glutamatergic dysfunction in the pathophysiology and treatment of autism has been proposed [48,49]. Glutamate, the primary excitatory amino acid neurotransmitter in the brain, is important in neuronal plasticity and higher cognitive functioning [50]. Evidence for the role of glutamate in autism comes from several areas including peripheral glutamate study, postmortem analysis, neuroimaging, and genetic studies [49]. Several reports have appeared that describe treatment of autistic individuals with drugs that affect the glutamate neurotransmitter system.

Lamotrigine

Lamotrigine, an anticonvulsant that attenuates glutamate release, resulted in improvement in "autistic symptoms" in 8 of 13 autistic children and adolescents during a study for intractable epilepsy [51]. Lamotrigine treatment of an 18-year-old female with profound mental retardation and a generalized seizure disorder led to improvement in irritability, sleep, social withdrawal, and emotional responsiveness [52]. Belsito and colleagues [53] conducted a double-blind, placebo-controlled trial of lamotrigine in 28 children with autism that was not as promising. In this study, lamotrigine (mean dose 5.0 mg/kg/d) was no better than placebo on any of the outcome measures, including the Autism Behavior Checklist [54], Autism Diagnostic Observation Schedule [55] (Lord and colleagues, 1989), ABC, or CARS.

D-cycloserine

D-cycloserine is an FDA-approved antibiotic used for the treatment of tuberculosis that also acts as a partial agonist at the N-methyl-D-aspartate (NMDA) subtype of glutamate receptor. Several studies in adults with schizophrenia found that D-cycloserine is beneficial for the treatment of the negative symptoms of schizophrenia [56,57]. However, a large multisite study has failed to confirm these finding [58].

Because of overlap between the negative symptoms of schizophrenia and that of social impairment in autism, our group recently published results of a single-blind study of D-cycloserine directed toward the core social impairment of subjects with autism [59]. Following a 2-week, single-blind placebo lead-in phase, 12 drug-free subjects with autism were given three different ascending doses (30 mg/d, 50 mg/d, 85 mg/d) of D-cycloserine during each of three 2-week periods. Two subjects withdrew from the study after completing only the 2-week placebo lead-in phase. The remaining 10 subjects (eight male, two female) (ages 5–28 years; mean age 10 years) completed all 8 weeks of the study. Response rates on the global CGI for the placebo, low-, medium-, and high-dose phases were 0%, 30%, 40%, and 40%, respectively. A statistically significant improvement was seen on the ABC Social Withdrawal subscale. Two subjects experienced adverse effects (a transient motor tic and increased echolalia) at the highest dose they received. Results from a double-blind, placebo-controlled study of D-cycloserine monotherapy are currently being analyzed [40].

N-methyl-D-aspartate antagonists

Amantadine, an uncompetitive antagonist at the NMDA subtype of glutamate receptor, has also been studied in autism. Open-label amantadine (dose range 3.7–8.2 mg/kg/d) led to improvement in four of eight children with developmental disabilities and associated aggression, hyperactivity, or impulsivity [60]. In a subsequent double-blind, placebo-controlled study, 39 subjects with autism (ages 5 to 19 years) were given amantadine (5.0 mg/kg/d) or placebo [61]. Clinician ratings of hyperactivity and inappropriate speech showed statistically significant improvement and there was a trend toward greater response in the amantadine group, based on ratings on the CGI. There was no statistical difference between amantadine and placebo on parent ratings; amantadine was well tolerated.

Memantine is another uncompetitive NMDA antagonist that is FDA-approved for the treatment of Alzheimer's disease. Memantine has been the subject of a case report [62], two retrospective reviews [63,64], and two open-label evaluations [65,66] in persons with autism and related PDDs. Over 8 weeks of treatment with memantine (10 mg/d), a 23-year-old man with autism exhibited significantly reduced irritable behavior and social withdrawal [62]. The effects of open-label memantine (mean dose 10.1 mg/d) over a mean duration of 19.3 weeks in 18 patients (ages 6–19 years) with PDDs were also examined by this group [63]. Eleven of 18 (61%) patients were judged responders based on ratings of "much improved" or "very much improved" on the CGI. Improvement was primarily seen in social withdrawal and inattention. In another retrospective review, 150 children and adolescents (mean age 9 years) with PDDs received memantine (mean dose 12.7 mg/d) for 4 to 8 weeks. On the CGI, 105 of 150 (70%) were "much improved" or "very much improved" in terms of language; 106 of 150 (71%) showed improvement in social behavior. In both of these reviews, memantine was frequently given as an adjunct to other medications.

Niederhofer [65] reported on an open-label trial of memantine (20 mg/d) in four persons with PDDs (mean age 17.2 years) who were medication-free for at least 2 weeks before the trial. After 4 weeks of treatment, the irritability, hyperactivity, and inappropriate speech subscales of the ABC had significantly improved. In another open-label trial, 14 children (ages 3–12 years) with PDDs were enrolled in an 8-week study of memantine (0.4 mg/kg/d) [66]. Four of 14 (29%) patients were continued on concomitant psychotropic medication during this trial. No patients were judged as "much improved" or "very much improved" on the CGI, although significant improvement was noted on the hyperactivity, social withdrawal, and irritability subscales of the ABC. The results of memantine studies in PDDs to date have been somewhat variable and warrant further, preferably placebo-controlled, study to further elucidate the effects of this compound in PDDs.

Dextromethorphan, an antitussive drug with NMDA antagonism, has also been the subject of one placebo-controlled trial employing an

ABAB design over 10 weeks in eight children (ages 9–17 years) with PDDs (seven with autism, one with PDD-NOS) [67]. The authors reported no group effect associated with use of dextromethorphan (30–60 mg/12 hours), but they did postulate that the drug was potentially more effective in children who exhibited significant inattention and hyperactivity.

Oxytocin

Oxytocin is a neuropeptide that has been implicated in social affiliation and attachment. Several lines of evidence suggest that it may also play a role in the pathophysiology of autism [68]. In a placebo-controlled crossover study, Hollander and colleagues [69] infused synthetic oxytocin into 15 adults with Asperger's disorder or autism during a comprehension task where they had to identify the affect (happy, indifferent, angry, and sad) of an audiotaped speaker making neutral statements. The majority of subjects had average to above-average IQ. The order of treatments was random; each treatment was conducted on separate days. The comprehension task was performed at baseline and at regular intervals during the 4-hour infusion. Both oxytocin and placebo infusions led to improvement in affective comprehension during the first of two trials. However, those receiving oxytocin first maintained this improvement at the time of the next baseline assessment, whereas those who received placebo first reverted back to their original baseline. This carryover effect makes interpretation of this crossover trial less straightforward, but suggests that further studies are warranted.

Summary

Identifying effective drugs to treat core social and communication impairment in autism presents many challenges. Currently, no drug has been consistently proven to be effective for the core social and communication impairment so central to the PDDs. Patients with autism exhibiting high levels of irritability may receive benefit in certain aspects of socialization and repetitive speech when prescribed risperidone. However, it is not clear whether this is an effect unique to risperidone or simply secondary to a reduction in irritability. A number of other drugs are promising and deserve further study. Most promising among these are the glutamatergic drugs and oxytocin. However, additional placebo-controlled trials are sorely needed before widely recommending these drugs for core symptom treatment. Conducting these trials is challenging, but significant progress toward the goal of identifying treatments for autism, particularly irritability, has been made over the past quarter century. The rate of progress should increase given the increased interest by society in studying the causes and treatments of autism.

References

[1] Lecavalier L. Behavioral and emotional problems in young people with pervasive developmental disorders: relative prevalence, effects of subject characteristics, and empirical classification. J Autism Dev Disord 2006;36(8):1101–14.

[2] Aman MG, Lam KS, Van Bourgondien ME. Medication patterns in patients with autism: temporal, regional, and demographic influences. J Child Adolesc Psychopharmacol 2005; 15(1):116–26.

[3] Bailey A, Le Couteur A, Gottesman I, et al. Autism as a strongly genetic disorder: evidence from a British twin study. Psychol Med 1995;25(1):63–77.

[4] Redcay E, Courchesne E. When is the brain enlarged in autism? A meta-analysis of all brain size reports. Biol Psychiatry 2005;58(1):1–9.

[5] Schultz RT, Chawarska K, Volkmar F. The social brain in autism: perspectives from neuropsychology and neuroimaging. In: Moldin SO, Rubenstein JLR, editors. Understanding autism: from basic neuroscience to treatment. Boca Raton (FL): CRC Press; 2006. p. 323–48.

[6] Lord C, Rutter M, Le Couteur A. Autism Diagnostic Interview–Revised: a revised version of a diagnostic interview for caregivers of individuals with possible pervasive developmental disorders. J Autism Dev Disord 1994;24(5):659–85.

[7] Chakrabarti S, Fombonne E. Pervasive developmental disorders in preschool children. JAMA 2001;285(24):3093–9.

[8] McDougle CJ, Scahill L, McCracken JT, et al. Research Units on Pediatric Psychopharmacology (RUPP) Autism Network. Background and rationale for an initial controlled study of risperidone. Child Adolesc Psychiatr Clin N Am 2000;9(1):201–24.

[9] Connolly HM, Crary JL, McGoon MD, et al. Valvular heart disease associated with fenfluramine-phentermine. N Engl J Med 1997;337(9):581–8.

[10] Geller E, Ritvo ER, Freeman BJ, et al. Preliminary observations on the effect of fenfluramine on blood serotonin and symptoms in three autistic boys. N Engl J Med 1982;307(3):165–9.

[11] Ritvo ER, Freeman BJ, Yuwiler A, et al. Fenfluramine treatment of autism: UCLA collaborative study of 81 patients at nine medical centers. Psychopharmacol Bull 1986;22(1): 133–40.

[12] Campbell M, Adams P, Small AM, et al. Efficacy and safety of fenfluramine in autistic children. J Am Acad Child Adolesc Psychiatry 1988;27(4):434–9.

[13] Sahley TL, Panksepp J. Brain opioids and autism: an updated analysis of possible linkages. J Aut Dev Disorders 1987;17(2):201–16.

[14] Campbell M, Anderson LT, Small AM, et al. Naltrexone in autistic children: behavioral symptoms and attentional learning. J Am Acad Child Adolesc Psychiatry 1993;32(6): 1283–91.

[15] Willemsen-Swinkels SH, Buitelaar JK, Weijnen FG, et al. Placebo-controlled acute dosage naltrexone study in young autistic children. Psychiatry Res 1995;58(3):203–15.

[16] Willemsen-Swinkels SH, Buitelaar JK, Nijhof GJ, et al. Failure of naltrexone hydrochloride to reduce self-injurious and autistic behavior in mentally retarded adults. Double-blind placebo-controlled studies. Arch Gen Psychiatry 1995;52(9):766–73.

[17] Guy W. ECDEU assessment manual for psychopharmacology, Publication No. 76-338. Washington, DC: U.S. DHEW, NIMH; 1976.

[18] Horvath K, Stefanatos G, Sokolski KN, et al. Improved social and language skills after secretin administration in patients with autistic spectrum disorders. J Assoc Acad Minor Phys 1998;9(1):9–15.

[19] McDougle CJ, Naylor ST, Cohen DJ, et al. A double-blind, placebo-controlled study of fluvoxamine in adults with autistic disorder. Arch Gen Psychiatry 1996;53(11):1001–8.

[20] McDougle CJ, Kresch LE, Posey DJ. Repetitive thoughts and behavior in pervasive developmental disorders: treatment with serotonin reuptake inhibitors. J Autism Dev Disord 2000;30(5):427–35.

[21] Hollander E, Phillips A, Chaplin W, et al. A placebo controlled crossover trial of liquid fluoxetine on repetitive behaviors in childhood and adolescent autism. Neuropsychopharmacology 2005;30(3):582–9.

[22] Scahill L, Riddle M, McSwiggin-Hardin M, et al. Children's Yale-Brown Obsessive Compulsive Scale: Reliability and validity. Journal of American Academy of Child and Adolescent Psychiatry 1997;36:844–52.

[23] Posey DJ, Erickson CA, Stigler KA, et al. The use of selective serotonin reuptake inhibitors in autism and related disorders. J Child Adolesc Psychopharmacol 2006;16(1–2):181–6.

[24] DeLong GR, Ritch CR, Burch S. Fluoxetine response in children with autistic spectrum disorders: correlation with familial major affective disorder and intellectual achievement. Dev Med Child Neurol 2002;44(10):652–9.

[25] McDougle CJ, Holmes JP, Carlson DC, et al. A double-blind, placebo-controlled study of risperidone in adults with autistic disorder and other pervasive developmental disorders. Arch Gen Psychiatry 1998;55(7):633–41.

[26] Research Units on Pediatric Psychopharmaology Autism Network. Risperidone in children with autism and serious behavioral problems. N Engl J Med 2002;347(5):314–21.

[27] Aman MG, Singh NN, Stewart AW, et al. The aberrant behavior checklist: a behavior rating scale for the assessment of treatment effects. Am J Ment Defic 1985;5:485–91.

[28] McDougle CJ, Scahill L, Aman MG, et al. Risperidone for the core symptom domains of autism: results from the study by the autism network of the research units on pediatric psychopharmacology. Am J Psychiatry 2005;162(6):1142–8.

[29] Freeman BJ, Ritvo ER, Yokota A, et al. A scale for rating symptoms of patients with the syndrome of autism in real life settings. J Am Acad Child Psychiatry 1986;25(1):130–6.

[30] Scahill L, McDougle CJ, Williams SK, et al. Children's Yale-Brown Obsessive Compulsive Scale modified for pervasive developmental disorders. J Am Acad Child Adolesc Psychiatry 2006;45(9):1114–23.

[31] Shea S, Turgay A, Carroll A, et al. Risperidone in the treatment of disruptive behavioral symptoms in children with autistic and other pervasive developmental disorders. Pediatrics 2004;114(5):e634–41.

[32] Posey DJ, Walsh KH, Wilson GA, et al. Risperidone in the treatment of two very young children with autism. J Child Adolesc Psychopharmacol 1999;9(4):273–6.

[33] Nagaraj R, Singhi P, Malhi P. Risperidone in children with autism: randomized, placebo-controlled, double-blind study. J Child Neurol 2006;21(6):450–5.

[34] Schopler E, Reichler RJ, DeVellis RF, et al. Toward objective classification of childhood autism: Childhood Autism Rating Scale (CARS). J Autism Dev Disord 1980;10(1):91–103.

[35] Luby J, Mrakotsky C, Stalets MM, et al. Risperidone in preschool children with autistic spectrum disorders: an investigation of safety and efficacy. J Child Adolesc Psychopharmacol 2006;16(5):575–87.

[36] Potenza MN, Holmes JP, Kanes SJ, et al. Olanzapine treatment of children, adolescents, and adults with pervasive developmental disorders: an open-label pilot study. J Clin Psychopharmacol 1999;19(1):37–44.

[37] Malone RP, Cater J, Sheikh RM, et al. Olanzapine versus haloperidol in children with autistic disorder: an open pilot study. J Am Acad Child Adolesc Psychiatry 2001;40(8):887–94.

[38] Kemner C, Willemsen-Swinkels SH, de Jonge M, et al. Open-label study of olanzapine in children with pervasive developmental disorder. J Clin Psychopharmacol 2002;22(5):455–60.

[39] Hollander E, Wasserman S, Swanson EN, et al. A double-blind placebo-controlled pilot study of olanzapine in childhood/adolescent pervasive developmental disorder. J Child Adolesc Psychopharmacol 2006;16(5):541–8.

[40] ClinicalTrials.gov. Available at: http://www.clinicaltrials.gov. Accessed May 16, 2008.

[41] Niederhofer H. Treating autism pharmacologically: also tacrine might improve symptomatology in some cases. J Child Neurol 2007;22(8):1054.

[42] Hardan AY, Handen BL. A retrospective open trial of adjunctive donepezil in children and adolescents with autistic disorder. J Child Adolesc Psychopharmacol 2002;12(3):237–41.

[43] Doyle RL, Frazier J, Spencer TJ, et al. Donepezil in the treatment of ADHD-like symptoms in youths with pervasive developmental disorder: a case series. J Atten Disord 2006;9(3): 543–9.

[44] Chez MG, Buchanan TM, Becker M, et al. Donepezil hydrochloride: a double-blind study in autistic children. J Pediatr Neurol 2003;1(2):83–8.

[45] Chez MG, Aimonovitch M, Buchanan T, et al. Treating autistic spectrum disorders in children: utility of the cholinesterase inhibitor rivastigmine tartrate. J Child Neurol 2004;19(3): 165–9.

[46] Nicolson R, Craven-Thuss B, Smith J. A prospective, open-label trial of galantamine in autistic disorder. J Child Adolesc Psychopharmacol 2006;16(5):621–9.

[47] Fish B. Children's Psychiatric Rating Scale. Psychopharmacol Bull 1985;21:753–70.

[48] Carlsson ML. Hypothesis: is infantile autism a hypoglutamatergic disorder? Relevance of glutamate—serotonin interactions for pharmacotherapy. J Neural Transm 1998;105(4–5): 525–35.

[49] Erickson CA, McDougle CJ, Stigler KA, et al. Glutamatergic function in autism. In: Heresco-Levy U, editor. Glutamate in neuropsychiatric disorders. Trivandrum, Kerala (India): Research Signpost, in press.

[50] Coyle JT, Leski ML, Morrison JH. The diverse role of L-glutamic acid in brain signal transduction. In: Davis KL, Charney D, Coyle JT, et al, editors. Neuropsychopharmacology: the fifth generation of progress. Philadelphia: Lippincott Williams & Williams; 2002. p. 71–90.

[51] Uvebrant P, Bauziene R. Intractable epilepsy in children. The efficacy of lamotrigine treatment, including non-seizure-related benefits. Neuropediatrics 1994;25(6):284–9.

[52] Davanzo PA, King BH. Open trial lamotrigine in the treatment of self-injurious behavior in an adolescent with profound mental retardation. J Child Adolesc Psychopharmacol 1996; 6(4):273–9.

[53] Belsito KM, Law PA, Kirk KS, et al. Lamotrigine therapy for autistic disorder: a randomized, double-blind, placebo-controlled trial. J Autism Dev Disord 2001;31(2):175–81.

[54] Krug DA, Arick J, Almond P. Autism behavior checklist record form. Austin (TX): PRO-ED; 1993.

[55] Lord C, Rutter M, Goode S, et al. Autism diagnostic observation schedule: a standardized observation of communicative and social behavior. J Autism Dev Disord 1989;19(2): 185–212.

[56] Goff DC, Tsai G, Levitt J, et al. A placebo-controlled trial of D-cycloserine added to conventional neuroleptics in patients with schizophrenia. Arch Gen Psychiatry 1999;56(1):21–7.

[57] Heresco-Levy U, Ermilov M, Shimoni J, et al. Placebo-controlled trial of D-cycloserine added to conventional neuroleptics, olanzapine, or risperidone in schizophrenia. Am J Psychiatry 2002;159(3):480–2.

[58] Buchanan RW, Javitt DC, Marder SR, et al. The Cognitive and Negative Symptoms in Schizophrenia Trial (CONSIST): the efficacy of glutamatergic agents for negative symptoms and cognitive impairments. Am J Psychiatry 2007;164(10):1593–602.

[59] Posey DJ, Kem DL, Swiezy NB, et al. A pilot study of D-cycloserine in subjects with autistic disorder. Am J Psychiatry 2004;161(11):2115–7.

[60] King BH, Wright DM, Snape M, et al. Case series: amantadine open-label treatment of impulsive and aggressive behavior in hospitalized children with developmental disabilities. J Am Acad Child Adolesc Psychiatry 2001;40(6):654–7.

[61] King BH, Wright DM, Handen BL, et al. Double-blind, placebo-controlled study of amantadine hydrochloride in the treatment of children with autistic disorder. J Am Acad Child Adolesc Psychiatry 2001;40(6):658–65.

[62] Erickson CA, Chambers JE. Memantine for disruptive behavior in autistic disorder. J Clin Psychiatry 2006;67(6):1000.

[63] Erickson CA, Posey DJ, Stigler KA, et al. A retrospective study of memantine in children and adolescents with pervasive developmental disorders. Psychopharmacology (Berl) 2007;191(1):141–7.

[64] Chez MG, Burton Q, Dowling T, et al. Memantine as adjunctive therapy in children diagnosed with autistic spectrum disorders: an observation of initial clinical response and maintenance tolerability. J Child Neurol 2007;22(5):574–9.

[65] Niederhofer H. Glutamate antagonists seem to be slightly effective in psychopharmacologic treatment of autism. J Clin Psychopharmacol 2007;27(3):317–8.

[66] Owley T, Salt J, Guter S, et al. A prospective, open-label trial of memantine in the treatment of cognitive, behavioral, and memory dysfunction in pervasive developmental disorders. J Child Adolesc Psychopharmacol 2006;16(5):517–24.

[67] Woodard C, Groden J, Goodwin M, et al. A placebo double-blind pilot study of dextrome-thorphan for problematic behaviors in children with autism. Autism 2007;11(1):29–41.

[68] Bartz JA, Hollander E. The neuroscience of affiliation: forging links between basic and clinical research on neuropeptides and social behavior. Horm Behav 2006;50(4):518–28.

[69] Hollander E, Bartz J, Chaplin W, et al. Oxytocin increases retention of social cognition in autism. Biol Psychiatry 2007;61(4):498–503.

ELSEVIER
SAUNDERS

Child Adolesc Psychiatric Clin N Am
17 (2008) 803–820

CHILD AND
ADOLESCENT
PSYCHIATRIC CLINICS
OF NORTH AMERICA

Complementary and Alternative Medicine Treatments for Children with Autism Spectrum Disorders

Susan E. Levy, MD[a],*, Susan L. Hyman, MD[b]

[a]Department of Pediatrics, University of Pennsylvania School of Medicine, The Children's Hospital of Philadelphia, 3405 Civic Center Boulevard, Philadelphia, PA 19104, USA
[b]Department of Pediatrics, University of Rochester School of Medicine, Golisano Children's Hospital at Strong, Box 671, 601 Elmwood Avenue, Rochester, NY 14642, USA

Autism spectrum disorders (ASD) are common disorders affecting 1 in 150 children [1] and are typically first recognized in early childhood. ASDs are characterized by core deficits in socialization, communication, and behavior [2] with a wide range of severity of symptoms. Disorders include autism, Asperger's disorder, childhood disintegrative disorder, Rett syndrome, and pervasive developmental disorder not otherwise specified (PDD-NOS). This article includes autism, Asperger's disorder, and PDD-NOS as the ASDs for discussion because childhood disintegrative disorder and Rett's disorder have different characteristics, outcome, and treatment. Function and outcome are affected not only by core deficits but frequently by associated comorbid behaviors [3,4] such as irritability, sensory abnormalities, hyperactivity, affective disorders, and others. Outcome is further affected by the presence or absence of language and by overall cognitive ability.

Although existing scientific data suggest the etiology is largely genetic with the plausibility of environmental factors, the specific causes are often not known. In addition, the symptoms are behaviorally defined, heterogeneous, and change with the acquisition of developmental skills. For these reasons, families of children with autism and related disorders may turn to therapies that are not based in the realm of conventional medical or psychologic practice.

Dr. Hyman was supported in part by grant PO1HD35466 from the National Institute of Mental Health and grant NIH UL1RR024160 from the National Center for Research Resources.

* Corresponding author.
E-mail address: levys@email.chop.edu (S.E. Levy).

This article discusses the common use of complementary and alternative medicine (CAM) by families of children with ASDs, investigates the reasons families seek CAM, reviews the commonly used CAM therapies for ASD, and describes the issues faced by conventional practitioners whose patients are interested in CAM use. The combination of conventional practice and complementary techniques which have some supportive evidence is often called "integrative medicine." Some interventions originally considered CAM are embraced into conventional practice as evidence supports their use.

Treatments for children with autism spectrum disorders

Research has shown that the most effective treatment is a combination of specialized and supportive educational programming, communication training (such as speech/language therapy), social skills support, and behavioral intervention [5,6]. Other treatments such as occupational therapy and physical therapy may promote progress because they address possible comorbid difficulties of motor coordination and sensory deficits. Progress may be slow, in part, owing to the pervasive nature of the core deficits and comorbid features.

Prevalence of use of complimentary and alternative medicine for symptoms of autism in children

The use of CAM is increasing for both adults and children. The National Center for Complementary and Alternative Medicine (NCCAM) reports that over three fourths of American adults use CAM for the treatment of disease or to maintain health (http://nccam.nih.gov/news/camsurvey_fs1. htm). The use of CAM in children mirrors the treatment choices of their parents. It is estimated that 2% to 50% of children in the United States are given CAM therapies [7]. This range is likely to be an underestimate.

Children with chronic illness such as cancer, asthma, rheumatoid arthritis, and neurodevelopmental disorders such as autism are treated with CAM therapies at even higher rates. As many as 50% to 75% of children with autism may be treated with CAM [8,9]. CAM use may be even more likely in children with comorbid intellectual disability. Levy and colleagues [10] reported that almost one third of young children referred for evaluation of ASD were being treated with dietary therapies by their parents even before confirmation of the diagnosis.

A wide range of CAM therapies are used in children. The NCCAM groups CAM therapies into four domains: (1) mind-body medicine, (2) biologically based practices, (3) manipulative and body-based practices, and (4) energy medicine. The most commonly used CAM treatments for ASD fall into the categories of biologically based practice and manipulative and body-based practices. Approximately half of families of children with ASD use a biologically based therapy, 30% a mind-body therapy, and 25% a manipulation or body-based method [8]. The range of reported response about usage is dependent upon the population queried and how the question is asked. Hanson [8] reported that 41% of respondents endorsed benefit with dietary and nutritional treatments, whereas Wong and Smith [9] found that 75% of respondents thought their treatments were helpful.

Who uses complementary and alternative medicine therapies and why

Conventional medicine has been directed at the goals of diagnosis, treatment, and, when possible, cure of disease states. CAM practices add promotion of health and involvement of the patient in a process of healing that must ultimately address the underlying cause of illness as interpreted by the practitioner [11].

CAM is often perceived as "natural," without the side effects of conventional medical treatments. The reasons why families use CAM have been studied in other chronic disorders of childhood. Adverse effects from conventional medication were the only significant predictors for CAM use in children with inflammatory bowel disease [12]. Similarly, for children with asthma, CAM use was predicted by older age, worse control of symptoms, more medications, more medical visits, and more side effects [13]. A survey in Italy identified the fear of side effects as the most common reason for parents to choose a CAM therapy for routine illness. Satisfaction was reported by 81% and successful symptom resolution attributed to the CAM therapy [11]. Adults who use CAM believe that a combined approach of CAM and conventional therapy is more likely to be successful than either treatment alone, and that nutritional support is an important part of health maintenance, preferring not to take prescription medications [14]. Among families of children with ASD surveyed by Hanson and colleagues [8], over 75% chose therapies based on their perception of safety, the absence of side effects, or prior experience with side effects. Despite the common use of CAM, two third of families report that they base their therapeutic choices on the recommendation of their health care provider or scientific support. Approximately 50% of families report that they desire more control over the therapies elected and that they choose CAM because of a hope for a cure or because of recommendations by friends or families of other children with ASD. Only 39% elect CAM because they prefer "natural" therapies, and 25% report choices based on media. CAM therapies are pursued to treat core symptoms of ASD, as well as to increase attention, to enhance relaxation, to decrease gastrointestinal symptoms, to regulate sleep, and to promote general health, in that order [9].

Patients who seek out CAM providers may be seeking the longer visits typically offered in CAM settings and perceive that the CAM provider pays more attention to the symptoms of concern to the family. Parents who use CAM for their children tend to use CAM for their own health and are better educated. It is not dissatisfaction with conventional care that leads families to employ CAM. The most commonly reported reasons are concern regarding side effects, the desire to include multiple approaches to address symptoms, and personal beliefs about health. With changes in society such as self-determination in health care, greater accessibility to information on the Internet, and a decline in faith in science and technology, people are seeking more control over their own medical decision making [14,15].

Complementary and alternative medicine therapies

All treatments should be based on principles of evidence-based medicine, integrating clinical expertise, patient (or family) values, and the best evidence for efficacy [16–18]. The selection of some treatments may reflect a bias affected by the caregiver's clinical experience, education or skills, and the families' unique concerns and expectations. Studies of efficacy of treatment should be judged by standards of scientific research, guiding study design and the hierarchy of types of study. The hierarchy of strength of evidence includes randomized controlled clinical trials, which are at the peak, followed by cohort studies, case-control studies, and then case reports. The most robust evidence would include meta-analyses, which thoroughly examine a number of valid studies on a topic. Meta-analysis combines results using accepted statistical methodology as if they were from one large study or a systemic review, which focuses on a clinical question and includes an extensive literature search to identify all studies with sound methodology. Unfortunately, even some commonly used medical treatments have not met these standards. For the purposes of this article, we have reviewed the existing literature and reported the strength of the evidence as grade A (randomized controlled trials, reviews, and/or meta-analyses), grade B (other evidence such as isolated well-designed controlled and uncontrolled studies), or grade C (case reports or theories). This grading refers to the strength of the evidence that supports or refutes the use of the intervention.

Mind-body medicine

Yoga–grade C

Decreasing anxiety through nonpharmacologic techniques has great attraction to both families and clinicians. Yoga is a mind-body approach that enjoys popular practice for increasing the sense of well-being and control with the potential to decrease anxiety. A trial of yoga for symptoms of attention-deficit hyperactivity disorder (ADHD) was underpowered to demonstrate effect but suggested some benefit in children on medication [19]. Relaxation therapy decreased symptoms of anxiety in inpatients with anxiety in a child psychiatry service [20] and in children with mental retardation [21]. No studies have been published related to symptoms of autism and the response to yoga techniques.

Music therapy–grade B

The use of music to reinforce communication is frequently applied in the context of educational interventions. The use of music in a discrete therapeutic format to enhance social skill and communication development in children with autism has been examined in small trials, with the potential for positive effects on spoken and gestural communication [22]. No effect on overall behavior was reported. Clinical practice often pairs music with other interventions with subjective benefit [23]. Further study of the neurobiology of music processing in persons with autism may provide additional rationale for music therapy as a discrete treatment or a part of other educational interventions [24,25].

Biologically based practices

Dietary supplements

Vitamin B_6/Mg^{2+}–grade B. Vitamin supplements to improve symptoms of mental health disorders have been in use for over 50 years, with vitamin B_6 and magnesium a popular treatment for autism over the past 20 years. This treatment has been the subject of reviews by several investigators [26–28]. Due to the small number of studies, methodologic deficits, and small sample sizes, meta-analysis could not be done, and the evidence was not adequate to support the use of these supplements.

The most recent Cochrane Review [26] identified three studies completed between 1993 and 2002 that compared outcomes to the findings in a placebo or nontreated group. A total of 28 subjects were treated in these trials. Findling and colleagues [29] studied 12 participants using a randomized, double-blind, placebo-controlled trial following a 2-week pre-randomization placebo lead-in period. No effects of treatment were seen in the 10 subjects who completed the study. More recently, Kuriyama and colleagues [30] reported improvement in IQ and social quotient scores in eight children treated with vitamin B_6 and Mg^{2+}. Despite the fact that these studies met criteria for Cochrane Review, they all suffered from significant methodologic weaknesses, including an inadequate description of the diagnosis, selection criteria, and outcome measures. One additional study with similar methodologic issues has been published since this review, describing an open study of 33 children with ASD who were reported to improve in symptoms after magnesium and vitamin B_6 treatment [31].

Dimethylglycine–grade B. Dimethylglycine and a related compound, trimethylglycine, are commonly used nutritional supplements. An older case series suggested improvement in language and attention in a group of children with intellectual disability treated with dimethylglycine. Two small, double-blind studies of dimethylglycine have not demonstrated positive effects on symptoms of autism in a comparison with placebo [32,33].

Melatonin–grade B. Some nutritional supplements have known pharmacologic properties. Melatonin is a hormone produced by the pineal gland that regulates sleep. Clinical studies have demonstrated abnormalities in melatonin production or release in individuals with ASD [34]. Clinical benefit in sleep onset and maintenance has been demonstrated in at least one large case series at doses ranging from 0.75 to 6 mg before bedtime [35]. This result would be predicted by the large effect size in small randomized trials [36]. Few side effects were reported. Andersen and colleagues [35] treated 107 children with autism with melatonin, many of whom were also being treated with psychotropic medications. Side effects of early morning sleepiness or enuresis were reported in three cases. No effect on seizures was noted.

Vitamin C–grade B. Vitamin C is not commonly used as an isolated treatment but is frequently added to vitamin mixtures used by children with ASD. Dolske and colleagues [37] reported positive results of decreased stereotyped behavior in a 30-week, double-blind, placebo-controlled trial in 18 children with ASD. To date, this study has not been replicated. Other reports have implicated vitamin C in its role with oxidative stress.

Amino acids–grade C and carnosine–grade B. Amino acids are precursors to neurotransmitters and act as neurotransmitters themselves [38]. As such, it is not surprising that some complementary approaches attempt to manipulate neurochemical actions by nutritional supplementation. The abnormalities in peripheral serotonin levels in persons with autism and their family members was one of the first biologic findings in autism [39]. Supplemental tryptophan might increase brain production of serotonin because the uptake across the blood-brain barrier is sensitive to the concentration in the bloodstream; however, no trials have examined the clinical effect of tryptophan supplementation on symptoms of autism. In adults with autism, tryptophan depletion exacerbated symptoms [40]. There are no peer-reviewed studies to date examining the effects of supplementation with other amino acids such as taurine, lysine, or GABA in children with autism, although they are often part of a CAM nutritional supplementation strategy. Taurine is a semi-essential sulfur-containing amino acid derived from methionine and cystine. It has antioxidant properties and has been associated with improved visual learning in rodents. L-carnosine is a dipeptide that was demonstrated in one double-blind, placebo-controlled trial in 31 children with autism to improve expressive and receptive vocabulary, with subjective improvement on the Gilliam Autism Rating Scale over an 8-week trial at 800 mg/d [41]. Lysine is an amino acid exogenously obtained from meat and milk products. With methionine, it can be endogenously made into carnitine [42]. Carnitine is involved in intracellular transport of long chain fatty acids and is important in energy generation. Although carnitine has documented usefulness in specific deficiency states and in the presence of certain medications such as valproic acid, it has never been evaluated as a treatment for motor or behavioral symptoms of autism. One case series of children with autism with elevated alanine and low carnitine suggests that some children with autism may have mitochondrial disease [43].

Omega 3 fatty acids–grade B. Polyunsaturated fatty acids, in particular omega 3 fatty acids, are crucial for brain development and cannot be manufactured in the body. Dietary consumption occurs through the ingestion of fish or fish oils. Oral supplementation with essential fatty acids has become popular for children with developmental differences including autism and ADHD [44]. Studies have examined differences in plasma levels of children with autism, which are decreased when compared with that in typical volunteers [45,46] without clinical correlations. Recently, Amminger and colleagues [47] reported improvement in behavior following a randomized double-blind, placebo-controlled, 6-week pilot trial of oral supplementation in 13 children with ASD with severe behavior difficulties. No side effects were noted beyond gastrointestinal symptoms.

Folate and oxidative stress–grade C. It has been hypothesized that exposure to toxic agents or endogenous abnormalities that lead to oxidative stress may cause neuronal insult and lead to the regression seen in as many as one third of children with autism [48]. Neuroanatomic differences in white and gray matter, cerebellar pathology (eg, Purkinje cell loss), and other evidence of cellular disruption [49] as well as functional abnormalities [50] led to the search for potential environmental causes of atypical brain development. Abnormal levels of antioxidants, transferrin, lipid peroxidases, methionine, and other biochemical intermediates have been reported in children with autism [51] without clinical correlation. James and colleagues [52] have described abnormal metabolic profiles in 20 children with autism compared with 33 controls, consistent with a presumed impaired methylation capacity. Laboratory findings normalized following a trial of folinic acid, betaine, and methylcobalamin; however, no clinical outcome data were reported. James and colleagues [53] also reported decreased measured indicators of methylation capacity in a larger population (80 with autism and 73 controls), also without clinical correlation. At present, there are no randomized controlled treatment trials reported in the scientific literature. These hypotheses require further study.

Gluten-free/casein-free diet–grade B

In addition to supplementation with vitamins or other nutritional supplements to address hypothetical deficiencies or to provide pharmacologic effect, modification of dietary intake has been a popular intervention for behavioral modification in children with ASD. It has been suggested that the elimination of the proteins gluten (found in barley, wheat, and rye) and casein (found in milk products), which either cause or aggravate symptoms of ASD after absorption across a damaged ("leaky") intestinal lining by acting as false opiate neuropeptides, will improve the behavior of children with ASD. The significance of reports of increased levels of metabolites of casein and gluten in the urine of persons with autism remains unclear [54]. Urinary peptides are not used in conventional practice to prescribe or monitor dietary restriction. Anecdotal reports and case series of dietary restriction leading to subjective improvement in the symptoms of autism have resulted in a report of a small single-blind trial that suggested some improvement [55] and a double-blind trial that did not identify objective improvement in language or behavior, although some parents reported subjective differences [56]. It is not yet clear whether some of the perceived improvements are due to elimination of lactose in children who are lactose intolerant or to other changes related to the alteration in protein source and food composition. Families who desire to try the gluten-free/casein-free diet must be counseled that adequate calcium and vitamin D intake must be maintained with supplements or supplemented foods. Attention to protein intake is also important because many young children obtain much of their protein through dairy products. Vegetable-based beverages including rice, potato, and almond "milk" do not contribute to protein sufficiency as soy-based products do. Consultation with a registered dietitian should be recommended.

Common dietary approaches to symptoms of inattention in children with ADHD are also often considered for children with ASD with hyperkinesis. Double-blind, placebo-controlled methods have consistently demonstrated no relationship of sugar to attention or related behaviors [57]. Although not specific for symptoms of ASD, there may be subgroups of children who do have a behavioral response to elimination of chemicals used as food colors [58].

Gastrointestinal medications–grade C

Dietary treatments are not the only gastrointestinal treatments that are pursued. Gastrointestinal symptoms of gastroesophageal reflux, constipation, diarrhea, feeding refusal, and others are frequently reported in clinical settings [44], although there is not yet documentation of an increased population-based prevalence of gastrointestinal abnormalities [59,60]. Given the frequent report of symptoms, digestive enzymes are used by some families [61]. No evidence-based studies are available to evaluate efficacy. Probiotics are also used to improve the microbial environment in the intestine [62].

Secretin–grade A

Secretin, a gastrointestinal hormone, has the distinction of being one of the most extensively studied pharmacotherapeutic agent for autism. It came to light as a potential treatment after a lay television show highlighted a report of a case series by Horvath [63] describing improvement in symptoms of autism after administration during endoscopy to examine pancreatic secretions. More than a dozen well-designed, well-executed studies have been published, failing to demonstrate the efficacy of secretin for symptoms of autism [44]. A recent Cochrane Review reported 14 randomized controlled trials with a total of 618 children. Nine studies used a crossover treatment design. It was concluded that there is no evidence that single- or multiple-dose intravenous secretin is effective for the treatment of ASD [64].

Hyperbaric oxygen therapy–grade C

Hyperbaric oxygen therapy (HBOT) is used in conventional practice to treat carbon monoxide poisoning, to enhance wound healing, and for pressure equalization after diving injuries [65,66]. HBOT provides pressurized oxygen at pressures greater than or equal to 2 atm. HBOT is generally considered to have few side effects other than a potential for exacerbation of ear pain or seizures, but limited data are available. Because of attributed properties of increasing blood flow or oxygen to the brain and decreasing inflammation, it has been evaluated therapeutically in disorders of the central nervous system, including cerebral palsy, dementia, and traumatic brain injury. Randomized controlled trials of HBOT in children with cerebral palsy at 100% O_2 at 1.75 atm compared with a control condition of room air at 1.3 atm reported no difference in motor and behavioral symptoms [67,68].

There is increasing popular interest in using HBOT for symptoms of autism because of hypotheses regarding inflammation of the gut or brain, brain hypoperfusion, and aberrant oxidative stress response, which proponents of HBOT suggest might be improved by up-regulation of the metabolic pathways by HBOT [69]. In an open clinical trial, 18 children with autism were given 40 sessions of HBOT at 1.3 atm and 24% O_2 (n = 6) or 1.5 atm and 100% O_2 (n = 12) in a nonrandom fashion [70]. Metabolic markers for oxidative stress, measurement of C reactive protein to evaluate inflammation, and parental report of behavior on the Aberrant Behavior Checklist, Social Responsiveness Scale, and Autism Treatment Evaluation Checklist (ATEC) were recorded before treatment and after each of 10 sessions. Each child received 40 sessions. Many children were already on antioxidant therapy, which was noted by the investigators when they reported no difference in markers of oxidative stress. C reactive protein decreased in the subgroup with the highest values. Parents reported subjective improvements in several areas; however, the subjective data and potential confounds make this study difficult to interpret. No randomized controlled trials of HBOT for the symptoms of ASD support the clinical use of this modality.

Chelation–grade C

Reports of an increased prevalence rate of autism, most likely due to multiple factors, have resulted in a search for potential environmental causes.

Questions of the relationship to vaccine administration came about in part because symptoms of autism are identified during late infancy and toddlerhood, and because a temporal relationship with immunizations is noted in some cases [71,72]. A report published in 2001 [73] developed a hypothesis relating symptoms of mercury intoxication to symptoms of autism. A meta-analysis completed by Ng and colleagues [74] of two studies concluded that there was not enough evidence to show that the hair mercury level was lower in autistic children than typical. Several epidemiologic studies have failed to confirm a link between the use of thimerosal as a vaccine preservative and elevated autism prevalence [72,75–86]. Despite the lack of scientific evidence of a link between the exposure to ethyl mercury in thimerosal (the mercury-containing preservative used in vaccines that has been largely eliminated in the United States since 2001), chemical chelation treatments are a popular intervention. Chelation is the process of administering either DMPS (2,3-dimercaptopropane-1-sulfonate) or DMSA (2,3-dimercaptosuccinic acid) to bind heavy metals such as mercury and facilitate elimination from the body. No controlled studies have examined the safety or efficacy of prescription or nonprescription chelation regimens for children with autism. More importantly, deaths have been reported from the inappropriate use of a chelator, EDTA, from hypocalcemia [87]. Proponents of this therapy suggest that mercury is poorly eliminated by children with autism and that it interferes with immune function and other biochemical systems.

Immune therapies–grade C

Increasing evidence suggests that the prenatal immune response may affect fetal brain development; however, the data regarding immune function in children with autism vary among reported populations [88,89]. Jyonouci and colleagues [90] found that dietary restriction did not alter immune findings in children with or without gastrointestinal symptoms. Three case series report trials of children who were infused with intravenous immunoglobulin G to treat purported immune deficits and symptoms of autism. One open trial reported improvement in subjective data [91], but subsequent trials with specific outcome measures and better subject characterization did not corroborate this finding [92]. Other treatments for immune function have been proposed but remain without support in the peer-reviewed literature [93]. In the absence of conventional symptoms of immune disorders, the work-up and treatment of immune status is not currently recommended in children with autism [6].

Antibiotics–grade C

Reports of frequent respiratory or gastrointestinal infections during the early years of development of children with autism have suggested that these exposures may be etiologic agents by promoting gut dysbiosis or are confirmation of immune dysfunction. Niehus and Lord [94,95] reported a cohort of young children with ASD who had a history of more frequent episodes of otitis media but no more illness-related fevers or use of antibiotics when compared with typically developing peers. Reports of frequency of gastrointestinal infection or colonization are inconsistent and suffer from methodologic difficulties such as small sample size, lack of clinical correlation to laboratory findings [96], and lack of a control group [97]. Sandler and colleagues [98] reported short-term behavioral improvement in 11 children treated with oral vancomycin. No further data or studies are available, and even the investigators suggested vancomycin should not be a routine clinical treatment.

Antifungal agents–grade C

Treatment with antifungal agents is based on an earlier report of presumed candidal overgrowth in two boys with autistic behavior who demonstrated what was interpreted as yeast metabolites in urine organic acids [99] and on reports suggesting yeast overgrowth due to antibiotic use or sugar ingestion [100]. Yeast overgrowth is conjectured to be secondary to intestinal dysbiosis or some other immune factors unique to autism. No controlled trials have tested this intervention to date despite the popularity of probiotic use and medications such as nystatin (Mycostatin) and fluconazole (Diflucan) for treatment of yeast overgrowth.

Manipulative and body-based practices

Chiropractic–grade C

The peer-reviewed literature does not include reports that specifically address either chiropractic manipulation or craniosacral massage for symptoms of autism. Chiropractic care is a common approach used by many families for general health issues. The potential for harm is low; however, it has been associated with injury from spinal manipulation and missed medical diagnoses [101].

Craniosacral massage–grade C

Physical manipulation of the skull and cervical spine has been used by chiropractors, osteopathic physicians, occupational therapists, and others for specific therapeutic purposes. Despite claims that practitioners can alter and sense cerebrospinal fluid flow or the cranial rhythm impulse, no movement of bony sutures or alteration of pressure could be demonstrated in a laboratory model [102] or in humans [103]. It is possible that perceived therapeutic response might be secondary to another aspect of the therapy such as touch. No studies are reported that examine this modality for use in autism.

Massage/therapeutic touch therapies–grade C

Sensory differences are frequently described by parents but do not figure prominently in the fourth edition of the Diagnostic and Statistical Manual of Mental Disorders criteria for the diagnosis of autism. Therapeutic approaches in this category include massage [104] and aroma therapy [105].

Auditory integration–grade B

The goal of auditory integration training is to ameliorate auditory processing deficits and improve concentration [106]. Many parents also report improved behaviors. Different methods of auditory integration training include listening through headphones to electronically modified music, voice, or sounds in an effort to improve function. Recent systematic reviews [106,107] included six randomized controlled trials, all of which showed significant methodologic weaknesses prohibiting meta-analysis. The authors of the Cochrane Review agreed with the recommendations of the American Academy of Pediatrics that auditory integration training should be considered an experimental treatment until evidence-based trials support its use [107,108].

Energy medicine

Transcranial magnetic stimulation–no grade

Transcranial magnetic stimulation involves placement of an electromagnetic coil on the scalp with the production of low level electrical currents in the cortex secondary to rapid magnetic pulses [109]. This research tool is currently being used to examine the potential overconnectivity of cortical neurons in autism [110] and to examine neurologic function in other disorders such as ADHD [111]. Treatment trials are underway for depression, pain syndromes, and motor function in other disease states. This technology is unrelated to the use of commercially obtained magnets applied topically as a type of community-based energy medicine. There are no reports of the therapeutic use of transcranial magnetic stimulation or other magnet therapy for the symptoms of autism to date.

When a patient elects complementary and alternative medicine

Traditionally trained clinicians know that many families they treat also elect to use CAM for their children with ASD. Although there is recent literature about the reasons why people choose CAM, the attitudes and response of traditional practitioners to the requests for information or the prescription of CAM is less well studied [11]. Although over half of families indicate that they would like to ask their physicians about CAM, many reasons are given for not disclosing CAM use. These reasons include a perceived lack of knowledge about CAM therapies on the part of the physician, the fact that the physician does not ask about such therapy, not seeing the necessity of reporting the use of other therapies, and concern regarding disapproval by the physician [9].

Although families often report that they use CAM because of a fear of side effects, there are limited data regarding the side effects of CAM practices themselves. Side effects may include direct systemic or topical toxicity, allergic reaction, the presence of contaminants, and interactions with prescribed medications [112]. Given the popularity of CAM, the interaction of CAM with prescription medication requires further study. CAM use may be underreported, and the dosage and type of exposure are often unknown [113]. Only if there is an open dialog about CAM will such practices be reported to the health care provider and the potential side effects and interactions adequately studied and monitored. Health care providers need to discuss the importance of continuing pharmacologic or other therapeutic interventions while CAM therapy is being used.

Nutritional supplements are not regulated as drugs but as foods; therefore, there is little oversight regarding quality control. Variability in response may be due to family or social factors or to variable delivery of the active compound.

Summary

As health care providers are increasingly looking toward the evidence for conventional medical practices, they should also be examining the evidence for CAM practices that patients may be using. They should encourage families to share all interventions that they are pursuing regardless of whether they are prescribed or endorsed by conventional practice. This approach is important for health monitoring of side effects and the potential for drug interactions. Some CAM practices have evidence to reject their use, such as secretin. Some CAM practices have emerging evidence to support their use in traditional medical practice, such as melatonin. Most treatments have not been adequately studied and do not have evidence to support their use. Although not direct effects of CAM practices, undesired side effects may relate to the delay or discontinuation of otherwise effective treatments.

References

[1] Autism and Developmental Disability Monitoring Network Surveillance Year 2002 Principal Investigators, Centers for Disease Control and Prevention. Prevalence of autism spectrum disorders–autism and developmental disabilities monitoring network, six sites, United States, 2000. MMWR Surveill Summ 2007;56:1–11.
[2] American Psychiatric Association. Diagnostic and statistical manual of mental disorders. 4th edition [text revised]. Arlington (VA): American Psychiatric Association; 2000.
[3] Gillberg C, Billstedt E. Autism and Asperger syndrome: coexistence with other clinical disorders. Acta Psychiatr Scand 2000;102:321–30.
[4] Matson JL, Nebel-Schwalm MS. Comorbid psychopathology with autism spectrum disorder in children: an overview. Res Dev Disabil 2007;28:341–52.
[5] Lord C, McGee J, editors. Educating children with autism [National Research Council]. Washington (DC): National Academy Press; 2001.
[6] Myers SM, Johnson CP. Management of children with autism spectrum disorders. Pediatrics 2007;120:1162–82.
[7] Davis MP, Darden PM. Use of complementary and alternative medicine by children in the United States. Arch Pediatr Adolesc Med 2003;157:393–6.
[8] Hanson E, Kalish LA, Bunce E, et al. Use of complementary and alternative medicine among children diagnosed with autism spectrum disorder. J Autism Dev Disord 2007;37: 628–36.

[9] Wong HH, Smith RG. Patterns of complementary and alternative medical therapy use in children diagnosed with autism spectrum disorders. J Autism Dev Disord 2006;36:901–9.

[10] Levy SE, Mandell DS, Merhar S, et al. Use of complementary and alternative medicine among children recently diagnosed with autistic spectrum disorder. J Dev Behav Pediatr 2003;24:418–23.

[11] Cuzzolin L, Zaffani S, Murgia V, et al. Patterns and perceptions of complementary/alternative medicine among paediatricians and patients' mothers: a review of the literature. Eur J Pediatr 2003;162:820–7.

[12] Heuschkel R, Afzal N, Wuerth A, et al. Complementary medicine use in children and young adults with inflammatory bowel disease. Am J Gastroenterol 2002;97:382–8.

[13] Shenfield G, Lim E, Allen H. Survey of the use of complementary medicines and therapies in children with asthma. J Paediatr Child Health 2002;38:252–7.

[14] McCaffrey AM, Pugh GF, O'Connor BB. Understanding patient preference for integrative medical care: results from patient focus groups. J Gen Intern Med 2007;22:1500–5.

[15] Simpson N, Roman K. Complementary medicine use in children: extent and reasons. A population-based study. Br J Gen Pract 2001;51:914–6.

[16] Kazdin AE. Evidence-based assessment for children and adolescents: issues in measurement development and clinical application. J Clin Child Adolesc Psychol 2005;34:548–58.

[17] Lilienfeld SO. Scientifically unsupported and supported interventions for childhood psychopathology: a summary. Pediatrics 2005;115:761–4.

[18] Sackett DL, Rosenberg WM, Gray JA, et al. Evidence based medicine: what it is and what it isn't. 1996. Clin Orthop Relat Res 2007;455:3.

[19] Jensen PS, Kenny DT. The effects of yoga on the attention and behavior of boys with attention-deficit/ hyperactivity disorder (ADHD). J Atten Disord 2004;7:205–16.

[20] Platania-Solazzo A, Field TM, Blank J, et al. Relaxation therapy reduces anxiety in child and adolescent psychiatric patients. Acta Paedopsychiatr 1992;55:115–20.

[21] Uma K, Nagendra HR, Nagarathna R, et al. The integrated approach of yoga: a therapeutic tool for mentally retarded children. A one-year controlled study. J Ment Defic Res 1989; 33(Pt 5):415–21.

[22] Gold C, Wigram T, Elefant C. Music therapy for autistic spectrum disorder. Cochrane Database Syst Rev 2006;2:CD004381.

[23] Kern P, Wolery M, Aldridge D. Use of songs to promote independence in morning greeting routines for young children with autism. J Autism Dev Disord 2007;37:1264–71.

[24] Heaton P. Interval and contour processing in autism. J Autism Dev Disord 2005;35:787.

[25] Whippell J. Music in intervention for children and adolescents with autism: a meta-analysis. J Music Ther 2004;41:90–106.

[26] Nye C, Brice A. Combined vitamin B_6-magnesium treatment in autism spectrum disorder. Cochrane Database Syst Rev 2005; CD003497.

[27] Nye C, Brice A. Combined vitamin B_6-magnesium treatment in autism spectrum disorder. Cochrane Database Syst Rev 2002;4:CD003497.

[28] Pfeiffer SI, Norton J, Nelson L, et al. Efficacy of vitamin B_6 and magnesium in the treatment of autism: a methodology review and summary of outcomes. J Autism Dev Disord 1995;25: 481–93.

[29] Findling RL, Maxwell K, Scotese-Wojtila L, et al. High-dose pyridoxine and magnesium administration in children with autistic disorder: an absence of salutary effects in a double-blind, placebo-controlled study. J Autism Dev Disord 1997;27:467–78.

[30] Kuriyama S, Kamiyama M, Watanabe M, et al. Pyridoxine treatment in a subgroup of children with pervasive developmental disorders. Dev Med Child Neurol 2002;44:284–6.

[31] Mousain-Bosc M, Roche M, Polge A, et al. Improvement of neurobehavioral disorders in children supplemented with magnesium-vitamin B_6. II. Pervasive developmental disorder-autism. Magnes Res 2006;19:53.

[32] Bolman WM, Richmond JA. A double-blind, placebo-controlled, crossover pilot trial of low dose dimethylglycine in patients with autistic disorder. J Autism Dev Disord 1999;29:191–4.

[33] Kern JK, Miller VS, Cauller PL, et al. Effectiveness of N,N-dimethylglycine in autism and pervasive developmental disorder. J Child Neurol 2001;16:169–73.

[34] Melke J, Goubran Botros H, Chaste P, et al. Abnormal melatonin synthesis in autism spectrum disorders. Mol Psychiatry 2008;13:90–8.

[35] Andersen IM, Kaczmarska J, McGrew SG, et al. Melatonin for insomnia in children with autism spectrum disorders. J Child Neurol 2008;23:482–5.

[36] Garstang J, Wallis M. Randomized controlled trial of melatonin for children with autistic spectrum disorders and sleep problems. Child Care Health Dev 2006;32:585–9.

[37] Dolske MC, Spollen J, McKay S, et al. A preliminary trial of ascorbic acid as supplemental therapy for autism. Prog Neuropsychopharmacol Biol Psychiatry 1993;17:765–74.

[38] McDougle CJ, Erickson CA, Stigler KA, et al. Neurochemistry in the pathophysiology of autism. J Clin Psychiatry 2005;66(Suppl 10):9–18.

[39] Ritvo ER, Yuwiler A, Geller E, et al. Increased blood serotonin and platelets in early infantile autism. Arch Gen Psychiatry 1970;23:566–72.

[40] McDougle CJ, Naylor ST, Cohen DJ, et al. Effects of tryptophan depletion in drug-free adults with autistic disorder. Arch Gen Psychiatry 1996;53:993–1000.

[41] Chez MG, Buchanan CP, Aimonovitch MC, et al. Double-blind, placebo-controlled study of L-carnosine supplementation in children with autistic spectrum disorders. J Child Neurol 2002;17:833–7.

[42] Crill CM, Helms RA. The use of carnitine in pediatric nutrition. Nutr Clin Pract 2007;22: 204–13.

[43] Filipek PA, Juranek J, Nguyen MT, et al. Relative carnitine deficiency in autism. J Autism Dev Disord 2004;34:615–23.

[44] Levy SE, Hyman SL. Novel treatments for autistic spectrum disorders. Ment Retard Dev Disabil Res Rev 2005;11:131–42.

[45] Sliwinski S, Croonenberghs J, Christophe A, et al. Polyunsaturated fatty acids: do they have a role in the pathophysiology of autism? Neuro Endocrinol Lett 2006;27:465–71.

[46] Vancassel S, Durand G, Barthelemy C, et al. Plasma fatty acid levels in autistic children. Prostaglandins Leukot Essent Fatty Acids 2001;65:1–7.

[47] Amminger GP, Berger GE, Schafer MR, et al. Omega-3 fatty acids supplementation in children with autism: a double-blind randomized, placebo-controlled pilot study. Biol Psychiatry 2007;61:551–3.

[48] Kern JK, Jones AM. Evidence of toxicity, oxidative stress, and neuronal insult in autism. J Toxicol Environ Health B Crit Rev 2006;9:485–99.

[49] Amaral DG, Schumann CM, Nordahl CW. Neuroanatomy of autism. Trends Neurosci 2008; 31(3):137–45.

[50] Glahn DC, Thompson PM, Blangero J. Neuroimaging endophenotypes: strategies for finding genes influencing brain structure and function. Hum Brain Mapp 2007;28:488–501.

[51] Pardo CA, Eberhart CG. The neurobiology of autism. Brain Pathol 2007;17:434–47.

[52] James SJ, Cutler P, Melnyk S, et al. Metabolic biomarkers of increased oxidative stress and impaired methylation capacity in children with autism. Am J Clin Nutr 2004;80: 1611–7.

[53] James SJ, Melnyk S, Jernigan S, et al. Metabolic endophenotype and related genotypes are associated with oxidative stress in children with autism. Am J Med Genet B Neuropsychiatr Genet 2006;141:947–56.

[54] Shattock P, Lowdon G. Proteins, peptides and autism. II. Implications for the education and care of people with autism. Brain Dysfunction 1991;4:323–34.

[55] Knivsberg AM, Reichelt KL, Hoien T, et al. A randomised, controlled study of dietary intervention in autistic syndromes. Nutr Neurosci 2002;5:251–61.

[56] Elder JH, Shankar M, Shuster J, et al. The gluten-free, casein-free diet in autism: results of a preliminary double blind clinical trial. J Autism Dev Disord 2006;36:413–20.

[57] Wolraich ML, Wilson DB, White JW. The effect of sugar on behavior or cognition in children: a meta-analysis. JAMA 1995;274:1617–21.

[58] Schab DW, Trinh NH. Do artificial food colors promote hyperactivity in children with hyperactive syndromes? A meta-analysis of double-blind placebo-controlled trials. J Dev Behav Pediatr 2004;25:423–34.

[59] Erickson CA, Stigler KA, Corkins MR, et al. Gastrointestinal factors in autistic disorder: a critical review. J Autism Dev Disord 2005;35(6):713–27.

[60] Kuddo T, Nelson KB. How common are gastrointestinal disorders in children with autism? Curr Opin Pediatr 2003;15:339–43.

[61] Brudnak MA, Rimland B, Kerry RE, et al. Enzyme-based therapy for autism spectrum disorders—is it worth another look? Med Hypotheses 2002;58:422–5.

[62] Brudnak MA. Probiotics as an adjuvant to detoxification protocols. Med Hypotheses 2002; 58:382–8.

[63] Horvath K, Stefanatos G, Sokolski K, et al. Improved social and language skills after secretin administration in patients with autistic spectrum disorders. J Assoc Acad Minor Phys 1998;9:9–15.

[64] Williams KW, Wray JJ, Wheeler DM. Intravenous secretin for autism spectrum disorder. Cochrane Database Syst Rev 2005;3:CD003495.

[65] Al-Waili NS, Butler GJ. Effects of hyperbaric oxygen on inflammatory response to wound and trauma: possible mechanism of action. ScientificWorldJournal 2006;6:425–41.

[66] Calvert JW, Cahill J, Zhang JH. Hyperbaric oxygen and cerebral physiology. Neurol Res 2007;29:132–41.

[67] McDonagh M, Carson S, Ash J, et al. Hyperbaric oxygen therapy for brain injury, cerebral palsy, and stroke. Evid Rep Technol Assess (Summ) 2003;85:1–6.

[68] McDonagh MS, Morgan D, Carson S, et al. Systematic review of hyperbaric oxygen therapy for cerebral palsy: the state of the evidence. Dev Med Child Neurol 2007;49:942–7.

[69] Rossignol DA, Rossignol LW. Hyperbaric oxygen therapy may improve symptoms in autistic children. Med Hypotheses 2006;67:216–28.

[70] Rossignol DA, Rossignol LW, James SJ, et al. The effects of hyperbaric oxygen therapy on oxidative stress, inflammation, and symptoms in children with autism: an open-label pilot study. BMC Pediatr 2007;7:36.

[71] Doja A, Roberts W. Immunizations and autism: a review of the literature. Can J Neurol Sci 2006;33:341–6.

[72] Parker SK, Schwartz B, Todd J, et al. Thimerosal-containing vaccines and autistic spectrum disorder: a critical review of published original data. Pediatrics 2004;114:793–804.

[73] Bernard S, Enayati A, Redwood L, et al. Autism: a novel form of mercury poisoning. Med Hypotheses 2001;56:462–71.

[74] Ng DK, Chan CH, Soo MT, et al. Low-level chronic mercury exposure in children and adolescents: meta-analysis. Pediatr Int 2007;49:80–7.

[75] DeStefano F. Vaccines and autism: evidence does not support a causal association. Clin Pharmacol Ther 2007;82:756–9.

[76] Hviid A. Postlicensure epidemiology of childhood vaccination: the Danish experience. Expert Rev Vaccines 2006;5:641–9.

[77] Hviid A, Stellfeld M, Wohlfahrt J, et al. Association between thimerosal-containing vaccine and autism. JAMA 2003;290:1763–6.

[78] Madsen KM, Lauritsen MB, Pedersen CB, et al. Thimerosal and the occurrence of autism: negative ecological evidence from Danish population-based data. Pediatrics 2003;112:604–6.

[79] McCormick MC. The autism "epidemic": impressions from the perspective of immunization safety review. Ambul Pediatr 2003;3:119–20.

[80] Nelson KB, Bauman ML. Thimerosal and autism? Pediatrics 2003;111:674–9.

[81] Offit P, Golden J. Thimerosal and autism. Mol Psychiatry 2004;9:644 [author reply: 645].

[82] Rutter M. Incidence of autism spectrum disorders: changes over time and their meaning. Acta Paediatr 2005;94:2–15.

[83] Stehr-Green P, Tull P, Stellfeld M, et al. Autism and thimerosal-containing vaccines: lack of consistent evidence for an association. Am J Prev Med 2003;25:101–6.

[84] Stokstad E. Epidemiology: vaccine-autism link dealt blow. Science 2003;301:1454–5.
[85] Thompson WW, Price C, Goodson B, et al. Early thimerosal exposure and neuropsychological outcomes at 7 to 10 years. N Engl J Med 2007;357:1281–92.
[86] Verstraeten T, Davis RL, DeStefano F, et al. Safety of thimerosal-containing vaccines: a two-phased study of computerized health maintenance organization databases. Pediatrics 2003;112:1039–48.
[87] Brown MJ, Willis T, Omalu B, et al. Deaths resulting from hypocalcemia after administration of edetate disodium: 2003–2005. Pediatrics 2006;118:e534–6.
[88] Stern L, Francoeur MJ, Primeau MN, et al. Immune function in autistic children. Ann Allergy Asthma Immunol 2005;95:558–65.
[89] Wills S, Cabanlit M, Bennett J, et al. Autoantibodies in autism spectrum disorders (ASD). Ann N Y Acad Sci 2007;1107:79–91.
[90] Jyonouchi H, Geng L, Ruby A, et al. Dysregulated innate immune responses in young children with autism spectrum disorders: their relationship to gastrointestinal symptoms and dietary intervention. Neuropsychobiology 2005;51:77–85.
[91] Gupta S, Aggarwal S, Heads C. Dysregulated immune system in children with autism: beneficial effects of intravenous immune globulin on autistic characteristics. J Autism Dev Disord 1996;26:439–52.
[92] DelGiudice-Asch G, Simon L, Schmeidler J, et al. Brief report: a pilot open clinical trial of intravenous immunoglobulin in childhood autism. J Autism Dev Disord 1999;29:157–60.
[93] Gupta S. Immunological treatments for autism. J Autism Dev Disord 2000;30:475–9.
[94] Niehus R, Lord C. Early medical history of children with autism spectrum disorders. J Dev Behav Pediatr 2006;27:S120–7.
[95] Rosen NJ, Yoshida CK, Croen LA. Infection in the first 2 years of life and autism spectrum disorders. Pediatrics 2007;119:e61–9.
[96] Finegold SM, Molitoris D, Song Y, et al. Gastrointestinal microflora studies in late-onset autism. Clin Infect Dis 2002;35:S6–16.
[97] Fernell E, Fagerberg UL, Hellstrom PM. No evidence for a clear link between active intestinal inflammation and autism based on analyses of faecal calprotectin and rectal nitric oxide. Acta Paediatr 2007;96:1076–9.
[98] Sandler RH, Finegold SM, Bolte ER, et al. Short-term benefit from oral vancomycin treatment of regressive-onset autism. J Child Neurol 2000;15:429–35.
[99] Shaw W, Kassen E, Chaves E. Increased urinary excretion of analogs of Krebs cycle metabolites and arabinose in two brothers with autistic features. Clin Chem 1995;41:1094.
[100] Crook WG. Nutrition, food allergies, and environmental toxins. J Learn Disabil 1987;20: 260–1.
[101] Vohra S, Johnston BC, Cramer K, et al. Adverse events associated with pediatric spinal manipulation: a systematic review. Pediatrics 2007;119:e275–83.
[102] Downey PA, Barbano T, Kapur-Wadhwa R, et al. Craniosacral therapy: the effects of cranial manipulation on intracranial pressure and cranial bone movement. J Orthop Sports Phys Ther 2006;36:845–53.
[103] Moran RW, Gibbons P. Intraexaminer and interexaminer reliability for palpation of the cranial rhythmic impulse at the head and sacrum. J Manipulative Physiol Ther 2001;24: 183–90.
[104] Silva LM, Cignolini A, Warren R, et al. Improvement in sensory impairment and social interaction in young children with autism following treatment with an original Qigong massage methodology. Am J Chin Med 2007;35:393–406.
[105] Williams TI. Evaluating effects of aromatherapy massage on sleep in children with autism: a pilot study. Evid Based Complement Alternat Med 2006;3:373–7.
[106] Sinha Y, Silove N, Wheeler D, et al. Auditory integration training and other sound therapies for autism spectrum disorders: a systematic review. Arch Dis Child 2006;91:1018–22.
[107] Sinha Y, Silove N, Wheeler D, et al. Auditory integration training and other sound therapies for autism spectrum disorders. Cochrane Database Syst Rev 2004;(1) CD003681.

[108] American Academy of Pediatrics. Committee on children with disabilities: auditory integration training and facilitated communication for autism. Pediatrics 1998;102:431–3.

[109] Frye RE, Rotenberg A, Ousley M, et al. Transcranial magnetic stimulation in child neurology: current and future directions. J Child Neurol 2008;23:79–96.

[110] Oberman LM, Ramachandran VS. The simulating social mind: the role of the mirror neuron system and simulation in the social and communicative deficits of autism spectrum disorders. Psychol Bull 2007;133:310–27.

[111] Hoeppner J, Wandschneider R, Neumeyer M, et al. Impaired transcallosally mediated motor inhibition in adults with attention-deficit/hyperactivity disorder is modulated by methylphenidate. J Neural Transm 2008;115(5):777–85.

[112] Cohen MH, Kemper KJ. Complementary therapies in pediatrics: a legal perspective. Pediatrics 2005;115:774–80.

[113] Fugh-Berman A. Herb-drug interactions. Lancet 2000;355:134–8.

ELSEVIER
SAUNDERS

Child Adolesc Psychiatric Clin N Am
17 (2008) 821–834

CHILD AND
ADOLESCENT
PSYCHIATRIC CLINICS
OF NORTH AMERICA

Applied Behavior Analysis Treatment of Autism: The State of the Art

Richard M. Foxx, PhD[a,b,*]

[a]*Psychology Program, Penn State University Harrisburg,
777 West Harrisburg Pike, Middletown, PA 17057, USA*
[b]*Department of Pediatrics, Penn State University School of Medicine,
500 University Drive, Hershey, PA 17033, USA*

The treatment of individuals with autism often involves the application of nonscientifically based practices, even though a scientifically validated and highly effective treatment, applied behavior analysis (ABA) is available [1]. ABA, sometimes called behavior therapy [2] or behavior modification [3], uses methods derived from scientifically established principles of behavior [4]. ABA has been applied successfully to a range of populations and areas including autism, developmental disabilities, education in all its many forms, business, mental health, counseling, marriage counseling, and child abuse, to name but a few [3].

The evidence for the effectiveness of ABA with autism is extensive. Box 1 lists much of this evidence.

In the past 20 years, there has been growing evidence that early intensive behavioral intervention (EIBI) by means of ABA results in improved developmental progress and intellectual performance in young children who have autism [13,15–17]. The effects with young children with autism under age 3 have been particularly gratifying.

Are other treatments effective?

Green [18] described the various types of evidence of effectiveness and detailed why subjective evidence such as testimonials, anecdotes, and personal accounts are not reliable. Nonbehavioral special education classes,

* Corresponding author. Psychology Program, Penn State Harrisburg, 777 West Harrisburg Pike, Middletown, PA 17057
E-mail address: rmf4@psu.edu

1056-4993/08/$ - see front matter © 2008 Elsevier Inc. All rights reserved.
doi:10.1016/j.chc.2008.06.007   *childpsych.theclinics.com*

Box 1. Evidence for the effectiveness of applied behavior analysis

Individuals of all ages have been successfully educated and treated for over 40 years and children for over 47 years [5].

ABA was identified as the treatment of choice for individuals with autism in the early 1980s [6].

Over 1000 peer-reviewed, scientific autism articles describe ABA successes [1].

No other educational or treatment approach to autism has the support of The State of New York Health Department [7] and United States Surgeon General [8].

The National Institute of Mental Health (NIMH) has been funding ABA autism research continuously for over 40 years.

All individuals who have autism receive some degree of benefit from ABA.

For over 35 years, agencies using ABA have provided successful nonresidential and residential autism services for thousands of school-aged children.

ABA is the only therapy recognized to treat young children who have autism.

No other educational or treatment approach to autism meets the standards of scientific proof that are met by ABA, and there are no other scientifically valid treatments that produce similar treatment, educational, or outcome results [9,10].

Competency guidelines regarding the delivery of ABA autism services are established [11], and certification of ABA practitioners has existed for several years [12].

Investing in early ABA intervention for young children [13] is financially worthwhile, whether the results lead to complete or partial effects [14].

---

individual therapies, and biological interventions (except antipsychotic medications) have not been established as effective treatments for children who have autism. Some treatments, especially facilitated communication and psychoanalysis, are quite harmful and should be avoided [19].

The New York State Department of Health [7] took a rigorous approach to guideline development and creation when it examined assessment and interventions for young children who have autism. To make recommendations regarding assessment and educational programming, a panel of professionals, service providers, and parents screened the literature and conducted an in-depth review of the most relevant articles. The selected studies had to meet high standards for quality, including adequate information concerning the intervention methods, controlled experimental designs, and the evaluation of functional outcomes [7,10]. The panel provided overall recommendations for early intervention programs, indicated the strength of the scientific evidence for each recommendation, and provided detailed summaries of the evidence on 18 types of interventions. ABA was the only intervention recommended. Interventions reviewed and not recommended included: auditory integration therapy, facilitated communication, floor time, sensory integration therapy, touch therapy, music therapy, hormones (corticotropin [ACTH] and Secretin), vitamin therapies, and special diets [7].

Criticisms of validated treatments such as ABA or traditional medicine often come from proponents of pseudoscientific interventions [20]. Consider that critics may suggest that ABA treatment or educational gains are specific to the setting where the intervention took place or may note that medications can cause adverse effects. These criticisms often are used to promote the adoption of unvalidated interventions. The push for early intensive behavioral (ABA) intervention (EIBI) with young children who have autism has met considerable resistance from several sources. The main resistance has come from educational and governmental agencies not wishing to pay for expensive individualized programs. Other opposition has come from professionals unfamiliar with autism, with philosophical perspectives antithetical to ABA, or with agendas that involve the promotion of competing approaches [9].

Eclecticism is not the best approach to the treatment and education of children with autism

Heward and Silvestri [21] discussed the thinking in special education that leads to eclecticism, wherein incorporating components from several different models into a program is designed to cover the gaps or deficiencies found in any single model. They pointed out that while the logic underlying such eclecticism may appear to have face validity, the problems inherent in eclecticism far outweigh its logical appeal. Heward [22] discussed several reasons why. Eclecticism is based in part on a misplaced egalitarian view that there is value in every approach, although not every model or theory is equally trustworthy and valuable. Indeed, the more models contained in the eclectic mix, the greater the probability that ineffective and potentially harmful components will be included. Practitioners sometimes do not choose the most important and effective parts of each model, but rather select weaker and perhaps ineffective components. Some components of a model can be ineffective when applied in isolation and without other essential elements of the model. Elements from different models are sometimes incompatible. An eclectic mix might prevent any single model from being implemented intensely enough to produce significant outcomes. Some of everything and a lot of nothing leave eclecticism as a recipe for failure. Teachers will not learn to implement any model with the fidelity necessary to achieve a good result. Eclectic practitioners typically are apprentices of many models but masters of none [22].

Heward and Silvestri [21] concluded that their wariness of eclecticism was

"based on (1) a commitment that students should only be taught with instructional tools that have empiric support for their effectiveness; (2) a research-derived knowledge that not all models are equally effective; and (3) the fact that some approaches have a harmful effect on student learning."

Adding ineffective treatment to an effective one may be detrimental

Adding an ineffective treatment to an effective one is at best not useful, and at worse detrimental [20]. The available evidence indicates that such combinations can be less effective than relying on a single validated treatment for individuals who have autism. For example, Eikeseth and colleagues [23] compared ABA with an eclectic treatment made up of ABA and unvalidated educational interventions. Although the interventions were of equal intensity, the performance of the ABA-only group was superior to that of the eclectic group.

Although no one yet had studied why combining treatments would reduce effectiveness, there are several possible explanations [20]. One, some of the combined treatments may be harmful. Two, ineffective treatments divert time and resources away from the effective interventions with which they have been combined. Three, treatments may interfere or counter each other's effectiveness. For example, while ABA emphasizes helping individuals follow a structured routine, other treatments may discourage this practice. Four, as noted by Heward [22], therapists may become "jacks of all trades and master of none" by implementing several interventions but none very well. In effect, combining treatments can present considerable risk, especially if any of the treatments have no empiric support [20].

Applied behavior analysis epitomizes effective intervention in autism

ABA programming follows the general guidelines for effective intervention for children who have autism spectrum disorders [9,24]:

Intervention should be started at the earliest possible age.
Intervention must be intensive.
Parent training and support are critical.
Intervention should focus on social and communication domains.
Treatment should be systematic, built upon individualized goals and objectives tailored to the child.
It is very important that effective intervention emphasize generalization.

ABA programming also incorporates all of the factors identified by the US National Research Council [25] as characteristic of effective interventions in educational programs for children who have autism. These factors included:

Early entry into intervention

Intensive instructional programming (defined as equivalent to a full school day, 5 or more days a week, 25 hours per week, year-round, 12 months per year)

Use of planned teaching in frequent brief instructional sessions

One-to-one or small group instruction to enhance the achievement of individualized goals

Use of specialized interventions such as discrete trial training and incidental teaching

Systematic and individualized instruction

Focus on the development of spontaneous social communication, adaptive skills, appropriate behaviors, play skills, and cognitive and academic skills

Major emphasis also was placed on monitoring progress, generalization of skills, use of skills in generalized settings, and the creation of opportunities to interact with typically developing peers [9,25].

The basics of the behavior analytic treatment of autism

Behavior analytic treatment of children and adolescents who have autism seeks to construct socially and educationally useful repertoires and decrease or reduce problem behaviors through the use of specific, carefully programmed environmental interventions [18]. Various behavior analytic methods are employed to strengthen the child's current skills and build new ones. Multiple, repeated opportunities are created each day for the child to gain new skills and practice mastered ones. Positive reinforcement is used generously to ensure that the child is motivated [26].

Often several steps are chained together to form a behavioral repertoire. Some of the ABA methods used include:

Positive reinforcement, in which appropriate behavior is followed by a pleasurable event such as praise, a hug, a check mark, a favorite activity

Shaping, rewarding the child for behavior that approaches the target behavior or goal

Fading, reducing the child's dependence on the therapist for help

Providing stimuli (prompting) that cue the child to try a behavior

Maintenance and generalization strategies to ensure that a recently learned behavior will last and be performed in other environments [26]

To treat inappropriate behaviors, several strategies are employed, including analyzing and altering the antecedents that trigger the behavior, ignoring the behavior, or providing undesired consequences [27]. The overall goal of ABA is to motivate the child to want to be successful.

Typically, teaching trials are repeated many times until mastery is obtained. Accurate records are kept so that progress can be assessed and programmatic changes made. Each child's program is unique to his or her needs and evolves with the child's progress. Teaching is done in several formats. The discrete trial format is characterized by a one-to-one interaction with the trainer/educator; short, clear instructions; careful use of prompting and fading; and immediate reinforcement for correct responding [28]. A less-structured format, incidental teaching, is used to help the child learn behaviors in less structured situations [18,29]. The overall teaching model is to move the individual's instruction systematically from one-to-one with a trainer/educator, to a small group and ultimately to a larger group [30].

ABA programming for children who have autism features the use of scientifically validated methods incorporated into a comprehensive but highly individualized package [31]. A defining feature of ABA programs is that they are applied consistently. This is accomplished: through the use of explicitly written programs for each skill to be taught or maladaptive behavior to be treated and by having the behavior analyst who is responsible for the child's program train everyone who works with the child to implement it. To increase the likelihood of the generalization of the treatment efforts, it is critical for therapists/parents to be trained to implement the programs across situations, settings, and people. Maladaptive behaviors such as aggression and self-injury are not reinforced, whereas specific, appropriate alternative behaviors are either taught or maintained through positive reinforcement [27].

Before treatment, an evaluation is conducted to assess the child's skill and developmental levels. This evaluation assists in the selection of therapeutic goals. The treatment regimen that is developed considers all pertinent domains, including academic, communication, leisure, play and self-care, and social in determining which skills will be taught. The next step is to break down each skill into smaller and more easily taught component skills or steps. As the child progresses, the skills that are taught are increased in complexity. Attention is given to the achievement of developmental milestones. The overall goal is to provide the kind of regimen that will ensure that each child reaches his or her highest potential and level of independence [28,29,31,32].

Critical to the therapeutic process is the direct and frequent measurement of the child's progress. The data from these observations are graphed to portray how each targeted skill and maladaptive behavior has responded to the treatment effort. The behavior analyst responsible for the child's program frequently checks the graphed and recorded data to determine if reasonable progress is occurring and to make any necessary programmatic adjustments

[31]. Ongoing review of the child's responsiveness to the intervention and treatment personnel allows problems to be identified and corrected quickly. Treatment consistency also is assured by having the responsible behavior analyst frequently observe the treatment efforts so that feedback can be provided to the program implementers [28].

Although the principles of ABA will guide programming efforts and activities, each child is seen as unique. High levels of consistency, repeated and consistent presentations of material, individually selected and strategically used motivators, careful use of prompting procedures, and systematic planning for generalization are used to establish and maintain a positive treatment environment. ABA programs strive to organize therapeutic experiences that will lead to enduring positive changes over time and across all settings in such crucial areas as toileting [33], feeding [34], social skills [35], and language [32].

All appropriate ABA interventions are directed by a professional with advanced formal training in behavior analysis. This person should have at least a master's degree and supervised experience in designing and implementing ABA programs for children who have autism and related disorders [11]. These professionals have either met the educational, experiential, and examination performance standards of the Behavior Analyst Certification Board (BACB) and are board-certified behavior analysts [12] or can document that they have equivalent training and experience. They adhere to the BACB's Guidelines for Responsible Conduct [12] and base all treatment decisions on the best available scientific evidence [31].

Applied behavior analysis in educational programs

Quality educational programs for children who have autism rely heavily on ABA principles, because eclecticism is not the best approach [21]. Effective school programs share several characteristics [36]:

Their interventions are based upon empirical evidence of effectiveness and are highly structured.

They do functional assessments and behavioral assessments of challenging behaviors, employ specificity in the development of objectives, have operationally defined targets, have criteria for the achievement of instructional objectives, feature the systematic use of instructional prompts, and have objective and ongoing measures of progress.

They identify specific skills to be taught, do direct teaching of social skills, employ peer tutoring, individualize reinforcement and lesson plans, and develop a tolerance for delay of reinforcement and an actively program for generalization.

Instructional objectives are determined without reference to disciplines. Services are wrapped around the child.

Parents whose children have success in school display several behaviors [36]. They:

> Do not rely on anecdotal information—they require accountability, make data collection a requirement, and seek frequent measures of success.
>
> Take their child's individualized education plan home and read it carefully, provide input on program design, relate instructional objectives to the child's home and community needs, have external monitoring of their child's school program, and have a behavior analyst accompany them to the IEP meeting
>
> Obtain training to allow replication at home and insist that successful relevant home programs be replicated at school
>
> They are active and spend time at the school.

Applied behavior analysis is the primary method of treating aberrant behavior in children and adolescents with autism

Although aberrant behavior represents a major obstacle to the successful treatment and education of individuals who have autism, ABA offers scientifically validated methods of overcoming it [27,37].

In most cases, aberrant behavior is an acquired behavior or set of behaviors. This means that the child has learned that a desired outcome can be achieved by behaving aberrantly. Typically, this desired outcome is to either gain attention from others or escape or avoid an unpleasant situation or demand [37]. Although aberrant behavior is learned, there can be antecedent or precipitating factors that increase the probability that it will occur. These factors can be environmental, physiologic, or social changes. An example of physiologic factors could include hunger and physical pain caused by illness or allergies. The treatment of aberrant behavior typically involves two initial considerations.

First, an attempt is made to identify the antecedent or precipitating factors, because changing or correcting them may eliminate the behavior. For example, a child who aggresses because of allergies can be given allergy medication, and one who aggresses because of hunger can be given snacks before the times when aggressive attacks typically occur. In school settings, a child's aberrant behavior often is related to the nature of the educational tasks being presented. If the task is too easy, the child may aggress, because doing so typically results in its termination by the teacher. Thus, aggression is reinforced by escape from the task. This problem can be avoided by establishing appropriate criterion levels of performance so that students are moved to the next step or program once they have demonstrated mastery. The same scenario can occur if the task is too difficult or if insufficient positive reinforcement is available for performing it. In the former case, a simpler task must be substituted or the task analyzed and broken down into more easily mastered steps, whereas sufficient positive reinforcement and other training procedures will solve the latter problem [27,38]. Second, a formal functional analysis or in-depth set of clinical observations [39] is conducted to determine the function or outcome of the aberrant behavior. At that point, a treatment program can be developed to help the child achieve the same outcome through more appropriate methods and alter the function and consequences of the aberrant behavior.

Several intervention strategies can be used to treat aberrant behavior, including withholding or withdrawing attention when aggression occurs, reinforcing appropriate behavior, teaching the child an appropriate way to communicate the desire to end or not participate in an activity, or not allowing the child's aberrant behavior to terminate or avoid the activity if it is critical to academic or life skills training [40].

The design of a successful treatment program to treat aberrant behavior

The overall successful treatment of aberrant behavior by ABA requires a consideration of the following strategies and factors.

First, a hypothesis-driven treatment model [37] is used, whereby interventions are designed after a formal functional analysis identifies the variables that control the behavior [41]. Because aberrant behavior is sometimes under multiple motivational and setting event controls and hence cannot be definitely linked to specific consequences, an in-depth analysis of antecedent and setting events is conducted to determine whether the occurrence or nonoccurrence of the behavior is correlated with environmental events that repeated themselves predictably with specific people or activities or across times of the day or days of the week.

Second, arrangements are made to ensure that the stimuli that can, at times, control appropriate behavior are present before, during, and after the aberrant behavior is treated. In order to determine what procedures, skills, and activities to implement when children are not misbehaving, all of their significant others can be surveyed for suggestions. Another tactic is to enhance the child's preexisting skills so that they can be displayed more frequently and with more variety.

Third, a skill-building strategy is employed wherein new behaviors are taught to serve the same function as the aberrant behavior. Behaviors are emphasized that access the same reinforcers, especially communicative ones. Requesting behaviors are taught that are functionally equivalent to the aberrant behavior but more effective in generating reinforcement. In effect, requesting behavior must be less effortful than aberrant behavior. For example, treatment personnel must respond consistently and rapidly to requests and be knowledgeable about the child's communication system.

Fourth, situations such as frustration, boredom, and protracted periods of inactivity are eliminated, because they are known to occasion aberrant behavior. This can be accomplished by varying tasks and activities, encouraging choice making, and increasing children's and adolescents' activity levels. In this way, problematic behaviors that produce attention or gain task or situation escape or avoidance will become unnecessary and thereby nonfunctional.

Fifth, the least restrictive treatment model is followed, wherein the least intrusive but effective procedure for a specific inappropriate behavior is selected based on a review of treatment literature [27]. Careful consideration is given to the intensity, severity, frequency, and topography (form) of the aberrant behavior.

Sixth, aberrant behavior is not allowed to produce escape from educational activities. The child is required to remain in the teaching situation and complete one or more requested tasks before ending the activity. This will prevent reinforcing escape-motivated problem behaviors and, instead, will provide escape for task completion.

Seventh, the complexity of social reinforcement and tasks are increased as the child's behavior becomes increasingly more appropriate [38,42]. Over time, the density of naturally occurring positive reinforcement will increase correspondingly as the child's behavior becomes more appropriate. The complexity and relevance of tasks also are increased.

Eighth, choice-making [40] and problem solving [43] are emphasized.

Ninth, treatment staff members are selected who are functional for the child, because they are associated with positive reinforcement. In other words, staff members are selected who are familiar and liked by the treated child, because a mutual affection exists.

Tenth, the participation of the child's significant others, typically parents, in every treatment decision is expected and encouraged. Parents and family are excellent and valuable sources of information, because they know the child's learning history, reinforcer preferences, communications skills, and history of inappropriate behavior.

Maintaining treatment effects

It is equally important to plan for the maintenance and long-term assessment of treatment effects. Maintenance refers to treatment effects or improvements that remain stable even after the intervention is removed [44]. Rarely are the effects of a treatment maintained in the absence of programming. As a result, careful planning is required to ensure that clinical effects will endure. Successful strategies for achieving maintenance effects are included, such as:

Actively programming for maintenance [45]
Ensuring similarity between the treatment and maintenance programs [46]
Ensuring that there is change agent and system accountability [37]
Following a functional approach by strengthening alternatives to the undesirable behavior and using naturally occurring positive reinforcers [47]
Ensuring that the program has social validity by being beneficial to the child and society [48]

Wherever possible, treatment should approximate the child's natural environment, because it permits potential maintenance-inferring problems to be identified and corrected and maintenance enhancing factors to be maximized. Some behavioral methods that approximate the natural environment and can be used to maintain therapeutic gains include:

Intermittent reinforcement
Reinforcement delay
Shifting to natural consequences
Fading therapist control
Teaching self-control
Developing peer or sibling support
Fading in situations and conditions that previously provoked the behavior before treatment [47]

All of these methods can fail, however, if treatment decisions are based on factors other than clinical progress, not individualized, or when sound ABA methods are stretched to the point where they cannot work effectively [47]. For example, fading therapist control cannot be made on the basis of expediency (eg, financial considerations rather than the child's progress).

The need for long-term follow-up assessment is particularly critical when treating aggressive behavior. Follow-up assessments should include repeated observations conducted over an extended period rather than a single behavioral sample. The contingencies in effect throughout the maintenance phase should be specified so that factors likely to have contributed to any durable effects can be identified [49].

Finally, generalization and maintenance of treatment gains are assessed independently, because they are separable and measurable. Doing so will prevent confounding generalization records with maintenance records. Maintenance and generalization differ in that maintenance refers to continued positive outcomes after the intervention ceases, whereas generalization refers to positive treatment effects being apparent even in the settings, situations, and behaviors not involved in the treatment. Addressing generalization and maintenance also facilitates inclusion, because it allows the determination of what are the existing functional and acceptable behaviors in the individual's social environment.

Behavior analysis has played a vital role in revolutionizing treatment and education in autism by freeing individuals from many behavioral, educational, and adaptive barriers that had kept them dependent and devalued. New research findings are being incorporated to enhance ABA [50]. It is important to distinguish between ABA and positive behavior support, because some individuals regard them as the same approach when in fact they are separate entities. They differ in the depth and breadth of their scientific base and their political correctness [51].

In closing, two conclusions reached by Metz and colleagues [9] in their discussion of fads and autism seem particularly relevant. One, few other medical or neurodevelopmental conditions have been as fraught with fad, controversial, unsupported, disproven, and unvalidated treatments as autism. Two, the only interventions that have been shown to produce comprehensive, lasting results in autism have been those based on the principles of ABA.

References

[1] Foxx RM. The critical importance of science based treatments for autism. Progress and challenges in the behavioral treatment of autism. Association for Behavior Analysis International Conference Proceedings February 2007;1:15–20.

[2] Lovaas OI, Koegel RL, Simmons JQ, et al. Some generalization and follow-up measures on autistic children in behavior therapy. J Appl Behav Anal 1973;6:131–65.

[3] Martin G, Pear JB. Behavior modification: what it is and how to do it. 8th edition. Upper Saddle River (NJ): Prentice Hall; 2007.

[4] Baer DM, Wolf MM, Risley TR. Some current dimensions of applied behavior analysis. J Appl Behav Anal 1968;1:91–7.

[5] Ferster CB. Positive reinforcement and behavioral deficits of autistic children. Child Dev 1961;32:437–56.

[6] DeMyer MK, Hingtgen JN, Jackson RK. Infantile autism reviewed: a decade of research. Schizophr Bull 1981;7:388–451.

[7] New York State Department of Health Early Intervention Program. Clinical practice guidelines; autism/pervasive developmental disorders, assessment, and intervention for young children (age 0–3 years). Albany (NY); 1999.

[8] US Surgeon General's Report on Mental Health—Autism Section 1999.

[9] Metz B, Mulick JA, Butter EM. Autism: a late 20th century fad magnet. In: Jacobson JW, Foxx RM, Mulick JA, editors. Controversial therapies for developmental disabilities: fads, fashion, and science in professional practice. Mahwah (NJ): Lawrence Erlbaum; 2005. p. 237–64.

[10] Newsom C, Hovanitz CA. The nature and value of empirically validated interventions. In: Jacobson JW, Foxx RM, Mulick JA, editors. Controversial therapies for developmental disabilities: fads, fashion, and science in professional practice. Mahwah (NJ): Lawrence Erlbaum; 2005. p. 31–44.

[11] Autism Special Interest Group. Association for Behavior Analysis—International. Available at: www.abainternational.org. Accessed August 1, 2008.

[12] Behavior Analyst Certification Board. Available at: www.BACB.com. Accessed August 1, 2008.

[13] Lovass OI. Behavioral treatment and normal educational and intellectual functioning in young autistic children. J Consult Clin Psychol 1987;55:3–9.

[14] Jacobson JW, Mulick JA, Green G. Cost-benefit estimates for early intensive behavioral intervention for young children with autism—general model and single state case. Behav Interv 1998;13:201–26.

[15] McEachin JJ, Smith TH, Lovass OI. Long-term outcome for children with autism who received early intensive behavioral treatment. Am J Ment Retard 1993;97(40):359–72.

[16] Perry R, Cohen I, DeCarlo R. Case study: deterioration, autism, and recovery in two siblings. J Am Acad Child Adolesc Psychiatry 1995;34:232–7.

[17] Sallows GO, Graupner TD. Intensive behavioral treatment of children with autism: four-year outcome and predictors. Am J Ment Retard 2005;110(6):417–38.

[18] Green G. Early behavioral intervention for autism: what does research tell us? In: Maurice C, Green G, Luce SC, editors. Behavioral intervention for young children with autism: a manual for parents and professionals. Austin (TX): Pro-Ed; 1996. p. 29–44.

[19] Smith T. Are other treatments effective? In: Maurice C, Green G, Luce SC, editors. Behavioral intervention for young children with autism: a manual for parents and professionals. Austin (TX): Pro-Ed; 1996. p. 45–62.

[20] Smith T. The appeal of unvalidated treatments. In: Jacobson J, Foxx RM, Mulick JA, editors. Controversial therapies for developmental disabilities: fads, fashion, and science in professional practice. Mahwah (NJ): Lawrence Erlbaum; 2005. p. 45–60.

[21] Heward WL, Silvestri SM. The neutralization of special education. In: Jacobson JW, Foxx RM, Mulick JA, editors. Controversial therapies for developmental disabilities: fads, fashion, and science in professional practice. Mahwah (NJ): Lawrence Erlbaum; 2005. p. 193–214.

[22] Heward WL. Ten faulty notions about teaching and learning that hinder the effectiveness of special education. J Spec Educ 2003;36(4):186–205.

[23] Eikeseth S, Smith T, Jahr E, et al. Intensive behavioral treatment at school for 4-7 year-old children with autism: a 1-year comparison-controlled study. Behav Modif 2002;26: 49–68.

[24] Kabout S, Masi W, Segal M. Advances in the diagnosis and treatment of autistic spectrum disorders. Prof Psychol Res Pr 2003;34:26–33.

[25] National Research Council. Education children with autism. Committee on educational interventions for children with autism. In: Lord C, McGee JP, editors. Washington, DC: National Academy Press; 2001.

[26] Foxx RM. Increasing the behaviors of persons with severe retardation and autism. Champaign (IL): Research Press; 1982.

[27] Foxx RM. Decreasing the behaviors of persons with severe retardation and autism. Champaign (IL): Research Press; 1982.

[28] Maurice C, Green G, Luce SC. Behavioral intervention for young children with autism: a manual for parents and professionals. Austin (TX): Pro-Ed; 1996.

[29] Maurice C, Green G, Foxx RM. Making a difference: behavioral intervention for autism. Austin (TX): Pro-Ed; 2001.

[30] Schreibman L. Autism. Newbury Park (CA): Sage; 1988.

[31] Green G. Applied behavior analysis for autism. Available at: www.behavior.org. Accessed August 1, 2008.

[32] Lovaas OI. Teaching developmentally disabled children: the me book. Austin (TX): Pro-Ed; 1981.

[33] Foxx RM, Azrin NH. Toilet training persons with developmental disabilities: a rapid program for day and nighttime independent toileting. Champaign (IL): Research Press; 1973.

[34] Williams KE, Foxx RM. Interventions for treating the eating problems of children with autism spectrum disorders and developmental disabilities. Austin (TX): Pro-Ed; 2007.

[35] Taylor BA. Teaching peer social skills to children with autism. In: Maurice C, Green G, Foxx RM, editors. Making a difference: behavioral intervention for autism. Austin (TX): Pro-Ed; 2001. p. 83–96.

[36] Anderson SR. Clinical Practice Guidelines: Methodology, Findings, and Implications. Presented at the Association for Science in Autism Treatment Conference. New York City; March 9, 2000.

[37] Foxx RM. Twenty years of applied behavior analysis in treating the most severe problem behavior: lessons learned. Behav Anal 1996;19(2):225–35.

[38] Foxx RM. The Jack Tizzard memorial lecture: decreasing behaviours: clinical, ethical, legal, and environmental issues. Australia and New Zealand Journal of Developmental Disabilities 1985;10:189–99.

[39] National Institutes of Health. Treatment of destructive behaviors in persons with developmental disabilities. Washington, DC: NIH Consensus Developmental Conference. US Department of Health and Human Services; 1991.

[40] Foxx RM. Thirty years of applied behavior analysis in treating problem behavior. In: Maurice C, Green G, Foxx RM, editors. Making a difference: behavioral intervention for autism. Austin (TX): Pro-Ed; 2001. p. 183–94.

[41] Romanczyk RG. Behavior analysis and assessment: the cornerstone to effectiveness. In: Maurice C, Green G, Luce SC, editors. Behavioral intervention for young children with autism: a manual for parents and professionals. Austin (TX): Pro-Ed; 1996. p. 195–217.

[42] Foxx RM. Social skills training: the current status of the field. Australia and New Zealand Journal of Developmental Disabilities 1985;10:237–43.

[43] Foxx RM, Bittle RG. Thinking it through: teaching a problem solving strategy for community living. Champaign (IL): Research Press; 1989.

[44] Foxx RM. Long term maintenance of language and social skills. Behav Interv 1999;14(3): 135–46.

[45] Stokes TF, Osnes PG. Programming the generalization of children's social behavior. In: Strain PS, Guralnick MJ, Walker H, editors. Children's social behavior: development, assessment, and modification. Orlando (FL): Academic Press; 1986. p. 407–40.

[46] Foxx RM, Livesay J. Maintenance of response suppression following overcorrection: a ten-year retrospective examination of eight cases. Analysis and Intervention in Developmental Disabilities 1984;4:65–79.

[47] Konarski EA Jr, Favell JE, Favell JE. Manual for the assessment and treatment of behavior disorders of people with mental retardation. Morganton (NC): Western Carolina Center Foundation; 1992.

[48] Wolf MM. Social validity: the case for subjective measurement, or how applied behavior analysis is finding its heart. J Appl Behav Anal 1978;11:203–14.

[49] Linscheid TR, Iwata BA, Foxx RM. Behavioral assessment. In: Jacobson JW, Mulick JA, editors. Manual of diagnosis and professional practice in mental retardation. Washington, DC: American Psychological Association; 1996. p. 191–8.

[50] Johnston JM, Foxx RM, Jacobson JW, et al. Positive behavior support and applied behavior analysis. Behav Anal 2006;29:51–74.

[51] Mulick JA, Butter EM. Positive behavior support: a paternalistic utopian delusion. In: Jacobson JW, Foxx RM, Mulick JA, editors. Controversial therapies for developmental disabilities: fads, fashion, and science in professional practice. Mahwah (NJ): Lawrence Erlbaum; 2005. p. 385–404.

ELSEVIER SAUNDERS

Child Adolesc Psychiatric Clin N Am
17 (2008) 835–856

CHILD AND
ADOLESCENT
PSYCHIATRIC CLINICS
OF NORTH AMERICA

Interventions to Improve Communication in Autism

Rhea Paul, PhD

Yale Child Study Center, 40 Temple Street #68, New Haven, CT 06510, USA

Communication deficits are one of the core symptoms of autism spectrum disorders (ASD). People who have ASD can be slow to begin talking or may not learn to talk at all; others may learn to produce words and sentences but have difficulty using them effectively to accomplish social interactive goals. Milestones in language and communication play major roles at almost every point in development for diagnosing and understanding autism. Most parents of children with ASD first begin to be concerned about their child's development because of early delays or regressions in the acquisition of speech [1]. Functional language use by school age has been shown to be related to better long-term outcomes in autism [2,3]. Fluency and flexibility of expressive language are key components of the distinction between "high-functioning" and "low functioning" autism in school age or adolescence [4]. A history of language delay can be particularly crucial in differentiating autism from other psychiatric disorders in high-functioning adults [5].

Because of the centrality of communicative deficits in the expression of ASD, the amelioration of communication problems in children with this syndrome is one of the most important areas of educational service. This discussion of intervention for communication disorders in ASD is divided into two broad sections: one discusses the development of early, prelinguistic communicative behaviors that lead to the emergence of language, and the

Preparation of this paper was supported by Research Grant P01-03008 funded by the National Institute of Mental Health (NIMH); the National Institute of Deafness and Communication Disorders R01 DC07129; MidCareer Development Award K24 HD045576 funded by NIDCD; the STAART Center grant U54 MH66494 funded by the National Institute on Deafness and Other Communication Disorders (NIDCD), the National Institute of Environmental Health Sciences (NIEHS), the National Institute of Child Health and Human Development (NICHD), the National Institute of Neurological Disorders and Stroke (NINDS); the National Alliance for Autism Research, and the Autism Speaks Foundation.

E-mail address: rhea.paul@yale.edu

doi:10.1016/j.chc.2008.06.011
childpsych.theclinics.com

second examines intervention for children who produce language but have difficulty using it appropriately for social interaction.

Communication intervention for children with prelinguistic communication and emerging language

Characteristics of early communication in autism spectrum disorders

Many studies have discussed the communicative characteristics of prelinguistic children who have ASD. Chawarska and Volkmar [6] reviewed this literature and identified several key characteristics of this group:

- Limited attention to speech, including failure to respond to name [7,8]
- Deficits in joint attention skills [9–13], including coordinating attention between people and objects, drawing others' attention to objects or events for the purpose of sharing experiences, following the gaze and point gestures of others, shifting gaze between people and objects for the purpose of directing another's attention, and directing affect to others through gaze
- Reduced rates of communication [13]
- Limitation in range of communicative intentions to those aimed at getting others to do or not do things for them (requests and protests) [13,14]
- Failure to compensate for lack of language with other forms of communication, particularly the more conventional forms, such as pointing or showing [13,15–18]
- Deficits in symbolic behaviors apart from language [19–21] and in imitation of vocal and other behaviors [22], both of which are closely related to language development in typical children

Intervention for communication in young children who have ASD attempts to address this range of difficulties.

Intervention methods for children with prelinguistic communication and emerging language

Goldstein [23], Paul and Sutherland [24], Rogers [25], and Wetherby and Woods [26] have reviewed interventions for early communication in autism, which are generally divided into three major categories. The first category is often referred to as didactic. Didactic methods are based on behaviorist theory and take advantage of behavioral technologies such as massed trials, operant conditioning, shaping, prompting, and chaining. Reinforcement is used to increase the frequency of desired target behaviors. Teaching sessions using these approaches involve high levels of adult control, repetitive periods of drill and practice, precise antecedent and consequent sequences, and a passive responder role for the client. The adult directs and controls all aspects of the interaction.

A second category of approaches is frequently called *naturalistic*. These attempt to incorporate behaviorist principles in more natural environments using functional, pragmatically appropriate social interactions instead of stimulus-response-reinforcement sequences. Naturalistic approaches focus on the use of "intrinsic" rather than tangible or edible reinforcers. Intrinsic reinforces include the satisfaction of achieving a desired goal through communication (the client says, "I want juice" and gets juice) rather than more contrived, extrinsic reinforcers, such as getting a token or being told "good talking." Finally, and perhaps most important, naturalistic approaches attempt to get clients to initiate communication rather than casting them always in a responder role.

The final orientation in this classification scheme is called *developmental* or *pragmatic*. These approaches emphasize functional communication, rather than speech, as a goal. As such, they encourage the development of multiple aspects of communication, such as the use of gestures, gaze, affect, and vocalization, and hold these behaviors to be necessary precursors to speech production. Activities provide multiple opportunities and temptations to communicate; the adult responds to any child initiation by providing rewarding activities. The child directs the interaction and chooses the topics and materials from among a range that the adult provides. Teachers strive to create an affectively positive environment by following the child's lead and react supportively to any behavior that can be interpreted as communicative (even if it was not intended in that way).

In the following sections, examples of each of these three types of intervention approaches, as applied to the prelinguistic and early language stages of communication in ASD, are presented.

Didactic approaches

A large body of research has demonstrated that didactic approaches are an effective means of initially developing attention to and understanding of language and initiating speech production in preverbal children who have ASD. Discrete trial instruction entails dividing the chosen skill into components and training each component individually using highly structured, drill-like procedures. Intensive training uses shaping, prompting, prompt fading, and reinforcement strategies. Trials continue until the child produces the target response with minimal prompting, at which point the next step in the hierarchy of behaviors (eg, correctly pointing to the named picture from among two pictures) is presented and trained.

Several group studies have shown that structured intervention based on behavioral principles is useful in improving expressive language in children who have ASD [27–29]. A relatively large literature based on single case studies has also demonstrated the efficacy of these approaches in eliciting vocal imitation [30] and speech from nonverbal children [29,31,32]. These approaches rely heavily on teacher direction, prompted responses, and contrived forms of reinforcement, however. An inherent weakness in didactic approaches lies in the fact that they often lead to a passive style of communication, in which children respond to prompts to communicate but do not initiate communication or transfer the behaviors acquired to situations outside the teaching context [33]. These difficulties in generalizing and maintaining behaviors taught through didactic approaches, along with changes in theoretic views of language learning that emphasized the central role of social exchanges in the acquisition of language, led to the introduction of more naturalistic methods of intervention.

Contemporary applied behavior analysis

Various practitioners of applied behavior analysis (ABA) [34–36] have confronted the major shortcoming of classic behavioral approaches: the lack of generalization. Hart and Risley [37] were the first to attempt to apply operant principles to more functional communicative situations. Their major insight concerned the importance of making access to the object of the child's interest contingent on the child's initiating some communicative exchange about it. These contemporary ABA, or naturalistic methods, share some aspects of the didactic approaches from which they are an outgrowth. They are moderately teacher-directed, address goals specified by the adult and rely on reinforcement, although the reinforcement is more intrinsic (the attainment of the child's desire or a social reinforcement) than the tangible rewards used in more traditional discrete trial instruction methods. The effectiveness of these methods has been amply documented in the literature, at least in single case studies, both for initiating speech in previously nonverbal children [38] and increasing the complexity of spoken language [39]. Direct comparisons of didactic and naturalistic approaches have shown some advantage for the more natural techniques, including maintenance and generalization of new behaviors [40], although not all investigators accept this [41].

Several techniques that fall within the category of contemporary ABA approaches to communication intervention include prompt-free training [42], incidental teaching [37,43], and mand-modeling [44]. *Milieu teaching* is an umbrella term that refers to this range of methods that is integrated into a child's natural environment [23]. The early language skills of children with a range of developmental disorders, including autism, have been shown to be enhanced through milieu teaching methods [34,45–47]. Milieu teaching approaches include

- Training in everyday environments
- Creating activities that take place throughout the day rather than only at "therapy time"
- Including preferred toys and activities so that participation in activities is self-reinforcing

- Encouraging spontaneous communication by using "expectant waiting" and refraining from prompting
- Waiting for the child to initiate teaching episodes by gesturing or indicating interest in a desired object or activity
- Providing prompts and cues for expansion of the child's initiation
- Rewarding child responses with access to a desired object or activity

In general, milieu approaches like these have been shown to be associated with increased ability to initiate communication in children who did not show this ability previously [48,49]. Nonverbal children have developed speech using these methods [50], and increases in the frequency, spontaneity, and elaboration of language have been documented [23,40,51]. Yoder and Stone [47] showed that children with autism who have some communicative behavior before intervention were more likely to develop speech in this program than were children with fewer communication behaviors at baseline.

In addition to the specific techniques described in this article, several comprehensive intervention programs have been designed within the contemporary ABA format. Some examples are listed in Table 1. A few studies have shown these programs to be more effective in improving language and cognitive outcomes—short-term and over the course of 2 years—than eclectic community interventions [27,28].

There is one significant problem with the naturalistic ABA methods, however. Because of their reliance on allowing children to initiate, which requires interventionists to make more on-line decisions, they involve a significant level of training for interventionists and rely to some degree on clinician sensitivity and skill. Although it has been demonstrated that both parents and peers can be taught to deliver naturalistic interventions successfully [31,52,53], these methods require more moment-to-moment decision making than didactic programs in which adult actions are clearly specified, unambiguous, and easily trained. Unlike didactic approaches, few materials are available that outline comprehensive curricula, and no training opportunities make it possible to master the approach from independent study of published manuals or through in-service training. Currently, it is difficult to disseminate these methods faithfully and efficiently to interventionists beyond those who created the approaches and their direct trainees.

Developmentally based, social-pragmatic strategies

This approach is based on the assumption that children who have autism develop language in the same way and following the same sequence as do typically speaking children. This means that children who do not speak are first encouraged to use other means of communicating to get intentions across to discover the value of communication in the ability to regulate others' behavior and control interactions. Proponents of this approach

Table 1
Examples of comprehensive programs

Program	Source	Description
Douglass Developmental Center	[114]	Developmentally sequenced program using behavioral approaches, beginning with discrete trials and moving toward more naturalistic methods
Learning Experiences and Alternative Program (LEAP)	[115]	Preschool program that blends behavioral and developmental approaches and incorporates peer-mediated social skills training and individualized curricula
Denver Model	[116]	Developmental, relationship-based program with home program that incorporates natural contexts
Pivotal Response Training	[117]	Parent education aimed at providing skills that enable the child to function in inclusive settings; aims at identifying pivotal skills, such as initiation and self-management; employs naturalistic behavioral methods
Treatment and Education of Autistic and Related Communication Handicapped Children (TEACCH)	[118]	Statewide program in North Carolina. Regional centers provide consultation and training to parents and schools; based on a structured teaching approach; includes parents as co-therapists; communication curriculum makes use of behavioral and naturalistic approaches and alternative communication strategies for nonverbal children
Walden Early Childhood Program	[34]	Comprehensive program for children through kindergarten age; makes use of inclusive classrooms, incidental teaching approaches, with developmentally selected goals; goals include functional language use, responsiveness, participation with peers, and daily living skills

advocate the use of a variety of nonverbal forms of communication as "stepping stones" to speech. The central tenets of this group of approaches include

- Following the child's attentional lead and allowing the child to choose the course of the interaction and use of materials
- Using the normal sequence of communicative development to provide the best guidelines for determining intervention goals
- Providing intensified opportunities for children who have ASD to engage in activities that are similar to those in which typically developing peers engage, in the belief that these are the most effective contexts for learning social and communication skills

- Exploiting learning opportunities ("teachable moments") that naturally arise in the course of interactions rather than relying on a predetermined curriculum; intervention is performed in the context of natural daily routines, such as bathing, dressing, and feeding
- Targeting *functional* goals for intervention (ie, targeted behaviors should be applicable to daily, meaningful activities in a variety of contexts apart from the one in which they were originally learned)
- Assuming the "prerequisite" role of nonverbal communication, including gestures, gaze, vocalization, and other nonvocal means, in the development of language.

Floor time

The developmental, individual-difference, relationship-based model [54], often referred to as "floor time," aims to develop symbolic, interactive communication through shared play and affect. Parents are trained to provide multiple, daily "floor time" sessions in which the adult follows the child's lead, comments on the child's actions, and provides many opportunities for reciprocal action and challenges and obstacles to "stretch" the child's capacities. The method uses "circles of communication" in which the adult follows the child's lead in attending to objects of interest to the child, then invites the child to interact in increasing complex and challenging ways with the chosen object. Few empiric reports of results of this intervention have appeared in the literature, although the authors give anecdotal reports of improvement [55,56].

Relationship development intervention

Gutstein and Sheeley [57] also present a program in which parents are trained to deliver intervention. In relationship development intervention, parents are taught a variety of strategies to use in providing scaffolded opportunities for their child to respond in more flexible ways to challenging and increasingly unpredictable activities throughout daily routines. The approach's authors, Gutstein, Burgess, and Montfort [58], reported reductions in autistic symptoms and increased mainstream school placements in an uncontrolled study of 16 children between 3 and 9 years who received this intervention and were followed for 2 years.

More than words

Another child-centered program, developed by Sussman [59], is derived from approaches developed by the Hanen Center for training parents and teachers to facilitate language development by providing enriched, contingent, and stimulating input to children with a range of disabilities. The focus of *More Than Words*—and the Hanen approach to autism in general—is on training the parents and teachers of preschool-aged children who have ASD to promote communication and social skills within ordinary interactions throughout the child's day. Although there is a good deal of research to support the use of the Hanen approach in elaborating language for children with typical and delayed development , there is as yet little empiric support for its use with children who have ASDs [60–62]. One case study provided promising data showing increases in vocabulary and initiations in children whose mothers underwent responsiveness training [63].

Augmentative and alternative communication strategies

For children who have ASD with significantly delayed development of speech, alternative methods of communication are often introduced. Originally developed to assist individuals with severe sensory or motoric impediments to speech production, these strategies, commonly referred to as augmentative and alternative communication, provide nonvocal options for communication. The main tenet of this approach is that all children have a need to communicate, and if speech is not present, communication need not wait for it to develop. Instead, the child is taught other ways to express intentions. The following sections provide some examples of augmentative and alternative communication methods that have been used with children who have ASD.

Sign language

Manual signs have been used frequently as a communication modality for children who have ASDs who do not talk. Seal and Bonvillian [64] reported that the acquisition of signs is related to fine motor abilities, suggesting that children with low levels of fine motor development are less likely to benefit from this form of augmentative and alternative communication. Goldstein [23] reviewed a range of studies using manual signs combined with speech, called total communication, and concluded that it can be effective for teaching early vocabulary receptively and expressively. Lord and McGee [15] argued that although signs may support children in making a transition to first words, they are not generally an entry into a fully functional language system. Use of signs has not been found to preclude the production of speech, but at least one study suggested that teaching signs does not accelerate speech development, either [32].

Picture exchange communication system

The picture exchange communication system (PECS) [65] begins with teaching single word requests by means of exchanging a picture for an object and then moves on to building sentence structure. Like milieu teaching approaches, PECS incorporates child initiation of communicative acts by requiring the child to initiate an exchange by handing a picture to an adult to obtain the desired object. Direct verbal prompts such as "what do you want?" are avoided to help increase the spontaneity of requests. Once a powerful reinforcer is identified, the child is required to exchange a picture card with the trainer for the desired item. It is recommended that two trainers be used, with one guiding the child through the picture exchange when he or she reaches toward the reinforcer. Spontaneity and generalization of the picture exchanges are addressed by

- Gradually increasing the distance between the child and the pictures
- Using the system in different environments
- Involving a variety of people
- Focusing on different reinforcers.

Charlop-Christy et al [66] conducted a study to examine the use of PECS with three preschool children who have ASD and its effects on speech development. Results from this study indicated that all the children met the learning criteria for PECS and showed increases in use of speech. Tincani [67] compared instruction in sign language and PECS and found that both increased production of independent requesting, but sign language training produced a higher percentage of vocalizations. He suggested that the child's ability to produce motor imitations was also related to outcome. Howlin and colleagues [68] showed modest effectiveness in terms of increasing children's rates of initiations by training teachers to use PECS, although there was no evidence of improvement in the children's speech or general communication development.

Aided augmentative and alternative communication

There is some limited evidence that nonspeaking individuals who have autism also can benefit from exposure to "high-tech" communication aids. In a study by Romski and Sevcik [69], two youths with autism showed increased expression using spoken language and a computerized voice output communication device over the course of a 2-year study, in which naturalistic teaching methods were used to teach the use of the device. This approach also resulted in an increased use of communicative behaviors to request objects, respond to questions, and make comments among the children who have autism in another study. A case study by Light et al [70] of one child who has autism also reported positive language outcomes when a voice output communication device was included as a component of a comprehensive communication system. Other components included gestures, natural speech, and a communication book.

Olive and colleagues [71] showed that three children with ASD learned to use a voice output communication device to request items during play when taught using a milieu teaching approach. Bernard-Opitz et al [72] used feedback from an IBM Speech Viewer to increase vocal imitation in children with autism. Shane and Weiss-Kapp [73] proposed that a comprehensive visual language system that includes pictures, symbols, and video clips presented on electronic devices be taught to children who have ASD. The program is aimed at providing nonspeech methods of expression and supporting language comprehension and organizational skills. Although these methods are appealing and a few initial reports are promising, additional larger scale research is required to assess the efficacy of high-tech aids such as these in this population.

Summary

Developmental-pragmatic approaches are widely used and advocated by many prominent communication specialists. One problem with these methods is that to an even greater extent than naturalistic approaches, they require a high degree of sensitivity, creativity, and on-line decision making on the part of interventionists. Programs such as Hanen have demonstrated that parents, teachers, paraprofessionals, and others can learn these methods, but they require extensive training, practice, and ongoing support. Demonstration of child outcomes in response to adult training is weak. To some degree, the success of developmental-pragmatic programs may hinge on the careful training, follow-up, support, and talent of persons who deliver the intervention.

Currently, developmental-pragmatic approaches have a narrower base in empiric research than the other two approaches to communication intervention in ASD. Some studies have shown them to be effective for eliciting speech in children with other developmental delays [60,74]. Studies of child-centered methods have demonstrated their ability to increase imitation, gaze, turn-taking, and joint attention in preverbal children who have autism [75,76]. Kasari [77] and Whalen et al [78] reported on small sample studies showing improvement in communication after training that focused specifically on eliciting joint attention. Yoder and McDuffie [46] reviewed research that suggested that training children in play and nonverbal communication skills may improve their ability to acquire speech.

Conclusions: early communication intervention

Programs to elicit initial communication behaviors and first words range from highly structured behaviorist to open-ended, child-directed methods, with a range of naturalistic approaches in between. Didactic and naturalistic ABA methods are aimed specifically at eliciting speech from preverbal children who have ASDs and have established efficacy for doing so in single case studies, although controlled experiments with random assignment to treatments, the "gold standard" of scientific evidence, are still relatively few as of this writing. Developmental-pragmatic approaches are aimed more broadly at the improvement of social communication and interaction and have a less well-established, although emerging, empirical track record for eliciting first words in children who have ASDs. In small sample and case studies, they have been shown to increase preverbal behaviors, such as imitation and joint attention.

Developmental approaches that incorporate augmentative and alternative communication methods, such as signs and pictures, have been shown to be compatible with the development of speech, although their efficiency relative to straightforward speech treatment has not yet been established. Little research exists on the relationship between child characteristics and intervention efficacy, so we do not know which approach is the best match for a particular child. What does seem clear is that communicative deficits in preverbal children who have autism are amenable to treatment and that a range of treatments has been shown to be useful in enhancing communicative behavior.

Speakers with autism spectrum disorders

Core deficits

Once children who have autism begin using words, the course of language development is similar to that seen in other children with disabilities [79]. When children who have ASD acquire basic language skills, however, significant challenges to the development of communicative competence remain. Tager-Flusberg et al [80] pointed to two commonly observed characteristics of the communication of speakers with ASD: (1) echolalia, which is the imitation of what has been heard, either directly after it is spoken, or as a delayed echo at a later time, and (2) pronoun reversal, which is primarily the tendency to use "you" instead of "I." Although this was at one time thought to reflect difficulties in ego formation, it is now seen as another instance of echolalia, in which the child refers to himself or herself as "you" as he or she has heard others say [81].

Both of these characteristics tend to decrease as language skill increases, and both are seen as transitional behaviors in typical development [80]. Few programs have addressed pronoun reversal directly because it tends to abate naturally, but various case studies have reported using behavioral methods successfully to reduce echolalia and replace it with simple request and labeling behaviors [82–84].

Deficits in prosody or musical aspect of speech, including its rate, loudness, pitch, voice quality, and use of stress, are also frequently seen in speakers who have ASD [85]. Sheinkopf et al [16] and Dawson et al [86] showed that even prelinguistic vocalizations in young children who have autism contained a significantly higher proportion of atypical vocal characteristics than did those of normal children. Paul et al [87] found that approximately half of high-functioning speakers who have autism were rated as atypical in elements of prosodic production. When these differences are present they tend to be persistent and show little change over time, even when other aspects of language improve [88–90]. Paul and colleagues [87,91] showed that ratings of social and communicative competence were related to ratings of prosody in speakers who have ASD, which suggests that difficulties in prosodic production affect listeners' attributions of competence to these individuals.

To date, little research has been conducted on the treatment of prosodic deficits in autism. Several commercially available programs have been developed for addressing prosodic difficulties in nonautistic speakers, but no research is available on their use with children with autism [92,93]. Addressing prosodic deficits remains a largely unmet need in this population.

Pragmatics, or appropriate use of language in social situations, is the most prominent aspect of communicative deficit in this population [94]. Children who have autism are less likely than children with typical development to initiate communication, particularly with peers [95]. Overall rates of communication are low, even in children who speak [96]. These children show reduced interest in language spoken to them; they are less likely to respond in a reciprocal fashion to the communicative bids of peers and more likely to produce self-directed, noncommunicative speech [94]. Paul and colleagues [97] reported that the following areas of pragmatics were most consistently impaired in speakers who have ASD:

- Use of irrelevant detail
- Inappropriate topic shifts
- Topic preoccupation/perseveration
- Unresponsiveness to partner cues
- Lack of reciprocal exchange
- Inadequate clarification
- Vague references
- Scripted, stereotyped discourse
- Excessively formal style (for speakers with Asperger syndrome only)

For children who have autism who develop speech, the conversational skills involved in managing turns and topics in discourse, flexibly adopting an appropriate style of speech keyed to the characteristics, setting and conversational partners, and inferring what information is relevant and interesting to others constitute the greatest difficulties. Unfortunately, few comprehensive, sequenced curricula are designed to address these pragmatic deficits. The following discussion reviews a range of programs available for addressing language issues in speakers who have ASD using the same tripartite scheme as discussed previously.

Intervention methods for speakers who have autism spectrum disorders

Didactic approaches

ABA programs have been developed to address the expansion of early symbols into more elaborated forms of expression. They focus primarily on improvement of language form (ie, vocabulary and sentence structures). One example is *Teach Me Language* [98], a comprehensive language program that provides a step-by-step guide with in-depth detail on intervention activities targeting language areas such as grammar, syntax, concepts, and advanced narrative skills. *Teach Me Language* methodology is behaviorally based. Children are expected to follow a teacher's lead, and regular repetition of drills is a key feature in the program.

The *Verbal Behavior* program takes a Skinnerian approach to language learning, based on the research of Michael et al [99,100]. The program, like *Teach Me Language,* provides a carefully sequenced curriculum for teaching language to children just emerging into symbolic communication and carries the curriculum through to children learning more advanced language forms. It uses a highly structured behavioral approach and incorporates techniques such as errorless teaching, specific quick-transfer (prompting and fading) procedures, and the use of discrete trial training during both intensive teaching sessions and in more naturalistic contexts. Language goals are structured in terms of Skinnerian categories of verbal behaviors, which include (hierarchically ordered)

- Echoes: practice in imitating verbal behavior
- Mands: verbal behaviors that produce an immediate benefit for the speaker (eg, requests)
- Tacts: labels
- Reception by feature, function, and class: responding to commonly used verbal stimuli (words)
- Intraverbals: verbal, nonechoic responses to the speech of others

Just as in the case of didactic approaches for children at prelinguistic communication levels, these highly behavioral language teaching programs have the potential weakness of leading to passive styles of communication and limited levels of generalization. A search of reference databases found no reports of empiric evidence to support the specific use of the *Teach Me Language* program. Partington et al [100–102] published data indicating increases in verbal production using their method. Still, little research is available on the functional effects of these programs on real-world communication or on their consequences for adaptive communication and independence. Although they may result in the achievement of target behaviors within the behavioral framework, as most ABA programs do, few data are available on their general, long-term effects on a child's functioning or independence.

A slightly less traditionally behaviorist approach, the PECS program, also provides a curriculum for children who have acquired basic symbolic communication skills. Once single-word exchanges have been mastered, sentence structure is targeted. The aim is for the child to combine an "I want" picture with a picture of a desired item or activity. A "sentence strip" is used to attach the pictures, which is passed to the communication partner. The sentences are further extended by the addition of other words (eg, adjectives such as "red"). Sentence strips are often color coded; for instance, there may be a green area for noun pictures that are framed in green, a blue area for verb pictures framed in blue, and a red area for adjective symbols framed in red. The next phase of the PECS moves from using the picture exchanges for requesting to encouraging commenting, which is done by introducing picture cards that represent phrases such as "I see," "I smell," and "I hear." Research on the efficacy of this stage of the program or its generalization to functional communication has not been reported.

Naturalistic approaches

There is much less research on the effectiveness of naturalistic ABA programs in improving communication for speakers who have ASD than there is for prelinguistic children. McClannahan and Kranz [103] provided an approach with empiric support that uses scripts—either pictured or written—to guide children with autism on what to say in given social situations. The scripts are developed by teachers with the students to address particular social settings. As the children continue to rehearse the scripts with various adults and peers, pieces of script are removed, or faded, so the child is required to provide longer and longer portions of the language on his or her own. Krantz and McClannahan [104] presented data suggesting that this method leads to improvement in conversation for children who have ASD.

Video modeling is a similar procedure. Short videos illustrate the language used in particular social situations, such as asking for a book from a librarian. The student watches the video with the instructor, discusses and verbally rehearses the scene, then practices it by role playing with an instructor and eventually trying it in a real setting. Charlop-Christy and colleagues [105] showed that this procedure is more effective than simply modeling the desired behaviors in vivo for children who have ASD.

Brinton and colleagues [106] developed a method for improving conversational turn-taking and topic maintenance. In a case study, they reported on work over a 2-year period with a boy with social disability who was taught a set of explicit rules for finding topics of common interest with peers and engaging in conversation about them. Brinton and colleagues stressed that change was slow, but they did report improvement in social acceptance as conversational skills improved.

Focused stimulation is a naturalistic means of increasing receptive language skills in children with various disabilities. This technique involves providing an interesting set of play materials and using simple, repetitive language to talk about the ongoing action in concrete, here-and-now terms, using many examples of forms the child needs to acquire. One single case study [107] provided preliminary support for this strategy in children who have ASD. Many of the comprehensive naturalistic ABA programs outlined in Table 1 provide examples of intervention methods for children who begin speaking.

Developmental-pragmatic approaches

Few examples of detailed programs take a child-centered approach to expanding basic language in speakers who have autism. Prizant and

Wetherby [108] advocated using the SCERTS (social communication, emotional regulation, transactional support) model, a comprehensive approach that allows the incorporation of an eclectic range of treatment methods and focuses on overarching goals that include improving social communication, encouraging behavioral self-regulation, and providing transactional supports to children who have autism. This program has not yet been subjected to empiric study.

Quill [109] presented another comprehensive curriculum for developing social and communicative skills in young children who have autism at various levels of functioning. The curriculum is also eclectic and advocates the full range of highly structured, naturalistic approaches and child-centered methods. It suggests focusing on the child's responsiveness to typical peers rather than promoting initiations. Intervention guidelines include organization of the environment to facilitate participation and cooperation, careful selection of materials, and activities structured to foster the target child's participation. Empiric support has not appeared for this program.

Child-centered methods discussed at the prelinguistic level, including "floor time" [54] and relationship development intervention [57], also contain components that can be used at higher language levels. Sussman [59] - developed a companion volume to *More than Words,* called *Talkability* [110], which is aimed at children who speak. No empiric validation of these methods for improving language skills in children who have ASD is available as of this writing.

Increasing social communication

As we have seen, a major difficulty for children who have ASD who speak and perhaps the central problem for students with high-functioning autism and Asperger syndrome concerns not the forms of language but its use in social contexts, particularly with peers. Apart from elaborating the form and increasing the frequency of language use, an additional important goal of communication intervention for children who have ASD is to provide supports that allow these children to engage in peer interactions, including pretend play, games, and conversations. Some of the naturalistic approaches discussed already, such as script fading and video modeling, go some distance to addressing this issue. McClannahan and Krantz [103] provided what comes closest to a comprehensive, sequential program for teaching conversational skills to this population.

Much of the literature that addresses the more comprehensive problem of increasing social communication opportunities and skills in speakers who have ASD is discussed under the rubric of "social skills training," a topic addressed in detail elsewhere in this issue. The main point, however, is that for children who have ASD who speak, speaking is not—in itself— sufficient. These children need supports aimed not only at increasing basic vocabulary and sentence structure but also at the pragmatic aspects of language use in the context of social interactions to address deficits such as those identified by Paul et al [97]. Studies of the effects of various approaches to social skills intervention [111] generally concur that trained peers are more effective agents of this intervention than are adults [112] and that the interventions are more effective when they take place in a child's natural environment, such as the classroom, than in a clinical setting [113].

Conclusions: language intervention

The most elaborated curricula for developing language at this level are highly behavioral. Although they have some demonstrated efficacy, behavioral programs maintain weaknesses in terms of the development of passive communication styles and failures of generalization. Naturalistic approaches have been developed to address aspects of social communication and have some demonstrated empiric support, but there are few comprehensive curricula. Developmental approaches for this stage of development have less fully elaborated curricula and limited empiric support.

Summary

Intervention for children who have ASD at prelinguistic and early language stages has been shown to make a dramatic difference, at least in short-term outcome [11]. Intervention methods that draw from a range of philosophies and make use of varying degrees of adult direction have been shown to be effective in increasing language and communicative behaviors, although direct comparisons among methods, controlled studies with random assignment to treatments, and long-term outcome studies are still lacking. Despite the gaps in our current knowledge, it is clear that children who have autism benefit from intensive, early intervention that focuses on increasing the frequency, form, and function of communication. Available evidence shows that highly structured behavioral methods have important positive consequences for these children, particularly in eliciting first words. The limitation of these methods in maintenance and generalization of skills suggests that many children with autism need to have these methods supplemented with more child-centered activities to increase communicative initiation and carry over learned skills to new settings and communication partners.

A review of programs aimed at language development in speakers who have ASD points out the importance of thinking beyond words and sentences to the social functions of communication and language use when developing interventions. Although a range of adult-mediated programs is reviewed in this article, providing opportunities for mediated peer interactions with trained peers in natural settings seems to be especially important in maximizing the effects of this intervention.

References

[1] Short A, Schopler E. Factors relating to age of onset in autism. J Autism Dev Disord 1988; 18:207–16.

[2] DeMyer M, Hingtgen J, Jackson R. Infantile autism reviewed: a decade of research. Schizophrenia Review 1981;7(3):388–451.

[3] Paul R, Cohen D. Outcomes of severe disorders of language acquisition. J Autism Dev Disord 1984;14(4):405–21.

[4] Venter A, Lord C, Schopler E. A follow-up study of high-functioning autistic children. J Child Psychol Psychiatry 1992;33(3):489–507.

[5] American Psychiatric Association. Diagnostic and statistical manual. 4th edition. Washington, DC: APA Press; 1994.

[6] Chawarska K, Volkmar F. Autism spectrum disorders in infants and toddlers. New York: Guilford; 2008.

[7] Osterling J, Dawson G. Early recognition of children with autism: a study of first birthday home videotapes. J Autism Dev Disord 1994;24(3):247–57.

[8] Paul R, et al. Dissociations of development in early communication in autism spectrum disorders. In: Paul R, editor. Language disorders from a developmental perspective. Mahwah (NJ): Lawrence Erlbaum Associates; 2007.

[9] Dawson G, et al. Affective exchanges between young autistic children and their mothers. J Abnorm Child Psychol 1990;18(3):335–45.

[10] Kasari C, et al. Affective sharing in the context of joint attention interactions of normal, autistic, and mentally retarded children. J Autism Dev Disord 1990;20(1):87–100.

[11] Lord C, McGee J. Social development. In: Lord C, McGee J, editors. Educating children with autism. Washington, DC: National Academy of Sciences; 2001. p. 66–81.

[12] Sigman M, Norman K. Continuity and change in the development of children with autism. In: Broman S, Fletcher J, editors. The changing nervous system: neurobehavioral consequences of early brain disorders. New York: Oxford University Press; 1999. p. 274–91.

[13] Wetherby A, Prizant B, Hutchinson T. Communicative, social/affective, and symbolic profiles of young children with autism and pervasive developmental disorders. Am J Speech Lang Pathol 1998;7(2):79–91.

[14] Mundy P, Stella J. Joint attention, social orienting, and nonverbal communication in autism. In: Wetherby AM, Prizant BM, editors. Autism spectrum disorders: a transactional developmental perspective communication and language intervention series. Vol. 9. Baltimore: Paul H. Brookes; 2000. p. 55–77.

[15] Lord C, McGee J. Educating children with autism. Washington, DC: National Research Council; 2002.

[16] Sheinkopf J, et al. Vocal atypicalities of preverbal autistic children. J Autism Dev Disord 2000;30:345–54.

[17] Schoen L, et al. Phonological behaviors in toddlers with autism spectrum disorders. Presented at National convention of the American Speech-Language-Hearing Association. November, 2003: Chicago.

[18] Schoen L, et al. Acoustic measurements of prelinguistic vocalizations in toddlers with ASD. Presented at Symposium for research in child language disorders. June, 2007: Madison.

[19] Stone WL, et al. Nonverbal communication in two- and three-year-old children with autism. J Autism Dev Disord 1997;27(6):677–96.

[20] Rogers S, Cook I, Meryl A. Imitation and play in autism. In: Volkmar F, et al, editors. Handbook of autism and pervasive developmental disorders. New York: Wiley; 2005. p. 382–405.

[21] Wetherby A, Prutting C. Profiles of communicative and cognitive-social abilities in autistic children. J Speech Hear Res 1984;27:364–77.

[22] Charman T, et al. Predicting language outcome in infants with autism and pervasive developmental disorder. Int J Lang Commun Disord 2003;38(3):265–85.

[23] Goldstein H. Communication intervention for children with autism: a review of treatment efficacy. J Autism Dev Disord 2002;32:373–96.

[24] Paul R, Sutherland D. Enhancing early language in children with autism spectrum disorders. In: Volkmar FR, et al, editors. Handbook of autism and pervasive developmental disorders. New York: Wiley & Sons; 2005. p. 946–76.

[25] Rogers S. Evidence-based intervention for language development in young children with autism. In: Charman T, Stone W, editors. Social and communication development in autism spectrum disorders: early identification, diagnosis, and intervention. New York: Guilford Press; 2006. p. 143–79.

[26] Wetherby A, Woods J. Effectiveness of early intervention for children with autism spectrum disorders beginning in the second year of life. Topics in Early Childhood Special Education 2006;26:67–82.

[27] Howard J, et al. A comparison of intensive behavior analytic and eclectic treatments for young children with autism. Res Dev Disabil 2005;26:359–83.

[28] Remington B, et al. Early intensive behavioral intervention: outcomes for children with autism and their parents after two years. Am J Ment Retard 2007;112:418–38.

[29] Tsiouri I, Greer R. Inducing vocal verbal behavior in children with severe language delays through rapid motor imitation responding. Journal of Behavioral Education 2003;12(3):185–206.

[30] Ross DE, Greer R. Generalized imitation and the mand: inducing first instances of speech in young children with autism. Res Dev Disabil 2003;24(1):58–74.

[31] Jones E, Carr D, Feeley K. Multiple effects of joint attention intervention for children with autism. Behav Modif 2006;30:282–834.

[32] Yoder P, Layton TL. Speech following sign language training in autistic children with minimal verbal language. J Autism Dev Disord 1988;18(2):217–29.

[33] Stokes KS. Planning for the future of a severely handicapped autistic child. J Autism Child Schizophr 1977;7(3):288–302.

[34] McGee G, Morrier M, Daly T. An incidental teaching approach to early intervention for toddlers with autism. J Assoc Pers Sev Handicaps 1999;24:133–46.

[35] Koegel LK, et al. Pivotal response intervention. I. Overview of approach. J Assoc Pers Sev Handicaps 1999;24(3):174–85.

[36] Anderson S, Romanczyk R. Early intervention for children with autism: continuum-based behavioral models. J Assoc Pers Sev Handicaps 1999;24:162–73.

[37] Hart B, Risley T. Incidental teaching of language in the preschool. J Appl Behav Anal 1975;8:411–20.

[38] Koegel RL, O'Dell M, Koegel LK. A natural language teaching paradigm for nonverbal autistic children. J Autism Dev Disord 1987;17(2):187–200.

[39] Laski KE, Charlop MH, Schreibman L. Training parents to use the natural language paradigm to increase their autistic children's speech. J Appl Behav Anal 1988;21(4):391–400.

[40] Delprato DJ. Comparisons of discrete-trial and normalized behavioral language intervention for young children with autism. J Autism Dev Disord 2001;31(3):315–25.

[41] Smith T. Discrete trial training in the treatment of autism. Focus Autism Other Dev Disabl 2001;16:86–92.

[42] Mirenda P, Santogrossi J. A prompt-free strategy to teach pictorial communication system use. Augment Altern Commun 1985;1:143–50.

[43] McGee G, et al. A modified incidental teaching procedure for autistic youth: acquisition and generalization of receptive object labels. J Appl Behav Anal 1983;16:329–38.

[44] Rogers-Warren A, Warren S. Mand for verbalization: facilitating the generalization of newly trained language in children. Behav Modif 1980;4:230–45.

[45] Kaiser A, Yoder P, Keetz A. Evaluating milieu teaching. In: Reichle SWJ, editor. Causes and effects in communication and language intervention. Baltimore (MD): Paul H. Brookes; 1992. p. 9–47.

[46] Yoder P, McDuffie A. Teaching young children with autism to talk. Semin Speech Lang 2006;27:161–72.

[47] Yoder P, Stone W. Randomized comparison of two communication interventions for preschoolers with autism spectrum disorders. J Consult Clin Psychol 2006;74(3):426–35.

[48] Matson JL, et al. An evaluation of two methods for increasing self-initiated verbalizations in autistic children. J Appl Behav Anal 1993;26(3):389–98.

[49] Yoder P, Warren SF. Effects of prelinguistic milieu teaching and parent responsivity education on dyads involving children with intellectual disabilities. J Speech Lang Hear Res 2002;45(6):1158–74.

[50] Koegel RL, Koegel LK, Surratt A. Language intervention and disruptive behavior in preschool children with autism. J Autism Dev Disord 1992;22(2):141–53.

[51] Koegel L. Interventions to facilitate communication in autism. J Autism Dev Disord 2000; 30:383–91.

[52] McGee GG, et al. Promoting reciprocal interactions via peer incidental teaching. J Appl Behav Anal 1992;25(1):117–26.

[53] Wetherby A, Woods J. Developmental approaches to treatment. In: Chawarska K, Volkmar F, editors. Autism in infancy. New York: Guilford; 2008. p. 170–206.

[54] Weider S, Greenspan S. Climbing the symbolic ladder in the DIR model through floor time/interactive play. Autism 2003;7:425–35.

[55] Greenspan S, Wieder S. Developmental patterns and outcomes in infants and children with disorders in relating and communicating: a chart review of 200 cases of children with autistic spectrum diagnosis. The Journal of Developmental and Learning Disorders 1997;1(1): 87–139.

[56] Greenspan S, Weider S. A functional developmental approach to autism spectrum disorders. J Assoc Pers Sev Handicaps 1999;24:147–61.

[57] Gutstein S, Sheely R. Relationship development intervention with children, adolescents, and adults. London: Jessica Kingsley Publishers; 2002.

[58] Gutstein S, Burgess A, Montfort M. Evaluation of the relationship development intervention program. Autism 2007;11:397–411.

[59] Sussman F. More than words. Toronto: The Hanen Center; 2001.

[60] Girolametto L, Pearce P, Weitzman E. Effects of lexical intervention on the phonology of late talkers. J Speech Lang Hear Res 1996;40:338–48.

[61] Clements-Baartman L, Girolametto L. Facilitating the acquisition of two-word semantic relations by pre-schoolers with Down syndrome: efficacy of interactive vs. didactic therapy. Canadian Journal of Speech-Language Pathology 1995;19:103–11.

[62] Girolametto L. Improving the social-conversation skills of developmentally delayed children: an intervention study. J Speech Hear Disord 1988;53:156–67.

[63] Girolametto L, Sussman F, Weitzman E. Using case study methods to investigate the effects of interactive intervention for children with autism spectrum disorders. J Child Psychol Psychiatry 2007;40:470–92.

[64] Seal B, Bonvillian J. Sign language and motor functioning in students with autistic disorder. J Autism Dev Disord 1997;27:437–66.

[65] Bondy AS, Frost LA. The picture exchange communication system. Semin Speech Lang 1998;19(4):373–88, quiz 389; 424.

[66] Charlop-Christy MH, et al. Using the picture exchange communication system (PECS) with children with autism: assessment of PECS acquisition, speech, social-communicative behavior, and problem behavior. J Appl Behav Anal 2002;35(3):213–31.

[67] Tincani M. Comparing the picture exchange communication system and sign language training for children with autism. Focus Autism Other Dev Disabl 2004;19:152–63.

[68] Howlin P, et al. The effectiveness of picture exchange communication system training for teachers of children with autism: a pragmatic, group randomized controlled trial. J Child Psychol Psychiatry 2007;48:473–81.

[69] Romski MA, Sevcik RA, Adamson LB. Communication patterns of youth with mental retardation with and without their speech-output communication devices. Am J Ment Retard 1999;104(3):249–59.

[70] Light JC, et al. Augmentative and alternative communication to support receptive and expressive communication for people with autism. J Commun Disord 1998;31(2):153–78, quiz 179–80.

[71] Olive M, et al. The effects of enhanced milieu teaching and a voice output communication aid on the requesting of three children with autism. J Autism Dev Disord 2007;37: 1503–13.

[72] Bernard-Opitz V, Sriram N, Nakhoda-Sapuan S. Enhancing social problem solving in children with autism and normal children through computer-assisted instruction. J Autism Dev Disord 2001;31(4):377–84.

[73] Shane H, Weiss-Kapp S. Visual language in autism. San Diego (CA): Pluarl Publishing; 2008.

[74] Fey M, Proctor-Williams K. Elicited imitation, modeling and recasting in grammar intervention for children with specific language impairments. In: Bishop D, Leonard L, editors. Specific speech and language disorders in children. London: Psychology Press; 2000. p. 177–94.

[75] Hwang B, Hughes C. The effects of social interactive training on early social communicative skills of children with autism. J Autism Dev Disord 2000;30(4):331–43.

[76] Pierce K, Schreibman L. Increasing complex social behaviors in children with autism: effects of peer-implemented pivotal response training. J Appl Behav Anal 1995;28(3):285–95.

[77] Kasari C, Freeman SF, Paparella T. Early intervention in autism: joint attention and symbolic play. In: Glidden LM, editor. International review of research in mental retardation: autism. Vol. 23. San Diego (CA): Academic Press; 2001. p. 207–37.

[78] Whalen C, Schreibman L, Ingersoll B. The collateral effects of joint attention training on social initiations, positive affect, imitation, and spontaneous speech for young children with autism. J Autism Dev Disord 2006;36:655–64.

[79] Tager-Flusberg H, et al. A longitudinal study of language acquisition in autistic and Down syndrome children. J Autism Dev Disord 1990;20(1):1–21.

[80] Tager-Flusber H, Paul R, Lord C. Language and communication in autism. In: Volkmar AKF, Paul R, editors. Handbook of autism and pervasive developmental disorders. New York: Wiley; 2005.

[81] Fay W. Personal pronouns and the autistic child. J Autism Dev Disord 1979;9(3):247–60.

[82] Ross D. Replacing faculty conversational exchanges for children with autism by establishing a functionally equivalent alternative response. Education & Training in Mental Retardation and Developmental Disabilities 2002;37:343–62.

[83] Karmali I, et al. Reducing palilalia by presenting tact corrections to young children with autism. Anal Verbal Behav 2005;21:145–53.

[84] Foxx R, et al. Replacing the echolalia of children with autism with functional use of verbal labeling. J Dev Phys Disabil 2004;16:307–20.

[85] Shriberg L, et al. Speech and prosody characteristics of adolescents and adults with high functioning autism and Asperger syndrome. J Speech Lang Hear Res 2001;44:1097–115.

[86] Dawson G, et al. Case study of the development of an infant with autism from birth to two years of age. J Appl Dev Psychol 2000;21(3):299–313.

[87] Paul R, Chawarska K, Fowler C, et al. Listen my children and you shall hear: auditory preferences in toddlers with autism spectrum disorders. Journal of Speech, Language, and Hearing Research 2008;50:1350–64.

[88] DeMyer M, Bryson C, Churchill D. The earliest indicators of pathological development: comparison of symptoms during infancy and early childhood in normal, subnormal, schizophrenic, and autistic children. In: for Research in Nervous and Mental Disorders Association, editor. Biological and environmental determinants of early development. 1973. p. 298–332.

[89] Kanner L. Follow-up study of eleven autistic children originally reported in 1943. J Autism Child Schizophr 1971;1:119–45.

[90] Rutter M, Greenfeld D, Lockyer L. A five to fifteen year follow-up study of infantile psychosis. II. Social and behavioural outcome. Br J Psychiatry 1967;113(504):1183–99.

[91] Paul R, Shriberg L, McSweeney J, et al. Patterns of prosody and social communicative skills in high functioning autism and Asperger syndrome. Presented at Symposium for research in child language disorders. June, 2002. Madison (WI).

[92] Awad S, Corliss M, Merson R. Prosidy. The speech bin. Vero Beach (FL); 2003.

[93] Ray B, Baker B. Hypernasality modification program. Austin (TX): ProEd; 2000.

[94] Tager-Flusberg H. Dissociation in form and function in the acquisition of language by autistic children. In: Tager-Flusberg IH, editor. Constraints on language acquisition: studies of atypical children. Hillsdale (NJ): Erlbaum; 1995. p. 175–94.

[95] McHale SM, et al. The social and symbolic quality of autistic children's communication. J Autism Dev Disord 1980;10(3):299–310.

[96] Stone WL, Caro-Martinez LM. Naturalistic observations of spontaneous communication in autistic children. J Autism Dev Disord 1990;20(4):437–53.

[97] Paul R, et al. Conversational behaviors in youth with high-functioning autism and Asperger syndrome. J Autism Dev Disord, in press.

[98] Freeman S, Dakes L. Teach me language: a language manual for children with autism, Asperger's syndrome and related disorders. Langley (Canada): SKF Books; 1996.

[99] Sundberg ML, Michael J. The benefits of Skinner's analysis of verbal behavior for children with autism. Behav Modif 2001;25(5):698–724.

[100] Sundberg M, et al. The role of automatic reinforcement in early language acquisition. Anal Verbal Behav 1995;13:21–37.

[101] Partington JW, et al. Overcoming an autistic child's failure to acquire a tact repertoire. J Appl Behav Anal 1994;27(4):733–4.

[102] Sundberg ML, et al. Contriving establishing operations to teach mands for information. Anal Verbal Behav 2001;18:15–29.

[103] McClannahan L, Krantz P. Teaching conversation to children with autism: scripts and script fading. Ethesda (MD): Woodbine House; 2005.

[104] Krantz PJ, McClannahan LE. Social interaction skills for children with autism: a script-fading procedure for beginning readers. J Appl Behav Anal 1998;31(2):191–202.

[105] Charlop-Christy MH, Le LL, Freeman KA. A comparison of video modeling with in vivo modeling for teaching children with autism. J Autism Dev Disord 2000;30(6):537–52.

[106] Brinton B, Robinson LA, Fujiki M. Description of a program for social language intervention: "if you can have a conversation, you can have a relationship." Lang Speech Hear Serv Sch 2004;35:283–6.

[107] Grela B, McLaughlin K. Focused stimulation for a child with autism spectrum disorder: a treatment study. J Autism Dev Disord 2006;36:753–6.

[108] Prizant B, et al. The SCERTS model: a comprehensive educational approach for children with autism spectrum disorders. Baltimore (MD): Brookes; 2005.

[109] Quill K. Do watch listen say: social and communication intervention. Baltimore (MD): Brookes; 2000.

[110] Sussman F. Talkability. Toronto: The Hanen Centre; 2008.

[111] Paul R. Promoting social communication in high functioning individuals with autistic spectrum disorders. Child Adolesc Psychiatr Clin N Am 2003;12(1):87–106, vi–vii.

[112] Goldstein H, Schneider N, Thiemann K. Peer-mediated social communication intervention. Topics in Language Disorders 2007;27:182–99.

[113] Bellini S, et al. A meta-analysis of school-based social skills interventions for children with autism spectrum disorders. Remedial and Special Education 2007;28:153–62.

[114] Harris S, et al. The Douglass developmental disabilities center: two models of service delivery. In: Handleman J, Harris S, editors. Preschool education programs for children with autism. Austin (TX): Pro-Ed; 2000. p. 233–60.

[115] Strain PS, Hoyson M. The need for longitudinal, intensive social skill intervention: LEAP follow-up outcomes for children with autism. Topics in Early Childhood Special Education 2000;20(2):116–22.

[116] Rogers SJ. Interventions that facilitate socialization in children with autism. J Autism Dev Disord 2000;30(5):399–409.

[117] Koegel R, Koegel L. Pivotal response treatments for autism. Baltimore (MD): Brookes; 2006.

[118] Marcus LM, Garfinkle A, Wolery M. Issues in early diagnosis and intervention with young children with autism. In: Schopler E, Yirmiya N, Shulman C, et al, editors. The research basis for autism intervention. New York: Kluwer Academic/Plenum Publishers; 2001. p. 171–85.

ELSEVIER
SAUNDERS

Child Adolesc Psychiatric Clin N Am
17 (2008) 857–873

CHILD AND
ADOLESCENT
PSYCHIATRIC CLINICS
OF NORTH AMERICA

Social Skills Training for Youth with Autism Spectrum Disorders

Scott Bellini, PhD[a],*, Jessica K. Peters, MS[b]

[a]*Indiana Resource Center for Autism, Indiana University,*
2853 East Tenth Street, Bloomington, IN 47408, USA
[b]*School of Education, Indiana University,*
201 N. Rose Avenue, Bloomington, IN 47404, USA

Social skill deficits are a pervasive and enduring feature of autism spectrum disorders (ASD) [1–5]. Deficits in social functioning are prominent in childhood and persist throughout adulthood. According to the *Diagnostic and Statistical Manual of Mental Disorders, Fourth Edition* (*DSM-IV*) [6], essential diagnostic criteria in the social domain include:

(a) marked impairment in the use of multiple nonverbal behaviors such as eye-to-eye gaze, facial expression, body postures, and gestures to regulate social interaction; (b) failure to develop peer relationships appropriate to developmental level; (c) a lack of spontaneous seeking to share enjoyment, interests, or achievements with other people; and (d) lack of social and emotional reciprocity.

Qualitative impairments in reciprocal social interaction are also a diagnostic imperative according to the *International Statistical Classification of Diseases, 10th Revision* (*ICD-10*) [7]. *ICD-10* lists difficulties interpreting socio-emotional cues, including failure to adapt behavior and emotion to social context and deficits in nonverbal communication, as essential social features of autism spectrum disorder (ASD). Social skill deficits have been linked to other deleterious outcomes, such as poor academic performance, peer rejection, isolation, social anxiety, depression, and other forms of psychopathology [8–10]. As such, there is a significant need for clinicians to develop effective, empirically tested social skill interventions. The purpose of this article is to provide a review of social skills training (SST) procedures that have been empirically tested via research. In addition, the article discusses social skills assessment procedures

* Corresponding author.
E-mail address: sbellini@indiana.edu (S. Bellini).

available to clinicians serving youth with ASD. The article concludes by presenting recommendations elucidated by meta-analytic reviews of social skill interventions.

An overview of social skills training

SST refers to instruction designed to improve or facilitate the acquisition or performance of social skills. Social skills are "socially acceptable learned behaviors that enable a person to interact with others in ways that elicit positive responses and assist in avoiding negative responses" [11]. Social skills are distinguished from social competence, in that social skills represent social behaviors, and social competence represents judgments or perceptions of those behaviors by others [12]. The distinction between social skills and social competence has important implications for the selection of outcome measures and the monitoring of treatment progress (the assessment of social functioning is discussed more comprehensively in a later section of this article). SST typically addresses three primary objectives: to promote skill acquisition, to enhance existing skills, and to facilitate the generalization of skills across settings and persons. Though SST programs vary considerably, most SST programs incorporate one or more of the following treatment modalities: modeling, coaching, social problem solving, behavior rehearsal, feedback, and reinforcement-based strategies [13].

Elliot and Gresham [11] discuss five factors that contribute to social skills deficits: (1) lack of knowledge, (2) lack of practice or feedback, (3) lack of cues or opportunities, (4) lack of reinforcement, and (5) the presence of interfering problem behaviors. These five factors are highly salient to the social skill deficits in youth with ASD. Youth with ASD often exhibit lack of knowledge regarding basic social functioning, such as how to initiate interactions, respond to the initiations of others, read nonverbal cues, infer the thoughts and feelings of others, and regulate their physiologic response to stressful situations. Youth with ASD also lack opportunities to perform social skills because of a high degree of social withdrawal. Intense isolation may preclude the child from practicing newly learned skills. Poor social skills may also lead to negative peer interactions. As such, youth with ASD may receive little to no reinforcement from peers in social situations or, worse, experience frequent aversive interactions with peers. Finally, youth with ASD may exhibit interfering problem behaviors that significantly derail social interactions, such as behaving aggressively, making inappropriate comments, talking out of turn, or violating the personal space of others. Effective SST entails designing assessment practices to identify the factors contributing to the social failure of the child with ASD, and then delivering SST strategies to ameliorate the specific areas of deficiency.

Specific social skills training strategies

McConnell [14] provides a taxonomy of social skill interventions that forms a helpful guide for synthesizing strategies. According to McConnell, social skill interventions can be divided into five categories: (1) environmental modifications, (2) child-specific interventions, (3) collateral skills interventions, (4) peer-mediated interventions, and (5) comprehensive interventions. Environmental modifications involve modifications to the physical and social environment that promote social interactions between youth with ASD and their peers. Child-specific interventions involve the direct instruction of social behaviors, such as initiating and responding. Collateral skill interventions involve strategies that promote social interactions by delivering training in related skills, such as play behaviors and language, rather than training in specific social behaviors. Peer-mediated interventions involve training nondisabled peers to direct and respond to the social behaviors of youth with ASD. Finally, comprehensive interventions involve social skill interventions that combine two or more of the aforementioned intervention categories.

This section reviews SST strategies that have been empirically supported by research. The review does not represent an all-inclusive list of treatment modalities available for individuals with ASD. Instead, we focus exclusively on child-specific interventions or strategies that directly target the social behaviors of youth with ASD. Child-specific interventions were chosen because this category of intervention is delivered most commonly by practitioners in clinical settings. McConnell [14] stated that child-specific interventions include:

> (a) general instructional interventions to increase knowledge and improve social problem solving (including social stories), (b) high density reinforcement to 'prime' social responding, (c) social skills training, (d) adult-mediated prompting and reinforcement, [and] (e) various generalization promotion techniques, (particularly self-monitoring).

The following section summarizes SST strategies from each of these areas of programming, including social stories, video modeling interventions, social problem solving, pivotal response training, scripting procedures, computer-based interventions, priming procedures, prompting procedures, and self-monitoring. The section provides a summary of each intervention modality and a sampling of research studies that have documented their use with youth with ASD.

Social stories

A social story [15] is a commonly used strategy to teach social skills and social rules to youth with ASD. A social story presents social concepts and rules to children in the form of a brief story. A social story may be used to teach a number of social and behavioral concepts, such as initiating interactions, making transitions, attending a birthday party, or going on a field trip. Gray emphasizes that the story should be written in response to the child's personal need and that the story should be something the child wants to read on his or her own (depending upon ability level). She also stresses that the story should be commensurate with the child's ability and comprehension level.

Sansosti and colleagues [16] conducted a research synthesis of eight social story intervention studies. The researchers concluded that a social story is an effective intervention strategy for addressing the social, communicative, and behavioral functioning of youth with ASD. Kuoch and Mirenda [17] created social stories for three young males with ASD. The researchers wrote individual social stories for each child, and these stories were read to the children before situations where problem behavior typically occurred. Interventionists responded to problem behaviors by providing corrective, verbal feedback. All three children immediately reduced their rate of problem behaviors when the social story was implemented. Hagiwara and Myles [18] implemented an intervention using computer-based social stories for three individuals with ASD. During the school day, the elementary school children read and listened to stories targeting specific tasks on the computer screen, and then watched a brief movie clip showing them performing the task.

Video modeling interventions

A video modeling intervention typically involves an individual watching a video demonstration of positive behavior and then imitating the behavior of the model. Video modeling interventions integrate a powerful learning modality for children with ASD (visually cued instruction) with a widely investigated intervention strategy (modeling). Video self-modeling (VSM) is a specific application of video modeling where the individual learns by watching his or her own efficacious behavior. Video modeling and VSM have been used across multiple disciplines and populations to teach a wide variety of skills, including motor behaviors, social skills, communication skills, self-monitoring, functional skills, vocational skills, athletic skills, and skills related to emotional regulation [19].

Results of a recent meta-analysis suggest that video modeling and VSM are highly effective intervention strategies for addressing social-communication skills, behavioral functioning, and functional skills in youth with ASD [20]. Results demonstrate that video modeling and VSM effectively promote skill acquisition and that skills acquired via video modeling and VSM are maintained over time and transferred across persons and settings. A number of studies examined the efficacy of video modeling and VSM interventions in teaching social skills and play behaviors to youth with ASD. In one case, Bellini and colleagues [21] used VSM to increase social engagement of preschool children with ASD. The researchers recorded the children in a free play activity within their preschool classroom. Teachers were instructed to prompt and cue the children with ASD to interact with peers. The prompts and cues delivered by the teacher were subsequently edited out of the video to depict the children effectively and independently interacting with peers. The children viewed one video each school day for 4 weeks. Increases in social engagement were substantial and rapid, and were maintained after the videos were no longer shown. Buggey [22] examined the effects of VSM across a variety of social behaviors including language, social initiations, tantrums, and pushing behaviors. The various interventions primarily involved scripted role-playing procedures and, in one case, the recording of naturalistic behaviors. All five participants exhibited immediate and significant gains in social-communication and behavioral functioning. In addition, gains were maintained after the interventions were withdrawn.

Social problem solving

Many youth with ASD have difficulties interpreting and analyzing social situations. These difficulties are due to a number of factors, including lack of self-awareness, failure to read nonverbal and contextual cues, difficulties with perspective taking, and failure to understand social rules. These difficulties also stem from a lack of necessary schema to effectively analyze social situations. Social problem solving (SPS) refers to analyzing and interpreting social situations. SPS requires the child to make inferences based on available contextual cues. Youth with ASD routinely struggle with SPS because of difficulties reading nonverbal behavior (eg, facial expression and body language) and their inability to simultaneously attend to multiple contextual cues in their environment.

Research has demonstrated that SPS can be taught to youth with ASD [23]. Many different methods and techniques have been used to facilitate the development of social reasoning in youth with and without ASD [24]. Bernard-Opitz and colleagues [23] had children with ASD perform SPS tasks on a computer program called "I can Problem-Solve." Children were presented with social problems and choices of possible solutions. After several sessions, the children improved at problem solving, and appeared to enjoy using the program. A meta-analysis conducted by Beelman and colleagues [25] found that SPS strategies were effective in increasing performance on social problem tasks. However, a major limitation noted by the researchers was that these increases in SPS ability had no carryover effect to other areas of social functioning, such as specific social behaviors or skills. That is, SPS strategies may increase SPS, but their impact on social skills and social competence is questionable.

Pivotal response training

Pivotal response training (PRT) [26] is an intervention program based on the principles of applied behavioral analysis. PRT is used in natural

environments and capitalizes on the availability of naturally occurring reinforcers. PRT targets pivotal behaviors, which are behaviors that lead to
widespread changes in other behaviors and that facilitate transfer of skills
to multiple settings and collateral improvements in nontargeted behaviors.
PRT targets four pivotal areas: responsiveness to multiple cues, initiation,
motivation, and self-management. PRT teaches children to attend and
respond to multiple cues in the environment. Intervention in this area
teaches the child to select cues that are relevant in a given context or situation. Intervention in the initiation area teaches the child to effectively initiate
interactions with others. Intervention in the motivation area addresses the
child's lack of motivation related to social situations. Intervention includes
giving the child a choice in activity, using natural reinforcers, and reinforcing reasonable attempts at interacting. Interventions in self-management
teach the child to be more independent and less reliant on prompts from
others in his or her environment.

The efficacy of PRT has been supported by numerous research studies.
Humphries [27] conducted a research synthesis of 13 studies that investigated the effectiveness of PRT. Humphries concluded that PRT is an effective strategy for addressing the behavior, communication, and social
functioning of youth with ASD. Stahmer [28] used PRT with seven preschool-aged males either in school or at home to teach them to engage in
symbolic play behaviors. The PRT occurred three times a week. After the
training, each of the children was able to engage in more symbolic play
and in more complex play. Symon [29] trained the parents of young males
with ASD to perform PRT techniques during a weeklong intervention program. After the parent intervention, children's social communication and
behaviors improved during their interactions with caregivers.

Scripting procedures

Scripting involves the presentation of a structured "script" to the child
that provides an explicit description of what the child will say or do during
a social interaction [30]. The script may provide a narrative of what to say
during a conversation, or what to do during an activity. The script may contain the entire sequence of the interaction, or only the initiation. For
instance, the child might be taught a script for joining in an activity with
a peer who is also taught to respond in a scripted fashion. The benefits of
scripting for individuals with ASD have been demonstrated in research
involving both conversational scripts [31] and play scripts [32].

A major limitation of scripting is that the child may become dependent
upon the script and be unable to engage in spontaneous, unscripted interactions. Script-fading is a research-based practice designed to address this limitation [33]. Script-fading involves the introduction of a script to facilitate an
increase in social interactions, and then a systematic fading of the script over
time to promote maintenance and generalization. Goldstein and Cisar [34]

used script-training with three boys with ASD in the preschool classroom. Each student was put into a group with two typical peers. The groups were taught one sociodramatic script at a time, each of which had three roles. The trainer prompted the students to complete each script, moving to the next script once students were 80% correct or had spent 10 training sessions on a script. Both the students with and without ASD involved in the intervention had significantly improved social and communicative behavior in free play following the intervention. Stevenson and colleagues [35] used audiotaped scripts with four boys with ASD ages 10 to 15. Each boy was trained on imitating four- and five-word audiotaped scripts. The scripts were introduced in the classroom and then systematically faded. Recipients of the interactions responded to the students with elaborations of their statements or questions. All students increased speech of both scripted and unscripted statements following the intervention.

Computer-based interventions

Several methods of computer-based instruction have been created and implemented to teach children with delays in theory-of-mind development to acquire social cognitive skills. Programs, techniques, and classes have demonstrated positive outcomes in regards to theory-of-mind and perspective-taking skills. Various virtual environments, including computer-based interventions, have been used effectively to teach social skills to individuals with ASD [36–38].

Silver and Oakes [39] looked at the effects of a computer intervention on emotion recognition and prediction in youth with ASD. The computer presented a sequential progression of exercises involving facial expression recognition, situations that trigger emotions, characters wanting something and receiving something (sometimes, but not always, the same thing), mental states that trigger emotions, and likes/dislikes and possibly related events. Children using the program showed significant improvement both in the program and also on other assessment measures, including emotion-recognition cartoons and strange stories. Two studies have examined the effectiveness of *Mind Reading,* an interactive computer software program designed to teach individuals to recognize emotions through the use of video clips, photographs, voice recordings, lessons, and games involving individuals displaying a range of emotions [40,41]. Golan and Baron-Cohen [40] found that adults with ASD that used the program independently for at least 10 weeks showed marked improvement in recognizing emotions in pictures and voices presented similarly to the computer program, but had little positive change when presented with photographs of individual's eyes or film clips. Lacava and colleagues [41] found that youth with ASD who used the software for an average of 10.5 hours over 10 weeks showed small but statistically significant improvements in emotion recognition for faces and voices.

Priming procedures

Priming refers to the "incidental activation of knowledge structures" [42], which facilitates memory recall or behavioral performance. Social cognitions and social behaviors can be primed by presenting cognitive or behavioral "primes" just before performance of the skill or behavior in the natural environment. Cognitive priming strategies can be either visual (eg, pictures, videos, modeling, or visual prompts) or verbal instruction (eg, verbal description of the behavior, discussion of the behavior, or verbal prompts). Behavioral priming strategies involve behavioral rehearsal, or practicing the skill or behavior just before performing it in the natural environment.

The positive effects of priming to facilitate social behavior is supported by researchers who used priming to increase the social initiations of preschool children with ASD [43] and to decrease problem behaviors in the classroom [44]. Video priming has been used to reduce problem behaviors during transitions for youth with ASD [45]. The researchers selected transitions in settings deemed most problematic by the children's parents. The researchers then videotaped the settings to show the environment just as the child would see it (eg, moving through the store, getting ready in the morning). The children were not depicted in the video. Priming procedures are useful because they activate knowledge structures and facilitate social cognition and social behaviors for children with ASD.

Prompting procedures

Prompts are highly effective in facilitating child–adult and child–child interactions for youth with ASD [5,14]. Prompts are supports and assistance provided to the child to help him or her acquire skills and successfully perform behaviors. Prompts can be used to teach new social skills (in the case of physical and modeling prompts) and to improve previously acquired skills. In addition, they may be used with novice or advanced performers, in clinical and group settings, with verbal children or with nonverbal children, and with preschoolers or with adults. Prompts may be delivered by adults or by other children. A limitation of prompting strategies is that the child with ASD may limit social interactions to only instances in which prompting is provided. As such, a prompt-fading plan is typically implemented to systematically fade prompts.

Research on prompting procedures highlights the effectiveness of this modality. A school-based study used teacher prompting to increase social interactions for two males with ASD [46]. Students were individually brought into a room with typical peers who had been trained to respond to the target student's initiations but not to initiate to the student. They were seated within reach of several toys and instructed to play. The teacher was instructed to use increasingly intrusive prompts to encourage the target students to initiate to peers. One of the males increased his initiations to peers, while the other student increased social interactions but failed to increase initiations. Taylor and Levin [47] used two different kinds of prompting with a 9-year-old boy with ASD. In the first phase, an adult prompted the student to initiate verbal statements every minute. In the second phase, the boy was given a vibrating pager set to vibrate every 60 seconds, and instructed to talk about his play activities when it vibrated. Tactile prompting through the use of the vibrating pager was found to be highly effective in increasing the student's verbal initiations.

Self-monitoring

Self-monitoring strategies have demonstrated considerable effectiveness for teaching youth with and without disabilities to both monitor and regulate their own behavior [48]. This is a particularly important area to address in youth with ASD because of their significant deficits in self-awareness. Lack of self-awareness diminishes the child's ability to regulate and evaluate the quality of his or her behavioral performance. The strength of self-monitoring strategies is that they support generalization of skills by requiring children to independently monitor their own behavior. The self-recording of behavior can be used during the behavioral performance or after the performance (or both). Strategies can target a number of externalizing behaviors, such as time-on-task, work completion, and disruptive behaviors, as well as internal processes, such as thoughts (self-talk) and feelings (both positive and negative affect). Self-monitoring strategies may involve having the child record occurrences, duration, and frequencies of behaviors (whether the behavior was performed, for how long, how frequently it was performed) and the quality of the behavioral performance (how well the behavior was performed).

Self-monitoring strategies have been the focus of a number of research studies investigating the social and behavioral functioning of youth with ASD [49–51]. Shearer and colleagues [49] and Strain and colleagues [50] effectively used self-monitoring to increase the social interactions of young children with ASD. Both studies reported maintenance and generalization of targeted skills. Coyle and Cole [51] used self-monitoring in combination with VSM to decrease off-task behavior in school-aged children with ASD. The researchers video-recorded the children while they engaged in classroom tasks, then edited the video to include only on-task behavior. The video was then used to train the children to use a self-monitoring procedure targeting on-task behavior. The intervention led to substantial decreases in off-task behavior, and results were maintained after the intervention was removed.

Assessment of social functioning

Evaluation of social skills and social competence is a critical element of SST [52]. The purpose of the social skills assessment is to identify skill deficits that will be the direct target of the intervention, and to monitor the outcomes of the SST program. Gresham [12] divides social skills assessment methods into three categories that measure different levels of social functioning.

Type I measures include rating scales and interviews designed to measure social competence or perceptions of social performance. Type I measures are the most socially valid assessment measures because they directly measure the impressions of key stakeholders. That is, the results of type I measures represent the judgments of parents and teachers. As such, treatment objectives developed from these measures are likely to be accepted and viewed as socially acceptable by these key stakeholders. A major advantage of type I measures is their ability to efficiently obtain information regarding social behavior from a variety of sources and across a variety of settings. A major disadvantage of type I measures is that they are often not sensitive to short-term changes in behavior. For instance, the child might demonstrate an increase in the target behaviors without key stakeholders noticing these changes.

Type II measures involve the direct assessment of the child's social skills or social behaviors. As such, these measures are valuable to progress monitoring and are used extensively in applied research studies involving single-subject methodology. Type II measures are sensitive to small changes in behavior because they are linked directly to the treatment objectives. For instance, if the clinician identifies "joining-in activities with peers" as a treatment objective, he or she would then observe the child to measure whether "joining-in" behavior has increased over the course of the intervention. Determination of treatment effectiveness would then be based on changes in the target behavior.

Type III measures are the least valid assessment measures, but they still have clinical utility. Type III measures involve conducting role-play scenarios or asking questions related to social cognition. For instance, for teaching a child to effectively respond to bullying, the clinician could set up a role-play scenario that requires the child to deal effectively with a bully; or, for teaching perspective taking to a child, the clinician could set up a role-play that requires the child to infer the thoughts or feelings of another person. Though these are important areas to address via intervention, and should be measured via assessment, research has demonstrated that these measures are not related to measures of social competence (type I measures) or measures of social skills (type II measures).

Available assessment tools

Social skills assessment often involves a combination of observations (both naturalistic and structured), interviews (eg, parents, teachers, child), and social skill rating forms (parent, teacher, and self reports). The following section focuses on the use of rating scales as these are most commonly used by researchers and clinicians to measure social competence in youth with ASD. A major advantage of rating scales is their ability to quickly and efficiently obtain large quantities of information regarding social behavior from a variety of sources and across a variety of settings [53]. This is especially important for clinicians who may not have the opportunity to monitor children in nonclinical settings. The use of rating scales can also increase the social validity of the social skills program when information gleaned from the assessment is linked directly to the development of treatment goals and objectives [12].

The Social Skills Rating System (SSRS) [13] is a widely used measure of social competence. This questionnaire provides information on the social competence of youth ages 3 to 18. The SSRS has been used in studies examining the social skills of individuals with ASD [52,54–56]. A limitation of the SSRS (and other well-established social competence measures) in its use with youth with ASD is that the measure was designed for a broad population of children. Thus, few of the items address the unique pattern of social behavior exhibited by youth with ASD, which limits the questionnaire's utility as an intervention planning tool. Another major disadvantage of most rating scales is that they are often insensitive to small changes in behavior [12,53]. Use of norm-referenced rating scales may not detect improvements in social behavior in youth with ASD, at least initially, because the normative group is comprised of a general population of children. Though the child with ASD might be making steady improvements in social behavior, his or her standard score on the rating scale may remain quite low because the child's behavior is being compared with that of a general population of children.

The Social Responsiveness Scale (SRS) [57] is currently the only commercially available social competency measure designed specifically for youth with ASD. The SRS is a well-studied instrument with sound psychometric properties [58,59]. The SRS was designed as a diagnostic tool and as a treatment-monitoring tool. The SRS is a 65-item measure that covers social behaviors in addition to items related to other areas of autistic symptomatology, such as preoccupations, and other repetitive, stereotypical behaviors. The SRS contains five subscales: Receptive, Cognitive, Expressive, Motivational Aspects of Social Behavior, and Preoccupations. The SRS is based on a normative sample of more than 1600 children (4–18 years of age) from the general population.

The Autism Social Skills Profile (ASSP) [60] is a new assessment tool that provides a comprehensive measure of social competence for youth with ASD. The ASSP was designed for use as an intervention planning and monitoring tool. The items on the ASSP represent a broad range of social behaviors typically exhibited by individuals with ASD, including initiation skills, social reciprocity, perspective-taking, and nonverbal communication skills. The ASSP was designed for use with youth with ASD between the ages of 6 and 17. A preliminary analysis of the psychometric properties of the ASSP with 340 youths with ASD indicated that the instrument has strong validity and reliability for this age group [61]. Factor analysis revealed three underlying dimensions, or subscales, for the ASSP: Social Reciprocity, Social Participation/Avoidance, and Detrimental Social Behaviors. Though it contains only 49 items, the ASSP provides a thorough and comprehensive assessment of social competence. For instance, the ASSP has over 10 items that measure different social initiation skills for youth with ASD (eg, "Joins in activities with peers," "Initiates greetings," "Asks others to join him/her in activities," "Asks questions about other persons"). This precision is essential to the elucidation of specific skills that will be the direct target of intervention.

Meta-analytic reviews of social skills training

Gresham and colleagues [12] concluded that meta-analytic reviews of SST have yielded a wide variety of results, ranging from ineffectual to highly effective interventions. Based on their review of the literature, the investigators provided a number of recommendations for promoting effective social skill interventions. First, the researchers recommended that SST should be implemented more frequently and more intensely than what is typically implemented. They concluded that 30 hours of instruction, spread over 10 to 12 weeks, is not enough. Second, they concluded that a major weakness of social skill interventions is a failure to produce adequate maintenance and generalization effects. Gresham and colleagues attributed this, in part, to the fact that social skills training often takes place in "contrived, restricted, and decontextualized" settings, such as resource rooms or other "pullout" settings. Third, the researchers posited that the ineffectiveness of many social skills programs is a result of the interventionists' failure to match the social skill strategy to the type of skill deficit presented. This information allows the interventionist to determine whether he or she should teach new skills to the child or enhance the performance of existing skills. In addition, the researchers concluded that the traditionally weak treatment effects of SST may be the result of interventions that fail to link assessment data with the development of intervention objectives. Assessments that lack reliability and validity hinder the clinician's ability to identify relevant and critical skills to teach and to accurately monitor progress. Finally, Gresham and colleagues found that few meta-analytic studies reported evidence that interventions were implemented as intended. This absence of fidelity data makes it extremely difficult to conclude whether a social skill intervention was ineffective due to an ineffectual intervention strategy or because it was implemented poorly.

Bellini and colleagues [62] conducted the only meta-analysis of SST for youth with ASD. The meta-analysis included 55 published research studies investigating school-based SST for youth with ASD. The reviewed studies included 147 students with ASD ranging from preschool to secondary school. The purpose of the meta-analysis was to measure the collective outcomes of school-based SST for youth with ASD, and to identify factors that lead to more beneficial outcomes. Results of the meta-analysis suggested that school-based SST is only minimally effective for children with ASD. Specifically, SST produced low treatment effects and low generalization effects across persons and settings. Moderate maintenance effects were observed, suggesting that when gains were made via SST, the gains were maintained after the intervention was withdrawn. The low treatment effects observed in the study are consistent with the results of previous meta-analyses conducted on SST for other populations of children [63–65].

Similar intervention, maintenance, and generalization effects were observed among interventions measuring collateral skills (eg, play skills, joint attention, and language skills) and interventions measuring specific social behaviors (eg, social initiations, social responses, and duration of interaction). There were no significant differences between the outcomes of studies that implemented group interventions and studies that implemented individual interventions, nor were there significant differences across the various types of interventions (eg, environmental modifications, child-specific interventions, collateral skills interventions, peer-mediated interventions, and comprehensive interventions). The length and duration of interventions varied considerably across studies. Hours of intervention ranged from 2.5 to 28 hours (median 7.25 hours), well below the dosage recommendation of Gresham and colleagues. Only 14 of the studies in the meta-analysis measured whether the intervention was implemented as intended, which makes interpretation of results problematic. Finally, only one study systematically matched the type of intervention strategy with the type of skill deficit exhibited by participants. An important finding of the study was that students receiving SST in their typical classroom setting had substantially higher treatment, maintenance, and generalization effects than did students who received services in a pullout setting. This finding supports the recommendation of Gresham and colleagues to deliver SST in the child's natural environment.

The results of the meta-analysis help to elucidate factors that lead to more beneficial social outcomes for youth with ASD. In addition, by synthesizing the results of the Bellini and colleagues meta-analysis and the Gresham and colleagues study, we are better able to determine the ingredients for effective SST, and thus make the following recommendations for programming: (1) Increase the dosage of social skill interventions, (2) provide instruction within the child's natural setting, (3) match the intervention strategy with the type of skill deficit, and (4) ensure intervention fidelity.

Gresham and colleagues noted that 30 hours of SST for 10 to 12 weeks is not enough for effective interventions. Though research has yet to identify specific dosage guidelines for SST for youth with ASD who exhibit significant social skill deficits, the recommendation by Gresham and colleagues should be considered a minimum dosage requirement for this population. This recommendation should not be interpreted as advocating for 30 hours of one-on-one SST with a clinician. On the contrary, SST should not stop the moment the child leaves the clinic facility; it should be ubiquitous. SST should be taught across many settings and with as many people as possible, including clinicians, family members, educators, and peers. Every setting the child enters provides an opportunity to teach social skills. Training across a variety of persons and settings avoids the common pitfall of many SST programs that train exclusively in contrived settings. It is also important to note that this recommendation does not preclude clinicians from implementing SST in clinical settings. However, as discussed previously, clinicians in these settings should look for opportunities to promote transfer of skills across other settings and persons. This is effectively done by partnering with parents, educators, and other service providers via a reciprocal exchange of information and resources. Matching strategy with type of skill deficit requires the clinician to discern between a skill acquisition deficit and performance deficit. A performance deficit refers to a skill or behavior that is present, but not demonstrated or performed, whereas a skill-acquisition deficit refers to the absence of a particular skill or behavior. This is a critical component of SST as it guides the clinician's selection of intervention strategies. For instance, if the child does not possess the requisite knowledge to join in an activity with peers (skill-acquisition deficit), then the clinician should select strategies designed to teach a new skill. If the child has the ability to join in activities, but fails to do so (performance deficit), then the clinician should select strategies to enhance the performance of this existing skill. Bellini [52] provides a comprehensive discussion of techniques for discerning between a skill-acquisition deficit and performance deficit and outlines a number of SST strategies for targeting these two types of deficits. Finally, researchers and clinicians should strive to collect data on treatment fidelity. Lack of treatment fidelity data makes it virtually impossible to determine if the low treatment effects were the result of ineffectual strategies, or of poorly implemented strategies. Given that few clinicians and educators receive adequate training in SST as part of their graduate or medical school training, it is probable that the failure of many SST programs is a result of poorly implemented strategies. Clinicians implementing SST program may also need to receive ongoing continuing education to develop and hone their skills in this area.

Summary

Social skill deficits are a pervasive and enduring feature of ASD. As such, SST should be a critical component of programming for youth with ASD. An essential first step of SST is to identify the skills that will be targeted during intervention. This is done through social skills assessment. The use of reliable and valid rating forms helps the clinician identify skills to target, and provides a measure of treatment progress. A number of SST strategies are available to clinicians with varying degrees of empiric support. The results of meta-analytic research suggest that SST programs should be intensive, be implemented in natural settings, include strategies that match type of skill deficit, and ensure intervention fidelity.

References

[1] Attwood T. Asperger's syndrome: a guide for parents and professionals. Philadelphia: Kingsley; 1998.
[2] Baron-Cohen S. The autistic child's theory of mind: a case of specific developmental delay. J Child Psychol Psychiatry 1989;30:285–97.
[3] Brown J, Whiten A. Imitation, theory of mind and related activities in autism: an observational study of spontaneous behaviour in everyday contexts. Autism 2000;4:185–205.
[4] Dawson G, Fernald M. Perspective taking ability and its relationship to the social behavior of autistic children. J Autism Dev Disord 1987;17:487–9.
[5] Rogers S. Interventions that facilitate socialization in children with autism. J Autism Dev Disord 2000;30:399–409.
[6] American Psychiatric Association. Diagnostic and statistical manual of mental disorders. 4th edition. Washington, DC: American Psychiatric Association; 2000. p. 75.
[7] World Health Organization. The ICD-10 classification of mental and behavioural disorders. Geneva (Switzerland): World Health Organization; 1992.
[8] Bellini S. The development of social anxiety in high functioning adolescents with autism spectrum disorders. Focus Autism Other Dev Disabl 2006;21:138–45.
[9] Tantam D. Psychological disorder in adolescents and adults with Asperger syndromeAutism 2000;4:47–62.
[10] Welsh M, Park RD, Widaman K, et al. Linkages between children's social and academic competence: a longitudinal analysis. J Sch Psychol 2001;39(6):463–81.
[11] Elliot SN, Gresham FM. Social skills interventions for children. Behav Modif 1993;17: 287–313.
[12] Gresham FM, Sugai G, Horner RH. Interpreting outcomes of social skills training for students with high-incidence disabilities. Teaching Exceptional Children 2001;67:331–44.
[13] Gresham FM, Elliot SN. Social skills rating system manual. Circle Pines (MN): American Guidance Service; 1990.
[14] McConnell SR. Interventions to facilitate social interaction for young children with autism: review of available research and recommendations for educational intervention and future research. J Autism Dev Disord 2002;32:351–72.
[15] Gray C. The new social story book: illustrated edition. Arlington (TX): Future Horizons; 2000.
[16] Sansosti FJ, Powell-Smith KA, Kincaid D. A research synthesis of social story interventions for children with autism spectrum disorders. Focus Autism Other Dev Disabl 2004;19: 194–204.
[17] Kuoch H, Mirenda P. Social story interventions for young children with autism spectrum disorders. Focus Autism Other Dev Disabl 2003;18(4):219–27.
[18] Hagiwara T, Myles BS. A multimedia social story intervention: teaching skills to children with autism. Focus Autism Other Dev Disabl 1999;14(2):82–95.
[19] Dowrick P. A review of self-modeling and related interventions. Appl Prev Psychol 1999;8: 23–39.
[20] Bellini S, Akullian J. A meta-analysis of video modeling and video self-modeling interventions for children and adolescents with autism spectrum disorders. Except Child 2007;73: 261–84.
[21] Bellini S, Akullian J, Hopf A. Increasing social engagement in young children with autism spectrum disorders using video self-modeling. School Psych Rev 2007;36:80–90.

[22] Buggey T. Video self-modeling applications with children with autism spectrum disorder in a small private school. Focus Autism Other Dev Disabl 2005;20(1):52–63.

[23] Bernard-Opitz V, Sriram N, Nakhoda-Sapuan S. Enhancing social problem solving in children with autism and normal children through computer-assisted instruction. J Autism Dev Disord 2001;31:377–84.

[24] Elias MJ, Butler LB, Bruno EM, et al. Social decision making/social problem solving: a curriculum for academic, social, and emotional learning. Champaign (IL): Research Press; 2005.

[25] Beelman A, Pfingsten U, Losel F. Effects of training social competence in children: A meta-analysis of recent evaluation studies. J Clin Child Adolesc Psychol 1994;213:260–71.

[26] Koegel RL, Koegel LK. Pivotal response treatment for autism: communication, social, academic development. Baltimore (MD): Paul Brookes; 2006.

[27] Humphries A. Effectiveness of PRT as a behavioral intervention for young children with ASD. Bridges practice-based research syntheses 2003;2(4):1–10.

[28] Stahmer AC. Teaching symbolic play skills to children with autism using pivotal response training. J Autism Dev Disord 1995;25(2):123–41.

[29] Symon JB. Expanding interventions for children with autism: parents as trainers. Journal of Positive Behavior Interventions 2005;7(3):159–73.

[30] Mayo P, Waldo P. Scripting: social communication for adolescents. Eau Claire (WI): Thinking Publications; 1994.

[31] Loveland KA, Tunali B. Social scripts for conversational interactions in autism and Down syndrome. J Autism Dev Disord 1991;21:177–86.

[32] MacDonald R, Clark M, Garrigan E. Using video modeling to teach pretend play to children with autism. Behav Interv 2005;20(4):225–38.

[33] Krantz PJ, McClannahan LE. Teaching children with autism to initiate to peers: effects of a script-fading procedure. J Appl Behav Anal 1993;26:121–32.

[34] Goldstein H, Cisar CL. Promoting interaction during sociodramatic play: teaching scripts to typical preschoolers and classmates with disabilities. J Appl Behav Anal 1992;25(2):265–80.

[35] Stevenson CL, Krantz PJ, McClannahan LE. Social interaction skills for children with autism: a script-fading procedure for nonreaders. Behav Interv 2000;15(1):1–20.

[36] Mitchell P, Parsons S, Leonard A. Using virtual environments for teaching social understanding to 6 adolescents with autistic spectrum disorders. J Autism Dev Disord 2007;37: 589–600.

[37] Moore D, Cheng Y, McGrath P, et al. Collaborative virtual environment technology for people with autism. Focus Autism Other Dev Disabl 2005;20(4):231–43.

[38] Parsons S, Leonard A, Mitchell P. Virtual environments for social skills training: comments from two adolescents with autistic spectrum disorder. Computers & Education 2006;47: 186–206.

[39] Silver M, Oakes P. Evaluation of a new computer intervention to teach people with autism or Asperger syndrome to recognize and predict emotion in others. Autism 2001;5(3):299–316.

[40] Golan O, Baron-Cohen S. Systemizing empathy: teaching adults with Asperger syndrome or high-functioning autism to recognize complex emotions using interactive multimedia. Dev Psychopathol 2006;18:591–617.

[41] Lacava PG, Golan O, Baron-Cohen S, et al. Using assistive technology to teach emotion recognition to students with Asperger syndrome. Remedial and Special Education 2007;28(3): 174–81.

[42] Bargh JA, Chen M, Burrows L. The automaticity of social behaviour: direct effects of trait concept and stereotype activation on action. J Pers Soc Psychol 1996;71:230–44.

[43] Zanolli K, Daggett J, Adams T. Teaching preschool age autistic children to make spontaneous initiations to peers using priming. J Autism Dev Disord 1996;2:407–22.

[44] Koegel LK, Koegel RL, Frea W, et al. Priming as a method of coordinating educational services for students with autism. Lang Speech Hear Serv Sch 2003;34:228–35.

[45] Schreibman L, Whalen C, Stahmer A. The use of video priming to reduce disruptive transition behavior in children with autism. Journal of Positive Behavior Interventions 2000;2:3–12.

[46] Gunter P, Fox JJ, Brady MP, et al. Nonhandicapped peers as multiple exemplars: a generalization tactic for promoting autistic students' social skills. Behav Disord 1988;13(2):116–26.

[47] Taylor BA, Levin L. Teaching a student with autism to make verbal initiations: effects of a tactile prompt. J Appl Behav Anal 1998;31(4):651–4.

[48] Carter JF. Self management: education's ultimate goal. Teaching Exceptional Children. 1993;25(3):28–33.

[49] Shearer DD, Kohler FW, Buchan KA, et al. Promoting independent interactions between preschoolers with autism and their nondisabled peers: an analysis of self-monitoring. Early Educ Dev 1996;7:205–20.

[50] Strain PS, Kohler FW, Storey K, et al. Teaching preschoolers with autism to self-monitor their social interactions. J Emot Behav Disord 1994;2:78–88.

[51] Coyle C, Cole P. A videotaped self-modeling and self-monitoring treatment program to decrease off-task behaviour in children with autism. J Intellect Dev Disabil 2004;29(1):3–15.

[52] Bellini S. Building social relationships: a systematic approach to teaching social interaction skills to children and adolescents with autism spectrum disorders and other social difficulties. Shawnee Mission (KS): Autism Asperger Publishing; 2006.

[53] Elliott SN, Malecki CK, Demaray MK. New directions in social skills assessment and intervention for elementary and middle school students. Exceptionality 2001;9:19–32.

[54] Bellini S. Social skills and anxiety in higher functioning adolescents with autism spectrum disorders. Focus Autism Other Dev Disabl 2004;19(3):78–86.

[55] Koning C, Magill-Evans J. Social and language skills in adolescent boys with Asperger syndrome. Autism 2001;5:23–36.

[56] Ozonoff S, Miller JN. Teaching theory of mind—a new approach to social skills training for individuals with autism. J Autism Dev Disord 1995;25(4):415–33.

[57] Constantino JN, Gruber CP. The Social responsiveness scale (SRS) manual. Los Angeles (CA): Western Psychological Services; 2005.

[58] Constantino JN, Davis SA, Todd RD, et al. Validation of a brief quantitative measure of autistic traits: comparison of the social responsiveness scale with the autism diagnostic interview—revised. J Autism Dev Disord 2003;33:427–33.

[59] Constantino JN, Gruber CP, Davis S, et al. The factor structure of autistic traits. J Child Psychol Psychiatry 2004;45:719–26.

[60] Bellini S. The Autism social skills profile. Shawnee Mission (KS): Autism Asperger Publishing, in press.

[61] Bellini S, Hopf A. Assessing the psychometric properties of the autism social skills profile. Focus Autism Other Dev Disabl 2007;22:80–7.

[62] Bellini S, Peters J, Benner L, et al. A meta-analysis of school-based social skill interventions for children with autism spectrum disorders. Remedial and Special Education 2007;28: 153–62.

[63] Forness SR, Kavale KA. Treating social skills deficits in children with learning disabilities: a meta-analysis of the research. Learn Disabil Q 1996;19:2–13.

[64] Mathur SR, Kavale KA, Quinn MM, et al. Social skills interventions with students with emotional and behavioral problems. A quantitative synthesis of single subject research Behav Disord 1998;23:193–201.

[65] Quinn MM, Kavale KA, Mathur SR, et al. A meta-analysis of social skills interventions for students with emotional and behavioral disorders. J Emot Behav Disord 1999;7:54–64.

ELSEVIER
SAUNDERS

Child Adolesc Psychiatric Clin N Am
17 (2008) 875–886

CHILD AND
ADOLESCENT
PSYCHIATRIC CLINICS
OF NORTH AMERICA

Behavioral Assessment and Treatment of Self-Injurious Behavior in Autism

Noha F. Minshawi, PhD[a,b,*]

[a]*Indiana University School of Medicine, 702 Barnhill Drive, Room 4300,
Indianapolis, IN 46202, USA*
[b]*Christian Sarkine Autism Treatment Center, James Whitcomb Riley
Hospital for Children, 702 Barnhill Drive, Room 4300, Indianapolis, IN 46202, USA*

Among one of the most challenging issues related to working with individuals who have autism is the presence of self-injurious behaviors (SIB). These behaviors warrant clinical and research attention because they place the individuals who have autism and people around them at risk for physical harm [1]. In addition, individuals who have maladaptive behaviors, such as SIB, aggression, and disruptions, are more likely to be placed in residential, as opposed to community, settings [2,3]. Therefore, accurate assessment and effective treatment are imperative [1,4]. The purpose of this article is to review the definition, prevalence, etiology, assessment, and treatment of SIB in individuals who have autism.

Definition of self-injurious behaviors

Self-injury is considered one of the most dangerous problems in individuals who have autism. The term, *SIB*, refers to a wide range of behaviors. The two most frequently occurring forms of SIB in individuals who have developmental disabilities are self-hitting or banging directed at the head or face and self-biting [5]. Other common topographies include scratching, pinching, and poking [6]. The *Diagnostic and Statistical Manual of Mental Disorders, Fourth Edition, Text Revision* [7] introduced a diagnostic code for SIB as a specifier for stereotypic movement disorder (SMD). SMD is diagnosed when an individual displays repetitive, nonfunctional motor behaviors (eg, body rocking, hand shaking, or self-hitting). This behavior must interfere significantly with normal activities or result in self-inflicted

* Christian Sarkine Autism Treatment Center, James Whitcomb Riley Hospital for Children, 702 Barnhill Drive, Room 4300, Indianapolis, IN 46202.
E-mail address: nminshaw@iupui.edu

1056-4993/08/$ - see front matter © 2008 Elsevier Inc. All rights reserved.
doi:10.1016/j.chc.2008.06.012   *childpsych.theclinics.com*

injury that requires medical attention. SMD should not be diagnosed when the behaviors are better accounted for by a compulsion, such as obsessive-compulsive disorder, a tic disorder, or trichotillomania. Additionally, the behavior cannot be a stereotypy that is associated with a pervasive developmental disorder, such as body rocking or hand flapping in autism, because these behaviors are part of the diagnosis. Finally, the behavior must be present for at least 4 weeks and cannot be the result of the direct physiologic effects of a substance or a general medical condition [7].

Prevalence

Individuals who have intellectual and developmental disabilities are susceptible to a wide range of destructive and problematic behaviors, including aggression, SIB, and property destruction [8]. Individuals who have intellectual disabilities (ID) are shown to engage in more disruptive and dangerous behavior than individuals who have normal intellectual and adaptive functioning [9]. Researchers have estimated that 17% of individuals in residential facilities engage in some form of SIB [10], whereas only 1.7% of individuals living in community settings engage in SIB [11]. Several studies have evaluated the relationship between SIB and level of intellectual functioning and found that they are negatively correlated [6,12]. Rojahn and colleagues [13] reported a sample in which 4% of individuals who had mild ID evinced SIB compared with 7% of those who had moderate ID, 16% who had severe ID, and 25% who had profound ID.

Researchers have concluded further that SIB is a greater problem in individuals who have autism as compared with those who have other developmental and ID. Bodfish and coworkers [14] reported that individuals who had autism engaged in more severe self-injury than their age-, gender-, and IQ-matched controls. Self-injury also is shown to be more common in children who have autism than in those who have language impairments alone [15]. In children who have autism, SIB has been found associated with deficits in adaptive and communicative skills [16,17].

Learning theory basis for self-injurious behaviors

Proponents of a learning theory basis of SIB suggest that these are behaviors that are shaped, strengthened, and maintained through positive and negative reinforcement [9,18]. Two hypotheses are proposed to account for the initial development and the maintenance of SIB and other maladaptive behaviors. Both hypotheses are based on the theoretic concept that maladaptive behaviors "function" as a means of obtaining reinforcement from the environment.

The first learning theory hypothesis states that SIB develops in response to a lack of environmental stimulation. When engaging in the behavior is met with positive consequences from the environment, positive reinforcement is believed to maintain the behavior for those individuals. This contingent positive reinforcement increases the likelihood that the behavior will reoccur in the future [19]. Lovaas and Simmons [20] demonstrated that in some individuals SIB ceased to engage in these behaviors when they were isolated from other people and, therefore, received no social attention. Common positive consequences for SIB are social attention [21,22] and access to preferred tangible items [23] that are provided contingent on the occurrence of SIB.

In some cases, SIB may provide sufficient sensory stimulation to make the behavior itself reinforcing [24–26]. For some individuals, SIB is shown to occur regardless of environmental consequences (eg, attention, escape from demands, or access to tangible items). Instead, SIB can be maintained by the sensory reinforcement that the behavior itself invokes [24]. This function typically is referred to as sensory or automatic reinforcement based on the lack of external stimulation and reliance on internal sensory stimulation.

A second learning hypothesis states that SIB reduces levels of stress, discomfort, or frustration [18]. This hypothesis is supported by research indicating an increase in the rate of problem behaviors after the induction of frustration [27]. Other researchers have shown that maladaptive behaviors, including SIB, can be increased or decreased based on the presentation or removal of difficult tasks [28–30]. Self-injury, therefore, may serve as a means of escaping or avoiding aversive internal and environmental stimuli [9]. Over time, these behaviors are shaped further through negative reinforcement, commonly in the form of escape or avoidance of demands [19].

In summary, learning theorists suggest that SIB and other problem behaviors are learned based on interactions that individuals experience in their environment. Self-injury, therefore, is believed to serve one or more specific functions for individuals. These functions are named based on the type of reinforcement individuals receive for engaging in a problem behavior. The primary types of reinforcement received aresocial attention from others, escape from demands, access to preferred tangible items, and sensory or automatic reinforcement. In addition, maladaptive behaviors can serve more than one of these functions for individuals and can be maintained by combinations of positive and negative reinforcement [31].

In a recent review of single-subject research studies, Hanley and colleagues [32] reported that 25.3% of studies found that problem behaviors were maintained by attention, 15.8% by nonsocial reinforcement and 10.1% by access to tangible items. In addition, 14.6% of studies identified multiple functions in that participants engaged in problem behaviors for more than one reason. Because the behavioral treatment of SIB is based on the functions that maintain an individual's SIB, accurate assessment of SIB is crucial to developing an effective behavioral intervention.

Behavioral assessment

The assessment of SIB in individuals who have developmental disabilities has received a great deal of attention from researchers. The majority of assessment research has been conducted using the learning theory model of the etiology and maintenance of SIB. The term, *functional assessment*, is used to describe methods of evaluating the function that a behavior serves for a particular individual. The purpose of a functional assessment is to determine the antecedents and consequences that support the occurrence of these behaviors. Functional assessment can be conducted with a variety of methods depending on individual needs of a client and the resources available to clinicians. The functional assessment of SIB can be grouped into three general categories: indirect assessments, descriptive analysis, and experimental functional analysis (EFA).

Indirect assessment

Rating scales

Several rating scales have been developed for the functional assessment of SIB and other maladaptive behaviors in individuals who have developmental disabilities. Two of the rating scales that have been thoroughly studied are the Motivation Assessment Scale (MAS) [33] and the Questions About Behavior Functions (QABF) [34]. The MAS assesses four categories of reinforcement: access to tangible items or activities, attention, escape from demands, and sensory or automatic reinforcement. Initial studies of small samples of children found high inter-rater and test-retest reliability, good factor structure, and good psychometrics [23]. Further studies failed to replicate these findings in a residential setting, however, and instead reported poor internal consistency and poor inter-rater reliability [35].

The QABF is an informant-based questionnaire that contains five subscales of behavior function: (1) attention, (2) escape from demand, (3) access to tangible reinforcers, (4) physical discomfort, and (5) automatic or sensory reinforcement [34]. Researchers have found that the QABF has good inter-rater and test-retest reliability for individuals who have ID in residential facilities [36]. Additionally, the five-factor structure of the QABF has been shown to account for 76% of score variance [36]. The QABF has been validated against functions derived from other assessment methods [37].

Interview

According to Iwata and coworkers [38], a functional assessment interview provides a description of the behavior, situations in which the behavior is most and least likely to occur, antecedents, and consequences. O'Neill and colleagues [39] are credited with designing one of the most comprehensive of these interviews. The interview usually is conducted with parents, teachers, and caregivers serving as informants. In O'Neill and colleagues' [39] framework, all undesirable behaviors are identified and operationally defined.

Environmental variables, such as medications, sleep cycles, daily routines and activities, and staffing patterns, also are considered. Clinicians evaluate the information obtained and develop hypotheses regarding the functions that behaviors serve for individuals. These hypotheses can be explored further through the use of additional functional assessment methods [39].

Descriptive analysis

The term, *descriptive analysis*, refers to the observation of target behaviors (eg, aggression or SIB) in the natural environment. The direct observation of target behaviors, their antecedents, and their consequences is a hallmark of functional assessment [40]. The descriptive analysis of aggression, SIB, and other maladaptive behaviors can include many methods of collection and presentation, such as frequency counts [19], partial interval recording [41], and scatter plot analysis [42].

Another commonly used form of descriptive analysis is antecedent-behavior-consequence (ABC) observations. ABC observations serve this purpose by collecting data regarding the frequency of the target behavior and information about the behavior's antecedents and consequences. Parents, teachers, and residential staff can conduct these observations using simple ABC checklists. Once this information is collected, an examiner is able to determine how many times a target behavior was preceded by a specific antecedent (eg, an instructional demand) or followed by a specific consequence (eg, access to a preferred item). These results then are summarized as probabilities or percentages of behavior occurring under certain antecedents and consequence conditions [43].

Experimental functional analysis

Although indirect and descriptive assessments provide valuable information, they are unable to establish direct cause-and-effect relationships between a behavior and the environment [43]. EFA was developed to address this limitation through the systematic, controlled experimental analysis of the impact of different conditions on the target behavior. The EFA methodology developed by Iwata and colleagues [5,22] consists of exposing individuals who have aggression, SIB, and other maladaptive behaviors to several potential maintaining conditions (consequences) in a controlled (analog) environment. The conditions are presented contingent on individuals engaging in the target behavior. The consequences used most commonly in EFA are attention, escape from demand, tangible objects, sensory or automatic reinforcement, and a control condition [5]. Conditions are presented in a multi-element or reversal design [40] and the frequency of the target behavior under each condition is recorded and graphed. Visual inspection of the graph is used to determine under which conditions the target behavior occurs most frequently. These conditions then are considered to be the function the target behavior serves for an individual.

Behavioral treatment

A variety of behavioral treatments for SIB have been proposed and are supported by empiric research. These techniques are based on their ability to increase positive, adaptive behavior or decrease undesirable behavior. The behavioral treatment of SIB can be divided into those based on the principles of reinforcement, extinction, punishment, and skill building. These procedures rarely are used in isolation, however, and often are combined within a treatment package.

Reinforcement-based treatments

Most researchers agree that when designing a behavioral intervention for SIB or other maladaptive behaviors, the first approach should be the least restrictive option available that still results in behavior reduction [44]. In most cases, this approach is the use of reinforcement principles. Several reinforcement schedules are empirically supported for use in severe behavior problems. Reinforcement can be scheduled to occur at a continuous interval without regard for whether or not individuals are engaging in appropriate behavior or SIB. This type of reinforcement is called noncontingent reinforcement (NCR) because the availability of reinforcement is not contingent on the behavior of an individual. Many schedules, however, are based on the concept of differential reinforcement. That is, the appropriate behaviors an individual engages in are reinforced and the target behaviors are ignored based on a pre-identified schedule. In the differential reinforcement of other behaviors (DRO), individuals are reinforced for not engaging in SIB for a set period of time [45].

Vollmer and colleagues [46] demonstrated the usefulness of NCR and DRO in two boys who had autism and ID who engaged in SIB. Functional analysis of both individuals' SIB indicated an escape function (ie, behaviors were maintained by negative reinforcement in the form of a break from demands). In the NCR condition, the participants received breaks from learning demands on a fixed-interval schedule regardless of whether or not they were engaging in SIB at the time reinforcement was delivered. In the DRO condition, the participants were provided with a break from learning demands for not engaging in SIB for a prespecified period of time. Vollmer and colleagues [46] reported that both reinforcement conditions resulted in significant decreases in SIB for both individuals.

Other variations include the differential reinforcement of incompatible behaviors (DRI) and the differential reinforcement of low rates of behavior (DRL). In a DRI schedule, individuals are provided with reinforcement for engaging in a behavior that is not compatible with the target behaviors. In a DRL schedule, a predetermined acceptable rate of SIB is established and individuals receive reinforcement for engaging in a rate at or lower than that predetermined rate. In reinforcement schedules, reinforcement can come in the form of social attention, access to preferred items or activities, or a brief break from demands [47].

Extinction-based treatments

Inherent in the differential reinforcement schedules is the concept of extinction. Extinction is defined as no longer providing reinforcement for a response that was previously reinforced [19]. By terminating the contingency between the response and the reinforcement, extinction procedures result in a decreased probability that the response will occur again. Extinction is a common component of many behavioral interventions and demonstrated as highly effective in the treatment of SIB and other maladaptive behaviors [48]. In addition, extinction is shown to be the crucial component in the efficacy of other interventions, such as functional communication training (FCT) [49].

Extinction procedures are selected based on the results of a functional analysis of SIB. Once the function of a behavior is determined, extinction procedures are implemented to address that function. For example, if SIB is shown to be reinforced by social attention from other people in the environment, then no longer providing attention contingent on SIB (ie, planned ignoring) is the extinction procedure selected. Furthermore, if escape from demands is maintaining SIB for an individual, then extinction comes in the form of continuously presenting demands regardless of the occurrence of SIB [50].

A form of extinction frequently used for severe forms of SIB that are maintained by sensory reinforcement is protective equipment. Protective equipment (eg, helmets, face shields, and gloves) frequently is recommended for dangerous forms of SIB that could result in tissue damage or severe injury. Protective equipment, however, also is used as a method of reducing behavior maintained by sensory reinforcement [51]. The rationale behind the use of protective equipment is that if the SIB functions to provide positive reinforcement in the form of sensory experiences, then protective equipment serves as an extinction procedure by blocking that positive reinforcement.

Moore and coworkers [52] recently demonstrated the effectiveness of protective equipment in a young girl who had multiple topographies of SIB. The participant's shoulders and legs were padded with foam and gloves placed on her hands. This padding provided protection from injury and blocked sensory reinforcement but did not restrict the participant's ability to engage in SIB (ie, equipment did not serve as a form of restraint). These researchers found that SIB decreased to a near-zero level when protective equipment was applied. In addition, if padding were removed from one area of the body, the participant engaged in SIB only to that area. The fact that SIB emerged only when body parts were exposed provides evidence that protective equipment may suppress SIB through the process of sensory extinction. In addition, extinction of sensory reinforcement sometimes can come in forms other than protective equipment. Kern and colleagues [53] reported the use of a topical anesthetic to reduce self-slapping in a 12-year-old who had autism and ID. When the topical anesthetic was applied to the skin, self-slapping reduced by 20% to 60% in this individual.

Punishment-based treatments

Although the first choice of behavioral interventions typically is the selection of reinforcement and extinction-based strategies, there are times when more invasive methods are necessary to gain control over dangerous behaviors, such as SIB. Punishment is defined as the presentation of an aversive stimulus or the removal of a positive stimulus contingent on engaging in a target behavior, such as SIB [19]. The key feature of the use of punishment in behavior intervention is that the punishing stimuli (eg, water mist) or event (eg, time out from positive reinforcement) must be strong enough to override the maintaining reinforcement for the behavior [38].

Several punishment methods have proved effective at reducing SIB in individuals who have autism. For example, when SIB is related to reinforcement in the form of contingent attention, time out from positive reinforcement has proved moderately successful in decreasing maladaptive behaviors [45]. Another punishment procedure used in the treatment of SIB is contingent physical exercise. Contingent physical exercise consists of having individuals engage in brief physical activity immediately after an occurrence of the target behavior [54]. This procedure originally was designed for use with aggressive and disruptive behaviors but recently has been applied to the treatment of SIB in individuals who have autism and ID [55,56].

The punishment procedure that has received the most debate is physical restraint. Physical restraint can range from complete immobilization on a bed, for example, to limiting the mobility of specific body parts (eg, rigid arm sleeves). Based on the limitation of movement provided by physical restraints, this option may be viewed as the most restrictive behavioral intervention. Furthermore, the application of physical restraints can make it difficult or impossible for individuals to engage in appropriate, adaptive behaviors. Despite these concerns, the programmatic use of physical restraint in severe instances of SIB has been shown effective. For example, rigid arm restraints have been used in many studies to reduce the frequency of SIB, especially hand-to-head SIB [56,57].

Use of restraints is not usually considered a final stage of intervention. The goal is to fade the use of restraints gradually over time so that individuals remain under the stimulus control of the restraints while not actually wearing them. The use of physical restraints always should be conducted in a systematic manner with careful consideration being given to providing the least amount of restraint necessary to reduce harm while inhibiting adaptive behaviors as little as possible [58].

Although punishment procedures continue to be controversial in the treatment of SIB, entirely dispensing with aversive interventions is troublesome. Some individuals who have ID engage in problem behaviors of sufficient severity to threaten their own lives. To eliminate the use of aversive interventions in these individuals is considered by some to be dangerous and unethical [44].

Skill-building

In most cases, decreasing the frequency or severity of SIB alone may not be sufficient. These behaviors must be replaced by more appropriate behaviors that allow individuals to obtain desired reinforcement in an adaptive manner. One successful method of training appropriate behaviors based on the function of SIB is FCT [21]. According to the functional communication theory, maladaptive behaviors are similar to other nonverbal behaviors, such as crying in an infant. For those who have limited communication skills, problem behaviors may provide a manner of expressing their wants or needs [59]. The goal of FCT is to teach a communicative behavior (eg, vocalization, sign language, or exchanging a picture) that is functionally equivalent to the SIB for an individual. This communicative behavior allows individuals to have control over the delivery of reinforcement and eliminating the need to engage in the maladaptive behavior [31]. FCT is a flexible, individualized treatment approach that allows for the training of any communicative response needed. Typically, chosen communication responses include teaching individuals to request a break (for escape-maintained behavior) or to request attention (for attention-maintained behavior). In addition, the form of the communicative response can be individualized based on individual communicative ability.

Researchers have shown the effectiveness of FCT in reducing a number of maladaptive behaviors, such as self-injury [21,60,61], aggression [62], and stereotypic behaviors [63]. Braithwaite and Richdale [63] demonstrated the use of FCT to reduce SIB and aggression in a boy who had autism. Because these maladaptive behaviors served multiple functions (ie, escape and tangible) for this child, many communicative responses were taught to replace them. The researchers taught the boy to verbally request help from adults and access to toys. As discussed previously, extinction also was used to ensure that engaging in SIB or aggression did not result in receipt of reinforcement. The researchers reported a rapid elimination of SIB and aggression after the training of functional communication responses.

Summary

SIB are among the most concerning problem behaviors seen in individuals who have autism and other developmental disabilities. In addition to the risk for physical harm to individuals, SIB can interfere with the social and adaptive development of these individuals, most of whom already have deficits in these areas. Through the use of a function-based, behavioral approach to assessment, clinicians can generate and test hypotheses regarding the antecedents and consequences that are most likely to produce SIB for individuals. The function of the behavior then can be used to design a treatment that reduces the rate of the maladaptive behavior while training more appropriate means of obtaining reinforcement.

References

[1] Gardner WI, Graeber-Whalen JL, Ford DR. Self-injurious behaviors: multimodal contextual approach to treatment. In: Dosen A, Day K, editors. Treating mental illness and behavior disorders in children and adults with mental retardation. Washington, DC: American Psychiatric Press, Inc; 2001. p. 323–57.

[2] Borthwick-Duffy SA, Eyman RK, White JF. Client characteristics and residential placement patterns. Am J Ment Defic 1987;92:24–30.

[3] Intagliata J, Willer B. Reinstitutionalization of mentally retarded individuals in residential facilities. Am J Ment Defic 1981;87:34–9.

[4] Mace FC, Lalli JS, Shea MC. Functional analysis and treatment of SIB. In: Luiselli JL, Matson JL, Singh NN, editors. Self-injurious behavior: analysis, assessment, and treatment. New York: Springer-Verlag; 1992. p. 122–52.

[5] Iwata BA, Pace GM, Dorsey MF, et al. The functions of self-injurious behavior: an experimental-epidemiological analysis. J Appl Behav Anal 1994;27:215–40.

[6] Rojahn J, Esbensen AJ. Epidemiology of self-injurious behavior in mental retardation: a review. In: Schroeder SR, Oster-Granite ML, Thompson T, editors. Self-injurious behavior: gene-brain-behavior relationship. Washington, DC: American Psychological Association; 2002. p. 41–77.

[7] American Psychiatric Association. Diagnostic and statistical manual of mental disorders. 4th edition. Washington, DC: American Psychiatric Association; 1994.

[8] Borthwick-Duffy S. Prevalence of destructive behaviors: a study of aggression, SIB and property destruction. In: Thompson T, Gray DB, editors. Destructive behavior in developmental disabilities: diagnosis and treatment. London: Sage Publications, Inc; 1994. p. 3–23.

[9] Carr EG. The motivation of self-injurious behavior: a review of some hypotheses. Psychol Bull 1977;84:800–16.

[10] Hill BK, Bruininks RH. Maladaptive behavior of mentally retarded individuals in residential facilities. American Journal of Mental Deficiency 1984;88:380–7.

[11] Rojahn J. Self-injurious and stereotypic behavior of noninstitutionalized mentally retarded people: prevalence and classification. American Journal of Mental Deficiency 1986;91:268–76.

[12] McClintock K, Hall S, Oliver C. Risk markers associated with challenging behaviours in people with intellectual disabilities: a meta-analytic study. J Intellect Disabil Res 2003;47:405–16.

[13] Rojahn J, Borthwick-Duffy SA, Jacobson JW. The association between psychiatric diagnoses and severe behavior problems in mental retardation. Ann Clin Psychiatry 1993;5:163–70.

[14] Bodfish J, Symons F, Parker D, et al. Varieties of repetitive behavior in autism: comparisons to mental retardation. J Autism Dev Disord 2000;30:237–43.

[15] Dominick KC, Davis NO, Lainhart J, et al. Atypical behaviors in children with autism and children with a history of language impairment. Res Dev Disabil 2007;28:145–62.

[16] Baghdadli A, Pascal S, Grisi S, et al. Risk factors for self-injurious behaviours among 222 young children with autistic disorders. J Intellect Disabil Res 2003;47:622–7.

[17] Saloviita T. The structure and correlates of self-injurious behavior in an institutional setting. Res Dev Disabil 2000;21:501–11.

[18] Guess D, Carr E. Emergence and maintenance of stereotypy and self-injury. Am J Ment Retard 1991;96:299–319.

[19] Kazdin AE. Behavior modification in applied settings. 6th edition. Belmont (CA): Wadsworth/Thomson Learning; 2001.

[20] Lovaas IO, Simmons JQ. Manipulation of self-destruction in three retarded children. J Appl Behav Anal 1969;2:143–57.

[21] Carr EG, Durand VM. Reducing behavior problems through functional communication training. J Appl Behav Anal 1985;18:111–26.

[22] Iwata BA. Toward a functional analysis of self-injury. Analysis and Intervention in Developmental Disabilities 1982;2:3–20.

[23] Durand VM, Crimmins DB. Identifying the variables maintaining self-injurious behavior. J Autism Dev Disord 1988;18:99–117.

[24] Favell JE, McGimsey JF, Schell RM. Treatment of self-injury by providing alternate sensory activities. Analysis and Intervention in Developmental Disabilities 1982;2:83–104.

[25] Wolery M, Kirk K, Gast DL. Stereotypic behavior as a reinforcer: effects and side effects. J Autism Dev Disord 1985;15:149–61.

[26] Vollmer TR. The concept of automatic reinforcement: implications for behavioral research in developmental disabilities. Res Dev Disabil 1994;15:187–207.

[27] Baumeister A, Forehand R. Effects of extinction of an instrumental response on stereotyped rocking in severe retardates. Psychol Rec 1971;21:235–40.

[28] Carr EG, Newsom CD, Binkoff JA. Stimulus control of self-destructive behavior in a psychotic child. J Abnorm Child Psychol 1976;4:139–53.

[29] Sailor W, Guess D, Rutherford G, et al. Control of tantrum behavior by operant techniques during experimental verbal training. J Appl Behav Anal 1968;1:237–43.

[30] Weeks M, Gaylord-Ross R. Task difficulty and aberrant behavior in severely handicapped students. J Appl Behav Anal 1981;14:449–63.

[31] Wacker D, Steege M, Northrup J, et al. Use of functional analysis and acceptability measures to assess and treat severe behavior problems: an outpatient clinic model. In: Repp AC, Singh NN, editors. Perspectives on the use of nonaversive and aversive interventions for persons with developmental disabilities. Sycamore (IL): Sycamore Publishing Company; 1990. p. 297–319.

[32] Hanley GP, Iwata BA, McCord BE. Functional analysis of problem behavior: a review. J Appl Behav Anal 2003;36:147–85.

[33] Durand VM, Crimmins DB. The Motivation Assessment Scale (MAS) administration guide. Topeka (KS): Monaco & Associates; 1992.

[34] Matson JL, Vollmer TR. The Questions About Behavior Functions (QABF) user's guide. Baton Rouge (LA): Scientific Publishers, Inc; 1995.

[35] Zarcone JR, Rodgers TA, Iwata BA, et al. Reliability analysis of the Motivation Assessment Scale: a failure to replicate. Res Dev Disabil 1991;12:349–60.

[36] Paclawskyj TR, Matson JL, Rush KS, et al. Questions About Behavioral Function (QABF): a behavioral checklist for functional assessment of aberrant behavior. Res Dev Disabil 2000; 21:223–9.

[37] Paclawskyj TR, Matson JL, Rush KS, et al. Assessment of the convergent validity of the Questions About Behavioral Function scale with analogue functional analysis and the Motivation Assessment Scale. J Intellect Disabil Res 2001;45:484–94.

[38] Iwata BA, Vollmer TR, Zarcone JR. The experimental (functional) analysis of behavior disorders: methodology, applications, and limitations. In: Repp AC, Singh NN, editors. Perspectives on the use of nonaversive and aversive interventions for persons with developmental disabilities. Sycamore (IL): Sycamore Publishing Company; 1990. p. 301–30.

[39] O'Neill RE, Horner RH, Albin RW, et al. Functional analysis of problem behavior: a practical guide. Sycamore (IL): Sycamore Publications; 1991.

[40] Gresham FM, Watson TS, Skinner CH. Functional behavioral assessment: principles, procedures, and future directions. School Psych Rev 2001;30:156–72.

[41] Pace GM, Iwata BA, Edwards GL, et al. Stimulus fading and transfer in the treatment of self-restraint and self-injurious behavior. J Appl Behav Anal 1986;19:381–9.

[42] Touchette PE, MacDonald RF, Langer SN. A scatter plot for identifying stimulus control of problem behavior. J Appl Behav Anal 1985;18:343–51.

[43] Feldman MA, Griffiths D. Comprehensive assessment of severe behavior problems. In: Singh NN, editor. Prevention and treatment of severe behavior problems: models and methods in developmental disabilities. Pacific Grove (CA): Brooks/Cole Publishing Company; 1997. p. 23–48.

[44] Foxx RM. Severe aggression and self-destructive behavior: the myth of the nonaversive treatment of severe behavior. In: Jacobson J, Foxx RM, Mulick J, editors. Controversial therapies for developmental disabilities: fads, fashion, and science in professional practice. Mahwah (NJ): Lawrence Erlbaum; 2005. p. 295–310.

[45] Harris SL, Ersner-Hershfield R. Behavioral suppression of seriously disruptive behavior in psychotic and retarded patients: a review of punishment and its alternatives. Psychol Bull 1978;6:1352–75.

[46] Vollmer TR, Marcus BA, Ringdahl JE. Noncontingent escape as treatment for self-injurious behavior maintained by negative reinforcement. J Appl Behav Anal 1995;28:15–26.

[47] Wacker D, Northrup J, Lambert LK. SIB. In: Singh NN, editor. Prevention and treatment of severe behavior problems: models and methods in developmental disabilities. Pacific Grove (CA): Brooks/Cole Publishing Company; 1997. p. 180–216.

[48] Thompson RH, Iwata BA, Hanley GP, et al. The effects of extinction, noncontingent reinforcement, and differential reinforcement of other behavior as control procedures. J Appl Behav Anal 2003;36:221–38.

[49] Kelly ME, Lerman DC, Van Camp CM. The effects of competing reinforcement schedules on the acquisition of functional communication training. J Appl Behav Anal 2002;35:59–63.

[50] Mace AB, Shapiro ES, Mace FC. Effects of warning stimuli for reinforcer withdrawal and task onset on self-injury. J Appl Behav Anal 1998;31:679–82.

[51] Dorsey MF, Iwata BA, Reid DH, et al. Protective equipment: continuous and contingent application in the treatment of self-injurious behavior. J Appl Behav Anal 1982;15:217–30.

[52] Moore JW, Fisher WW, Pennington A. Systematic application and removal of protective equipment in the assessment of multiple topographies of self-injury. J Appl Behav Anal 2004;37:73–7.

[53] Kern L, Bailin D, Mauk JE. Effects of a topical anesthetic on non-socially maintained self-injurious behavior. Dev Med Child Neurol 2003;45:769–71.

[54] Luce SC, Delquadri J, Hall RV. Contingent exercise: a mild but powerful procedure for suppressing inappropriate verbal and aggressive behavior. J Appl Behav Anal 1980;13:583–94.

[55] Foxx RM, Garito J. The long term successful treatment of the very severe behaviors of a preadolescent with autism. Behavioral Interventions 2007;22:69–82.

[56] Kahng S, Abt KA, Wilder DA. Treatment of self-injury correlated with mechanical restraints. Behavioral Interventions 2001;16:105–10.

[57] Fisher W, Piazza CC, Bowman LG, et al. Direct and collateral effects of restraints and restraint fading. J Appl Behav Anal 1997;30:105–20.

[58] Wallace MD, Iwata BA, Zhou L, et al. Rapid assessment of the effects of restraint on self-injury and adaptive behavior. J Appl Behav Anal 1999;32:525–8.

[59] Durand VM. Severe behavior problems: a functional communication training approach. New York: Guilford Press; 1990.

[60] Durand VM, Kishi G. Reducing severe behavior problems among persons with dual sensory impairments: an evaluation of a technical assistance model. J Assoc Pers Sev Handicaps 1987;12:2–10.

[61] Bird F, Dores PA, Moniz D, et al. Reducing severe aggressive and self-injurious behaviors with functional communication training. Am J Ment Retard 1989;94:37–48.

[62] Durand VM, Carr EG. Social influences on 'self-stimulatory' behavior: analysis and treatment application. J Appl Behav Anal 1987;20:119–32.

[63] Braithwaite KL, Richdale AL. Functional communication training to replace challenging behaviors across two behavioral outcomes. Behavioral Interventions 2000;15:21–36.

ELSEVIER
SAUNDERS

Child Adolesc Psychiatric Clin N Am
17 (2008) 887–905

CHILD AND
ADOLESCENT
PSYCHIATRIC CLINICS
OF NORTH AMERICA

Assessment and Behavioral Treatment of Feeding and Sleeping Disorders in Children with Autism Spectrum Disorders

Tiffany Kodak, PhD*, Cathleen C. Piazza, PhD

Munroe-Meyer Institute, University of Nebraska Medical Center, 985450 Nebraska Medical Center, Omaha, NE 68198-5450, USA

According to the *Diagnostic and Statistical Manual of Mental Disorders, 4th Edition* (*DSM-IV-TR*), autism and autism spectrum disorders (ASD) have three core characteristics: (1) qualitative impairments in social interactions, (2) marked communication deficits, and (3) repetitive, restrictive, or stereotyped activities, interests, and behavior [1]. In addition, autism may place the child at risk for a variety of other behavioral deficits or excesses. The specific behaviors of concern that are the focus of this article are problems relating to sleeping and feeding. Children with sleeping and feeding problems can pose a significant challenge for caregivers, and add to the stress that parents of children diagnosed with autism already may feel.

Media attention on autism has exploded in recent years as the result of a number of factors, including (but perhaps not limited to) the increasing number of children diagnosed with ASD. More federal and private dollars are being dedicated to understanding the cause of ASD and to identifying methods for ameliorating its symptoms. Arguably, interventions based on applied behavior analysis (ABA) have the most empiric support in terms of symptom amelioration of the behavioral deficits and excesses associated with ASD [2]. Thus, ABA has gained increasing acceptance among professionals and caregivers as a viable method of treatment. In this article, we focus exclusively on assessment and treatment techniques for sleeping and feeding difficulties from the perspective of ABA, which we call a behavioral approach.

---

* Corresponding author.
E-mail address: tkodak@umnc.edu (T. Kodak).

1056-4993/08/$ - see front matter © 2008 Published by Elsevier Inc.
doi:10.1016/j.chc.2008.06.005
childpsych.theclinics.com

There are a number of potential advantages of a behavioral approach for symptoms related to ASD, particularly for assessing and treating problems of sleeping and feeding. First, a primary focus of ABA is on behavior and behavior change, with a specific emphasis on behaviors that society believes are important. The emphasis of ABA on behavior and behavior change is not only appropriate, but also appealing to professionals and caregivers when the goal for a child diagnosed with ASD is to change behavior. We all can agree that sleeping and feeding are two important human behaviors and too much, too little, or dysfunctional sleeping or feeding warrants intervention.

A second important dimension of ABA is its focus on observable behavior. ABA emphasizes precise quantification of behavior with the assumption that precise quantification (measurement) of behavior allows us to track the level of the problem (the amount of behavior that is occurring), the stability of the behavior (Does behavior change moment to moment, hour to hour, day to day?), and the trend of behavior (Is behavior improving, worsening, or staying the same?). We know from the literature that direct observation of behavior provides a more precise quantification of behavior when compared with other methods of measuring behavior (eg, anecdotal report, recall, rating scales) [3]. ABA emphasizes the development of specific goals and objective measurement of progress toward those goals.

Third, as the name ABA implies, the field strives to be analytic. That is, applied behavior analysts place an emphasis on demonstrating "control" over behavior in a manner analogous to turning a light switch on and off [4]. For example, the applied behavior analyst seeks to show that behavior A improves in the presence and not the absence of treatment A. The advantage of this analytic focus is that the technology provides empiric evidence for the effects of a given treatment on a child's behavior, thus eliminating the guesswork and subjective judgment that sometimes accompanies interventions.

The applied behavior analyst attempts to establish functional relations between behavior, environmental events, and physiologic variables [5]. With respect to sleeping and eating, ABA research has sought to understand how these behaviors (sleeping and feeding) are influenced both by what goes on around the individual and what goes on "inside" the individual. As discussed below, physiology and environment often interact to alter the behaviors of sleeping and feeding in important ways.

Because ABA has a long history of incorporating the scientific literature into its assessment and treatment procedures, numerous empiric studies on sleeping and feeding problems in children have used the principles of ABA. In outlining the details of the studies, we identify those that include children diagnosed with ASD. We also indicate when procedures have not been tested specifically with children with ASD, and offer recommendations about the probability of success of a particular treatment with children with ASD.

Sleeping disorders

A good night's sleep can be one of the most satisfying experiences a person can have. By contrast, poor sleep, particularly over consecutive days or weeks, can be a most frustrating experience. Poor sleep at any age is associated with irritability, altered mood, difficulties concentrating, and, in children, learning and behavior problems [6,7]. In addition, children diagnosed with ASD and sleep problems show more affective problems and poorer social interactions than children diagnosed with ASD and no sleep problems [6].

When a child doesn't sleep well, it is likely that nobody in the family sleeps well [5]. In fact, poor sleep is associated with child maltreatment [8,9], possibly as a result of the caregiver's inability to contain the irritability that comes from chronic sleep deprivation [5].

Sleep problems are common in children. Approximately 30% of children have sleeping problems, according to reports from parents [10]. Rates of sleeping problems in children diagnosed with ASD may be even higher. For example, one survey of typically developing children, children diagnosed with autism, and children diagnosed with Asperger's disorder found a prevalence of sleep disorders of 50%, 73%, and 73%, respectively. The specific sleep problems that have been reported in children with ASD consist of difficulties falling asleep, difficulties remaining asleep, and early waking.

Sleep problems may represent an even greater hazard for the child who awakens at night and engages in problematic behavior while unsupervised (eg, leaving the house, turning on the stove). Patzold and colleagues [11] found that sleep problems in children diagnosed with ASD showed some improvements with age, but that children diagnosed with ASD still slept less than typically developing peers. This greater need for supervision throughout the day and night may leave the caregiver feeling exhausted with a sense that he or she "never gets a break." Thus, identification of effective treatment strategies for sleep disorders for children with ASD is critical for ensuring adequate sleep for the child and family; reducing sleep deprivation–related learning, affective, social, and behavior problems; and reducing the risk of child abuse.

Assessment

Brown and Piazza [12] suggested that it might be useful to assess the relation between environmental events (eg, parental responses to a child's inappropriate behavior) and bedtime problems in children. This type of assessment is referred to in ABA as functional analysis. Functional analysis strives for an understanding of why the behavior occurs (What is the motivation for the child's behavior?). Thus, the functional analysis focuses on (1) identification of the situations in which the behavior occurs, which is referred to as antecedents of the behavior (the child is placed in bed); (2) identification of events that occur after the behavior, which is referred to as the consequences of the behavior (the parents bring the child into bed with them when the child cries); and (3) identification of the relation between the behavior, its antecedents, and its consequences ("If I cry at bedtime, my parents will bring me into bed with them"). Functional analysis has been used widely in the assessment of behavior problems, such as self-injurious behavior, aggression, and destructive behavior, in children diagnosed with ASD [13,14]. In fact, functional analysis is considered the gold standard of assessment in ABA. Studies have shown that treatments based on the results of a functional analysis are more effective than treatments developed in the absence of a functional analysis [15].

Despite the demonstrated effectiveness of the functional analysis method for the assessment and treatment of behavior problems, this method has not been applied to the assessment of sleep problems [12]. However, it may be useful for the assessment of sleep problems, and Friman and Piazza [5] propose that some treatment failures for sleep problems may be a result of the lack of correspondence between the behavior and its function. For example, the treatment for a child who exhibited tantrums to gain parental attention would be different from the treatment for a child who exhibited tantrums at bedtime to delay his or her bedtime.

A functional approach to sleep attempts to use information about the causes of the child's disrupted sleep to inform treatment. Data collection during a functional analysis should include information about the child's behavior and information about the parent's response to child behavior. We typically help the parent develop a data sheet that is individualized for the child's specific sleep problem, but is still simple to design and complete. For example, we would have a parent record bedtime, sleep-onset time, wake time, and occurrence of crying for a child whose sleep problem consisted of tantrums with difficulty initiating and maintaining sleep. Information about parental behavior is critical to the analysis, so we have parents indicate what they did during the child's sleep-related tantrums (eg, rocked the child to sleep, allowed the child to get out of bed).

Table 1 shows a sample data sheet for one child who cried at bedtime, had prolonged sleep-onset times, and awakened at night. We had the parents write down each intervention they typically tried when the child would not go to sleep or awakened at night. These interventions are numbered from one to six. The columns on the far left indicate the time of day. Subsequent columns are for the parent to indicate if the child was in bed, asleep, or crying. The column on the far right is for the parent to indicate what he or she did when the child did not fall asleep or cried. Having the parents write down and number all the probable interventions they may use at the top of the data sheet then makes it easier for them to fill out the data sheet because they can simply write down the number of the intervention they used (eg, 1: turned on music), rather than having to write a narrative for each intervention.

Table 1
Sample functional analysis data sheet for sleep problems

	In bed	Sleeping	Crying	Parent's behavior
7:00 PM				
7:15 PM				
7:30 PM	√		√	1, 2
7:45 PM	√		√	3
8:00 PM	√			5
8:15 PM	√	√		
8:30 PM	√	√		
8:45 PM	√	√		
9:00 PM	√	√		
9:15 PM	√	√		
9:30 PM	√	√		
9:45 PM	√	√		
10:00 PM	√	√		
10:15 PM	√	√		
10:30 PM	√	√		
10:45 PM	√	√		
11:00 PM	√	√		
11:15 PM	√	√		
11:30 PM	√	√		
11:45 PM	√		√	2
Midnight		√		6

Write down what you do when your child cries at bedtime: 1 — Turn on music. 2 — Wait for 15 minutes to see if she will calm down. 3 — Pat her back for 15 minutes to see if she will calm down. 4 — Take her out of bed and give her a bottle. 5 — Take her out of bed and rock her until she falls asleep. 6 — Bring her into our bed.

The data sheet from the child in the example shows that the caregiver put the child to bed at 7:30 PM, at which time the child began to cry. The caregiver turned on the music and then waited 15 minutes to see if the child falls asleep. When the child was still crying at 7:45 PM , the caregiver patted the child on the back for 15 minutes. When this intervention did not result in the child falling asleep, the caregiver removed the child from bed and rocked the child to sleep. The child fell asleep, but then awakened at 11:45 PM and began to cry. The caregiver waited for 15 minutes to see if the child would fall back asleep. When the child failed to fall asleep by midnight, the caregiver brought the child into her bed.

The data produce a story of the child's bedtime problems that are captured with a relatively simple measurement procedure. If the data are similar for several nights, then they tell a story of a child who cannot fall asleep by herself. That is, even though the caregivers place her in her own bed, she is unable to fall asleep. She only falls asleep when the caregivers introduce some intervention to help her fall asleep, like rocking her to sleep or bringing her into their bed. The specific intervention for the child would need to address the issue of the child learning to fall asleep independently.

Treatment

A number of behavioral treatment procedures have been used with individuals exhibiting sleep disorders. Most studies of specific sleep treatments involve children with typical development or children with mental retardation, some of whom are diagnosed with ASD. Some treatments only have been evaluated for one type of sleep disorder (eg, bedtime tantrums [16–18]), whereas others have been shown to be effective for a variety of sleep disorders (eg, bedtime tantrums, repeated night awakenings, late onset to sleep, reduced total sleep time per day, daytime sleeping [19–24]). Behavioral treatments that have been evaluated in the literature and are reported in this article include (1) bedtime scheduling, (2) positive routines, (3) bedtime fading, (4) extinction and graduated extinction, and (5) chronotherapy.

Bedtime scheduling

One critical aspect of any treatment is teaching caregivers the importance of putting the child to bed at the same time every night, providing naps at the same time every day, and awakening the child at a consistent time in the morning and at naptime. Such advice can be onerous to hear because most parents are reluctant to awaken a child who has had insufficient sleep. However, allowing the child to "sleep in" in the morning or at naptime only will exacerbate the child's sleep problems over the long run. In addition, consistency is often difficult for parents to achieve when bedtimes and naptimes interfere with other scheduled activities (eg, doctor's appointments, grocery shopping).

Colville and colleagues [18] used sleep scheduling to treat the sleep disorders of five children diagnosed with Sanfilippo syndrome. Three children showed improvement following treatment, while no changes were observed in one child's behavior. Some children may not respond to a treatment involving sleep scheduling only [25]. Even so, the sleep schedule should form the foundation of any other sleep intervention. It is unlikely that any sleep intervention will be effective in the absence of a consistent sleep schedule.

Bedtime routines, positive routines

Establishing a consistent bedtime routine is one of the simplest components of establishing good sleep habits in a child. Yet it is often overlooked. Children with ASD typically respond well to routines. Thus, a bedtime routine is a simple, low-cost intervention that is reasonable to try for a child with a sleep problem. The advantage of a bedtime routine is that all of the activities involved in the intervention occur at bedtime. Thus, the caregiver is not required to implement procedures in the middle of the night when fatigue may affect protocol implementation.

The precise activities involved in the actual bedtime routine probably are less important than the schedule itself and the implementation of a routine.

The activities generally should be quiet and calming (eg, reading a book as opposed to watching a violent cartoon on television). Children with autism often show good response to routines, although some children with autism become overly fixated on routines and will not go to sleep unless the specific routine is followed. Therefore, it can be a good idea to introduce a small amount of variety into the bedtime routine (eg, having the child wear different pajamas each night; reading a different book) to help prevent the bedtime routine from becoming an unbreakable ritual for the child.

Most studies have incorporated a bedtime routine as one component of a multicomponent treatment package [16,17]. For example, Adams and Rickert [16] evaluated a treatment called "positive routines" that involved having the child engage in enjoyable behaviors before bedtime. In addition, the exact bedtime was adjusted to occur at the time the child naturally went to bed. Subsequently, the bedtime was progressively shifted earlier to the desired bedtime. In addition, bedtime tantrums following the positive routines were ignored (see section on "extinction" below). Results indicated that treatment was effective in reducing tantrums in preschool-aged children. It is not clear, however, whether the bedtime routine, the bedtime fading, the extinction, or a combination resulted in the treatment effects. None of the children in the Adams and Rickert study were identified as having ASD. However, a bedtime routine is generally considered to be an essential component to promoting good sleep hygiene [26]. In addition, as indicated above, bedtime routines are relatively easy to implement and have few negative side effects. Therefore, parents should be encouraged to incorporate a bedtime routine into their child's sleep schedule.

Bedtime fading

Bedtime fading is a treatment procedure for sleep disorders that has been tested in typically developing children as well as children with developmental disabilities, including children diagnosed with ASD. Bedtime fading involves initially setting a bedtime that is likely to result in a rapid onset of sleep [16,21,23,24]. The bedtime then is adjusted gradually when the data suggest that the child is falling asleep rapidly. It is important to note that this treatment is not the same as simply waiting for the child to become tired and fall asleep. All of the adjustments in the bedtime fading procedure described by Piazza and colleagues [21,23,24] involve the use of baseline data to set a bedtime when rapid sleep onset is highly likely. The data then are used to adjust the bedtime systematically (as opposed to waiting each night until the child is "tired").

Piazza and colleagues [21,23,24] showed that the bedtime fading treatment is effective in treating multiple types of sleep problems (eg, sleeping in the parents' bed, difficulty falling asleep, waking early, and waking multiple times per night). For example, Piazza and Fisher [23] collected baseline data on one child's sleep-wake cycle and identified a time when the child typically was asleep (eg, 11:30 PM). Treatment involved requiring the child to stay awake until 30 minutes past the average time identified in baseline (eg, midnight). The child also was not permitted to sleep during the day or outside of the prescribed period of sleep (eg, from 8:30 PM to 6:30 AM). When the child fell asleep within 15 minutes of the identified bedtime, the bedtime was shifted earlier by 30 minutes on the following night. However, if the child did not fall asleep within 15 minutes of the identified bedtime, the bedtime was shifted later by 30 minutes. Results indicated that the child (diagnosed with mental retardation) slept during 82% of her scheduled sleep time and had little to no daytime sleeping following treatment.

Piazza and colleagues [24,25] conducted additional studies to evaluate the bedtime fading procedure when a response-cost procedure was added to treatment. The inclusion of the response-cost procedure involved removing the child from the bed and keeping the child awake for 1 hour if the child had not fallen asleep within 15 minutes of the prescribed bedtime. Piazza and colleagues [24] evaluated bedtime fading plus response cost with children diagnosed with developmental delays, including some children diagnosed with ASD. Results indicated that sleep disturbances (waking during the night, sleeping during the day, decreased total sleep) improved for all participants.

Bedtime fading with and without response cost has been shown to be effective in decreasing sleep disturbances in children with mental retardation, including children diagnosed with ASD. The bedtime fading and bedtime fading with response-cost procedures consist of multiple components and it was not clear which component of the procedure was responsible for the changes in child sleep behavior. Therefore, Piazza and colleagues [25] conducted an evaluation to determine which component of treatment was responsible for the change in sleep behavior. The investigators compared a bedtime scheduling procedure (ie, placing the child in bed at the same time each night and waking them at the same time each morning, which is one component of the bedtime fading with response-cost procedure) to bedtime fading with response cost. Children in the bedtime fading with response-cost treatment group showed more improvement in their sleep than children in the bedtime scheduling group.

Bedtime fading is a relatively easy treatment procedure to implement. Although treatment may initially involve keeping the child awake until the prescribed bedtime, the scheduled bedtime can be altered relatively quickly such that, following just a few nights of treatment, the child is going to bed at a more reasonable time. Another advantage of the bedtime fading procedure is that all of the intervention components are implemented at bedtime rather than in the middle of the night when fatigue may impair a caregiver's ability to implement procedures with integrity. However, some parents may feel uncomfortable when they have to keep their child awake before the scheduled bedtime or if the child attempts to fall asleep during the day. Nevertheless, parents need to be reminded that this is a critical component to the procedure, and it is unlikely to be successful if the parent allows the child to sleep outside of the prescribed sleep times.

Extinction

Extinction (sometimes referred to as allowing the child to "cry it out") is a treatment procedure that has been evaluated for a number of behavioral disorders. Extinction has been shown to be a highly effective procedure when implemented correctly, but it can have a deleterious effect on behavior if used incorrectly. Extinction as a treatment for sleep problems has been shown to be effective in reducing bedtime tantrums [27]. For example, Didden and colleagues [19] instructed the parents of two children with developmental disabilities to place each child in bed and then leave the room during the night, even when one or both children exhibit bedtime tantrums. The procedure was effective in decreasing both children's sleep disturbances.

Even though extinction is a demonstrated effective treatment, particularly for nighttime tantrums and delayed sleep onset, we rarely recommend this treatment in clinic. Many parents feel uncomfortable with leaving their child to cry for an extended period without checking on the child [27], and parents feel uncomfortable allowing their child to cry if they live in an apartment building or other setting where neighbors might be disturbed by the child's crying [5]. In addition, extinction for bedtime problems may present some safety concerns for children with ASD who engage in self-injurious or destructive behavior when left unattended.

Another concern with extinction is that bedtime problems may actually worsen significantly if the procedure is implemented incorrectly. Parents often allow the child to cry for some period of time (eg, 15 or 30 minutes), decide that they cannot tolerate the crying any longer, and then intervene (eg, bring the child into bed with them). In these cases, the child learns that crying for long periods brings about the desired outcome ("Mom and Dad allow me to come into bed with them"). Thus, the next time the parents try to let the child cry it out, the child will cry even longer and harder. Thus, parents need to be well informed of the advantages and disadvantages of allowing the child to cry it out before they attempt this treatment.

An alternative to extinction is a procedure called graduated extinction, although children with ASD did not participate in these evaluations [16,21,28,29]. During graduated extinction, parents are permitted to respond to their child's problem behavior following increasing intervals of time. For example, on the first night of treatment, the parent places the child in bed and then allows the child to cry for 5 minutes. After 5 minutes, the parent enters the child's room, provides brief comforting (eg, patting the child on the back briefly), and exits the room. The parent re-enters the child's room every 5 minutes as long as the child is crying. The length of the wait time (amount of time the parent allows the child to cry before entering the room) is increased on subsequent nights (eg, 10 minutes, 15 minutes). Eventually, the child learns to fall asleep before the parent enters the room.

Durand and colleagues [20] used graduated extinction with two children diagnosed with mental retardation who exhibited tantrums and disruptive behavior at bedtime. Treatment resulted in decreases in nighttime problem behavior. Thus, graduated extinction may provide an effective and more acceptable alternative to traditional extinction as the graduated extinction procedure allows the caregiver to supervise and attend to the child when he or she is crying.

Chronotherapy

Finally, chronotherapy is a procedure that has been used with adults with sleep-cycle schedule disorder [30]. Piazza and colleagues [22] used chronotherapy to treat multiple sleep problems (ie, daytime sleeping, variable sleep and wake times, and reduced total sleep time per day) in one child diagnosed with mental retardation. Initially, the child was placed in bed at a time that was likely to result in rapid sleep onset. Each subsequent night, bedtime was delayed by 2 hours until the participant would fall asleep rapidly when placed in bed at an acceptable time (ie, 9:00 PM). Treatment resulted in an increase in the total amount of time spent sleeping (ie, an increase of 2 hours per night) as well as consistent bedtime and waking schedules. Obviously, chronotherapy is not a practical treatment for most children with sleep problems because it involves a complete disruption of both the child's and the caregiver's daily schedule. Nevertheless, it may be a treatment for consideration in cases where the child has not responded to other, less intrusive sleep treatments.

Conclusion

The literature suggests that sleep problems are common in children diagnosed with ASD. In fact, they may be more common than in children with typical development and appear to have approximately a similar prevalence in children with developmental disabilities. Sleep problems have been associated with irritability, learning and behavior problems, and poorer affect and social behavior in children diagnosed with ASD and sleep problems relative to children diagnosed with ASD without sleep problems. Sleep problems cause increased stress in the family and increase the risk for child maltreatment. A functional approach to assessment may improve the effectiveness of prescribed treatments, but this approach has not been applied to the assessment of sleep problems in children with ASD.

Good sleep hygiene procedures (ie, promoting appropriate sleep-wake patterns) generally involve initiating a consistent bedtime routine and consistent sleep-wake schedule. These procedures have demonstrated effectiveness for some children, but not all children with sleep problems. Bedtime fading (with and without response cost), extinction (allowing the child to cry it out), and graduated extinction also have support as effective treatments in the empiric literature. Extinction has been associated with some negative side effects, and inaccurate implementation of extinction may cause behavior to worsen. Chronotherapy has been used with only one child with sleep problems, so its suitability for children with ASD and sleep problems is unknown. All of the treatments reviewed above rely minimally on verbal interaction with the child, which may be an advantage when working with children with ASD whose communication skills are limited.

Feeding disorders

Parents typically find feeding their child to be a satisfying experience. However, for parents of children with feeding disorders, mealtime may be an extremely stressful experience, and parents with children with feeding disorders often feel frustrated and depressed when their child exhibits a feeding problem. In the most severe cases, feeding problems can have significant negative consequences for the child, including malnutrition, dehydration, learning and behavior problems, and even death.

Feeding problems, like sleep problems, represent one of the most common concerns that parents report about their children. Feeding problems are estimated to occur in approximately 25% to 35% of typically developing children. Prevalence of feeding problems is estimated to be as high as 90% in children with ASD [31]. Schreck and colleagues [32] conducted a survey of the feeding behaviors of typically developing children and children with ASD and found that feeding problems were more common in the group of children diagnosed with ASD. Specifically, the children diagnosed with ASD, compared to typical children, refused more foods, required more specific utensils to eat, required food presented in more specific ways, were more likely to consume foods at a lower texture (eg, pureed food), and ate a narrower range of foods. Thus, mealtime problems may be relatively common in individuals with developmental disabilities.

Assessment procedures

Rating scales

A number of assessment procedures can be used to identify variables that may be related to the child's feeding disorder. For example, rating scales are available to help identify whether a child is exhibiting behaviors that may be characterized within a feeding disorder. The Brief Autism Mealtime Behavior Inventory is a 21-item questionnaire with items related to limited variety of foods, food refusal, and disruptive mealtime behavior, and with items related to characteristics associated with autism (eg, short attention span, aggression, self-injurious behavior) [33]. Matson and Kuhn [34] developed the Screening Tool of Feeding Problems to identify feeding disorders in children diagnosed with mental retardation. This scale includes 23 questions that target specific feeding problems, such as food selectivity (by type or texture), eating too quickly, vomiting, and pushing food away; and measures five categories of feeding behaviors, including the risk of aspiration, food selectivity, problem behaviors during mealtimes, feeding skills, and nutrition.

Functional analysis

Past literature has indicated that the way a parent responds to the child during mealtime may affect inappropriate mealtime behavior. Thus, a behavioral evaluation of a feeding disorder may include conducting direct observations of the parents during mealtimes and recording consequences that are provided when the child engages in problem behavior. Piazza and colleagues [35] observed how parents responded to their child's inappropriate mealtime behavior (eg, batting at the spoon, head turning). Of the children who participated in the study, only one was diagnosed with ASD, although four others were diagnosed with a developmental disability. Results indicated that when children exhibited inappropriate behavior, parents responded by (1) providing a toy during mealtime or allowing access to a more highly preferred food, (2) allowing the child to stop eating, and (3) reprimanding the child or coaxing the child to eat ("This is good for you. You should eat your food."). Thus, the investigators designed assessment conditions to experimentally evaluate how the above-mentioned consequences influenced the child's inappropriate behavior during mealtime. The assessment conducted by Piazza and colleagues consisted of "test" conditions (called attention, escape, and tangible) and a "control" condition. The test conditions were designed to mimic the consequences that they observed parents using during meals.

During the attention condition, a therapist provided reprimands and coaxed the child to eat each time the child engaged in inappropriate behavior. During the escape condition, the therapist allowed the child to take a brief break from eating following inappropriate behavior. Finally, during the tangible condition, the therapist provided the child with a toy or another food item when the child engaged in inappropriate behavior. Results of this assessment indicated that providing one or more of these consequences following inappropriate mealtime behavior resulted in an *increase* in child inappropriate behavior for 67% of participants. The investigators then used the results of the functional analyses to develop treatment.

Treatment for feeding disorders

The literature on the prevalence of feeding disorders suggests that feeding problems are common in children with ASD and that children with ASD exhibit a variety of types of feeding problems (eg, refusal, limited variety). Thus, the types of intervention for the feeding problem depends on the type and function of the specific feeding problem exhibited by the child.

Many of the empirically validated behavioral treatment procedures have been developed to target food refusal behavior, and these treatments have been used to increase oral intake in children who refuse all or most foods and to increase variety of foods consumed for children who consume only a limited variety of foods. The treatment procedure with the most empiric evidence is based on extinction of inappropriate behavior and often is referred to as "escape extinction" [36–39]. The idea behind escape extinction is that most children with severe feeding problems have inappropriate meal-time behavior (crying, batting at the spoon, head turning to avoid or get out of (ie, escape) eating), as demonstrated by Piazza and colleagues [35]. When a child cries, bats at the spoon, or turns his or head during a meal, parents generally either stop presenting food briefly or end the meal altogether. Thus, children with feeding problems learn that "when I cry, turn my head, or bat at the spoon, it goes away," thus increasing the likelihood that this behavior will reoccur when the spoon is presented in the future. During an escape extinction procedure, the child's inappropriate behavior no longer results in the spoon "going away" (ie, the child no longer escapes the food by engaging in inappropriate behavior).

Two commonly used forms of escape extinction are nonremoval of the spoon [36–38] and physical guidance [36,40]. During nonremoval of the spoon, the spoon remains at the child's lips until the child opens his or her mouth, and the feeder deposits the bite into the child's mouth. During physical guidance, the therapist places gentle pressure on the child's man-dibular joint to open the child's mouth, and then the feeder deposits the bite into the child's mouth. Escape extinction procedures have been com-bined with differential reinforcement (the child receives adult attention or access to toys following acceptance or consumption of food [39]) and non-contingent reinforcement (adult attention, toys, or both are available throughout the meal). Generally, the addition of differential or noncontin-gent reinforcement helps to reduce inappropriate behavior, but escape extinction is necessary to produce increases in acceptance and consump-tion of food. Even though escape extinction procedures have demonstrated effectiveness, these procedures should be used only under direct supervi-sion of a trained therapist as feeding problems can worsen if the proce-dures are used incorrectly.

A treatment procedure that has been evaluated with children who exhibit both food selectivity and food refusal involves simultaneously presenting a preferred and nonpreferred food item [39,41]. Piazza and colleagues [39] compared the effects of simultaneous and sequential presentation of pre-ferred and nonpreferred foods with three children diagnosed with ASD. The simultaneous presentation procedure consisted of placing a preferred food (eg, a chip) on top of, next too, or beneath the nonpreferred food (eg, broccoli). The sequential presentation condition consisted of giving the child the preferred food (eg, chip) after he or she ate the nonpreferred food (eg, broccoli). Piazza and colleagues showed that the simultaneous pre-sentation procedure resulted in higher levels of acceptance compared with the sequential presentation procedure.

One variation of the simultaneous procedure described above involves blending a preferred and nonpreferred food together [42]. Mueller and col-leagues [42] showed that the blending procedure resulted in increased levels of acceptance relative to repeated presentation of a nonpreferred food. In the study, the investigators blended (mixed) the preferred food (eg, apple-sauce) with nonpreferred foods (eg, carrots) in a 90:10 ratio of preferred food to nonpreferred food. The ratio of preferred to nonpreferred foods was decreased gradually over time (ie, 80:20, 70:30) until the child was consuming the nonpreferred food by itself.

Patel and colleagues [43] used a similar procedure to increase consumption of milk with a high-calorie beverage, Carnation Instant Breakfast (CIB), in one child diagnosed with ASD. Before treatment, the child would drink water, but no other beverage. The authors blended small amounts of CIB into the water and then gradually replaced the water with milk until the child was drinking the milk with CIB. Similar blending procedures have been used to increase children's consumption of foods with varied textures [44].

Pica

Assessment procedures for pica

Pica is reported in up to 25% of the population of individuals diagnosed with mental retardation [45]. Pica may be considered one of the most severe forms of self-injurious behavior because ingesting inedible items may result in surgery to remove the item, repeated visits to hospital emergency rooms, lead poisoning, introduction of bacteria or disease into the body, or even death. In fact, the rate of death from pica is estimated to be higher than that of any other form of self-injurious behavior [46].

As indicated above, functional analysis is considered to be the gold standard of assessment for such behavior problems as pica. The goal of functional analysis is to identify the variables maintaining the behavior and then to use the results of the analysis to develop treatment. A most basic functional assessment would include an interview of the caregivers to construct a list of antecedents and consequences surrounding pica. However, interviews and questionnaires provide less definitive information about the function of problem behavior compared with an assessment in which the antecedents and consequences for behavior are manipulated directly [47].

For example, Chapman and colleagues [48] identified three consequences that occurred following 75% of instances of excessive pill ingestion (ie, attention from caregivers, escape from work, and attention from medical personnel) in one young man diagnosed with ASD. The investigators conducted a functional analysis in which the young man was alone in a room with a one-way mirror, classroom and work assignments, and four pill bottles containing placebos varied only by their label color. The consequences associated with swallowing pills from each bottle were: (1) The orange label resulted in parental attention for 30 minutes; (2) the red label resulted in medical attention for 30 minutes; (3) the blue label resulted in lying down for 30 minutes; and (4) the yellow label resulted in no consequences. Results of the assessment indicated that the participant consumed the most pills from the colored bottle associated with lying down and taking a break from work, suggesting that the young man ingested pills to gain a break (escape from working).

The basic format of a functional analysis of any form of pica (eg, ingestion of string, cigarette butts) would be similar to that described by Chapman and colleagues [48]. That is, a room is "baited" with items that are safe for consumption, but would simulate the unsafe or unhealthy items the individual typically consumes [49–52]. In addition, a prescribed set of consequences is delivered in a series of sessions following instances of pica. Typical consequences that are tested are attention from adults and escape from work. The assessment also would include a situation in which no consequence is "programmed" (ie, the adult does not respond or react when the individual engages in pica) to determine if the pica behavior is "self-stimulating," "automatically reinforced," or "stereotypical behavior." Finally, during the control condition, the adult interacts with the individual and ignores instances of pica. The results of the functional analysis are used to inform treatment. For example, if the results of the functional analysis suggest that the individual engages in pica to gain adult attention, then the adult might withhold attention for pica in treatment.

Treatment of pica

Before the development of functional analysis methodology, treatments for pica typically involved providing alternative forms of stimulation, such as food or toys [53]. Providing competing stimuli (alternative food items or toys that may compete with pica) may be effective in certain circumstances. If pica is maintained by some form of automatic reinforcement (eg, engaging in pica produces oral stimulation), providing more appropriate items that provide similar forms of stimulation (referred to as matched stimuli) may reduce pica. Piazza and colleagues [50] showed that two participants engaged in pica that was hypothesized to be maintained by oral stimulation. The investigators conducted a treatment comparing matched items (items that were hypothesized to produce the same type of stimulation as the pica items) and unmatched items (hypothesized to produce the same type of stimulation as the pica items). For example, with a child who engages in pica that is hypothesized to be maintained by stimulation to the mouth, matched items may include food items or nonfood items that can produce oral stimulation (eg, a toothbrush). Unmatched items would include those providing alternative forms of stimulation, such as visual (eg, a spinning top) or auditory stimulation (eg, music). Results indicated that matched stimuli were more effective in reducing pica.

Piazza and colleagues [49] assessed and treated one young man for consumption of cigarette butts. In a series of analyses, the investigators showed that the young man's cigarette butt pica was not influenced by social consequences (ie, attention from adults, escape from work), and that the young man was more likely to consume cigarette butts that contained nicotine relative to cigarette butts or components of cigarettes that did not contain nicotine. Treatment consisted of making highly preferred foods available and interrupting the young man's attempts to pick up cigarette butts. Goh and colleagues [54] evaluated a procedure that included differential re-inforcement of alternative behavior and response interruption in which participants could exchange cigarette butts for reward and a therapist or caregiver prevented (blocked) attempts to pick up cigarette butts. Treatment was effective in reducing pica for three of the four participants in the study.

Chapman and colleagues [48] used a similar treatment for a young man's ingestion of pills as described in the section on assessment of pica. Treatment involved giving the young man a break from work when he turned in pills he found and giving him a work task (polishing shoes) if he ingested or attempted to ingest pills.

Some pica, like the pill ingestion of the young man described above, may be so life-threatening, that a consequence for the behavior may be warranted [55]. Some consequences that have been used for pica include a visual screen (covering the child's eyes [55]), overcorrection [46], physical restraint [56], and time-out [57].

Thus, a number of effective treatment procedures exist for pica, and clinicians must help parents determine which form of treatment should be implemented with each child. If an assessment determines that pica is maintained by social consequences (eg, attention from adults), then a reinforcement-based treatment procedure may be the most appropriate choice of treatment. However, if pica is life-threatening and few items appear to compete with the occurrence of pica, consequences, such as those mentioned above, may be the treatment of choice to reduce the likelihood of successful instances of pica.

Conclusions

Feeding disorders occur quite often in individuals diagnosed with ASD. Understandably, rigid mealtime routines and food selectivity may be common among these individuals because many individuals with ASD exhibit repetitive activities, interests, and behaviors. Feeding disorders may be associated with poor nutrition, consumption of life-threatening substances (ie, pica), stress during mealtimes, and restricted family activities (eg, the family may not eat at restaurants because of problem behavior associated with eating novel foods). However, the field of ABA has identified assessment procedures to identify the antecedents and consequences that may maintain feeding disorders in children with ASD. The gold standard for assessment of feeding disorders includes use of functional analysis methodology.

The majority of effective treatments for children with feeding disorders involve function-based treatment procedures. That is, following the functional analysis, the consequence found to maintain problem behavior (eg, attention from an adult) is withheld when the child engages in inappropriate behavior (eg, screaming during mealtime), and is provided for an appropriate alternative behavior (eg, accepting a bite of a novel food). Extinction is an important component of treatment to ensure that the child's inappropriate behavior is no longer producing the reinforcing consequences. Blending preferred and nonpreferred foods has also been shown to be effective in increasing acceptance of nonpreferred foods in individuals with food selectivity. Finally, for life-threatening feeding disorders (eg, pica), such consequences as time-out, facial screen, and physical restraint have been found to be effective in reducing pica. Consequences that are empirically derived are preferred because they are more likely to effectively reduce problem behavior. As with any treatment procedure implemented in the home, parents should be informed of the potential side effects (eg, increased crying when treatment is first implemented) of treatment. In addition, clinicians should inform parents of the importance of following the treatment procedures with a high degree of integrity or treatment may not be effective.

Summary

Behavior problems related to sleeping and feeding disorders and pica are common in children diagnosed with ASD. It is unlikely that these disorders will remit without some form of programmed intervention. Children with ASD are unlikely to simply "grow out" of these behaviors. Parents of children who exhibit issues with sleeping, feeding, or pica may be very concerned for the health and safety of their child. In addition, these disorders may cause a great deal of stress among family members, and restrict the family from engaging in typical social activities in the community. Fortunately, the field of ABA has identified effective assessment and treatment procedures for these disorders. Studies have shown that parents can be trained to accurately implement treatment protocols in the home environment. Thus, clinicians working with children with ASD who exhibit problems with feeding, sleeping, and pica have a number of behavioral treatment options.

References

[1] American Psychiatric Association. Diagnostic and statistical manual of mental disorders. Washington, DC:1994.
[2] Green G. Early behavioral intervention for autism. In: Maurice C, Green G, Luce SC, editors. Behavioral interventions for young children with autism. Texas (TX): Pro-ed; 1996. p. 29–44.
[3] Miltenberger R. Understanding problem behavior through functional assessment. In: Miltenberger R, editor. Behavior modification principles and procedures. Belmont, CA: Wadsworth/Thomson Learning; 2004. p. 257–82.
[4] Baer DM, Wolf MM, Risley TR. Some current dimensions of applied behavior analysis. J Appl Behav Anal 1968;1:91–7.
[5] Friman PC, Piazza C. Behavioral pediatrics: a logical point of entry into pediatric medicine for applied behavior analysts. In: Fisher WW, Piazza CC, Roane HS, editors. Handbook of applied behavior analysis. Guilford Publications, Inc.: New York, in press.
[6] Kuhn DE, Matson JL. Assessment of feeding and mealtime behavior problems in persons with mental retardation. Behav Modif 2004;28:638–48.

[7]   Marlow BA, Marzec ML, McGrew SG, et al. Characterizing sleep in children with autism
      spectrum disorders: a multidimensional approach. Sleep 2006;12:1563–71.
[8]   Blampied NM, France KG. A behavioral model of sleep disturbance. J Appl Behav Anal
      1993;26:477–92.
[9]   Blum NJ, Carey WB. Bedtime problems among infants and young children. Pediatr Rev
      1996;17:87–93.
[10] Lozoff B, Wolf AW, Davis NS. Sleep problems seen in pediatric practice. Pediatrics 1985;75:
      477–83.
[11] Patzold LM, Richdale AL, Tongue BJ. An investigation into the sleep characteristics of
      children with autism and Asperger's disorder. J Paediatr Child Health 1998;34:528–33.
[12] Brown KA, Piazza CC. Enhancing the effectiveness of sleep treatments: developing a func-
      tional approach: commentary. J Pediatr Psychol 1999;24:487–9.
[13] Hanley GP, Iwata BA, McCord BE. Functional analysis of problem behavior: a review.
      J Appl Behav Anal 2003;36:147–85.
[14] Iwata BA, Pace GM, Dorsey MF, et al. The functions of self-injurious behavior: an
      experimental-epidemiological analysis. J Appl Behav Anal 1994;27:215–40.
[15] Iwata BA, Pace GM, Cowdery GE, et al. What makes extinction work: an analysis of pro-
      cedural form and function. J Appl Behav Anal 1994;27:131–44.
[16] Adams LA, Rickert VI. Reducing bedtime tantrums: comparison between positive routines
      and graduated extinction. Pediatrics 1989;84:756–9.
[17] Allison DB, Burke JC, Summers JA. Treatment of nonspecific dyssomnia with simple stim-
      ulus control procedures in a child with Down's syndrome. Can J Psychiatry 1993;38:274–6.
[18] Colville GA, Watters JP, Yule W, et al. Sleep problems in children with Sanfilippo syndrome.
      Dev Med Child Neurol 1996;38:538–44.
[19] Didden R, Curfs LMG, Sikkema SPE, et al. Functional assessment and treatment of sleeping
      problems with developmentally disabled children: six case studies. J Behav Ther Exp Psychi-
      atry 1998;29:85–97.
[20] Durand VM, Gernert-Dott P, Mapstone E. Treatment of sleep disorders in children with
      developmental disabiltities. J Assoc Pers Sev Handicaps 1996;21:114–22.
[21] Piazza CC, Fisher WW, Moser H. Behavioral treatment of sleep dysfunctions in patients
      with the Rett syndrome. Brain Dev 1991;13:232–7.
[22] Piazza CC, Hagopian LP, Hughes CR, et al. Using chronotherapy to treat severe sleep prob-
      lems: a case study. Am J Ment Retard 1998;102:358–66.
[23] Piazza CC, Fisher WW. Bedtime fading in the treatment of pediatric insomnia. J Behav Ther
      Exp Psychiatry 1991;22:53–6.
[24] Piazza CC, Fisher WW. A bedtime fading with response cost protocol for treatment of mul-
      tiple sleep problems in children. J Appl Behav Anal 1991;24:129–40.
[25] Piazza CC, Fisher WW, Sherer M. Treatment of multiple sleep problems in children with
      developmental disabilities: faded bedtime with response cost versus bedtime scheduling.
      Dev Med Child Neurol 1997;39:414–8.
[26] Ferber R. Solve your child's bedtime problems. New York: Simon & Schuster; 1985.
[27] Rickert VI, Johnson CM. Reducing nocturnal awakening and crying episodes in infants and
      young children: a comparison between scheduled awakenings and systematic ignoring. Pedi-
      atrics 1988;81:203–12.
[28] Pritchard A, Appleton P. Management of sleep problems in pre-school children. Early Child
      Dev Care 1988;34:227–40.
[29] Sadeh A. Assessment and intervention for infant night waking: parental reports and activity-
      based home monitoring. J Consult Clin Psychol 1994;62:63–8.
[30] Czeisler CA, Shanahan TL, Klerman EB, et al. Suppression of melatonin secretion in some
      blind patients by exposure to bright light. N Engl J Med 1995;332:6–11.
[31] DeMeyer MK. Parents and children in autism. New York: Wiley; 1979.
[32] Schreck KA, Williams K, Smith AF. A comparison of eating behaviors between children
      with and without autism. J Autism Dev Disord 2004;34:433–8.

[33] Lukens CT, Linscheid TR. Development and validation of an inventory to assess mealtime behavior problems in children with autism. J Autism Dev Disord 2008;38:342–52.

[34] Matson JL, Kuhn DE. Identifying feeding problems in mentally retarded persons: development and reliability of the Screening Tool of Feeding Problems (STEP). Res Dev Disabil 2001;22:165–72.

[35] Piazza CC, Fisher WW, Brown KA, et al. Functional analysis of inappropriate mealtime behaviors. J Appl Behav Anal 2003;36:187–204.

[36] Ahearn WH, Kerwin ME, Eicher PS, et al. An alternating treatments comparison of two intensive interventions for food refusal. J Appl Behav Anal 1996;29:321–32.

[37] Hoch TA, Babbitt RL, Coe DA, et al. Contingency contacting: combining positive reinforcement and escape extinction procedures to treatment of persistent food refusal. Behav Modif 1994;18:106–28.

[38] Piazza CC, Patel MR, Gulotta CS, et al. On the relative contributions of positive reinforcement and escape extinction in the treatment of food refusal. J Appl Behav Anal 2003;36:309–24.

[39] Piazza CC, Patel MR, Santana CM, et al. An evaluation of simultaneous and sequential presentation of preferred and nonpreferred food to treat food selectivity. J Appl Behav Anal 2002;35:259–70.

[40] Patel MR, Piazza CC, Martinez CJ, et al. An evaluation of two differential reinforcement procedures with escape extinction to treat food refusal. J Appl Behav Anal 2002;35:363–74.

[41] Kern L, Marder TJ. A comparison of simultaneous and delayed reinforcement as treatments for food selectivity. J Appl Behav Anal 1996;29:243–6.

[42] Mueller MM, Piazza CC, Patel MR, et al. Increasing variety of foods consumed by blending nonpreferred foods into preferred foods. J Appl Behav Anal 2004;37:159–70.

[43] Patel MR, Piazza CC, Kelly ML, et al. Using a fading procedure to increase fluid consumption in a child with feeding problems. J Appl Behav Anal 2001;34:357–60.

[44] Shore BA, Babbitt RL, Williams KE, et al. Use of texture fading in the treatment of food selectivity. J Appl Behav Anal 1998;31:621–33.

[45] Danford DE, Huber AM. Pica among mentally retarded adults. Am J Ment Defic 1982;87: 141–6.

[46] Foxx RM, Martin ED. Treatment of scavenging behavior (coprophagy and pica) by overcorrection. Behav Res Ther 1975;13:153–62.

[47] Thompson RH, Iwata BA. A comparison of outcomes from descriptive and functional analyses of problem behavior. J Appl Behav Anal 2007;40:333–8.

[48] Chapman S, Fisher W, Piazza CC, et al. Functional assessment and treatment of life-threatening drug ingestion in a dually diagnosed youth. J Appl Behav Anal 1993;26:255–6.

[49] Piazza CC, Hanley GP, Fisher WW. Functional analysis and treatment of cigarette pica. J Appl Behav Anal 1996;29:437–50.

[50] Piazza CC, Fisher WW, Hanley GP, et al. Treatment of pica through multiple analyses of its reinforcing functions. J Appl Behav Anal 1998;31:165–89.

[51] Piazza CC, Adelinis JD, Hanley GP, et al. An evaluation of the effects of matched stimuli on behaviors maintained by automatic reinforcement. J Appl Behav Anal 2000;33:13–27.

[52] Piazza CC, Roane HS, Keeney KM, et al. Varying response effort in the treatment of pica maintained by automatic reinforcement. J Appl Behav Anal 2002;35:233–46.

[53] Favell JE, McGimsey JF, Schell RM. Treatment of self-injury by providing alternate sensory activities. Analysis and Intervention in Developmental Disabilities 1982;2:83–104.

[54] Goh H, Iwata BA, Kahng S. Multicomponent assessment and treatment of cigarette pica. J Appl Behav Anal 1999;32:297–316.

[55] Fisher WW, Piazza CC, Bowman LG, et al. A preliminary evaluation of empirically derived consequences for the treatment of pica. J Appl Behav Anal 1994;27:447–57.

[56] Singh NN, Bakker L. Suppression of pica by overcorrection and physical restraint: a comparative analysis. J Autism Dev Disord 1984;14:331–41.

[57] Ausman J, Ball TS, Alexander D. Behavior therapy of pica with a profoundly retarded adolescent. Mental Retardation 1974;12:16–8.

**ELSEVIER
SAUNDERS**

Child Adolesc Psychiatric Clin N Am
17 (2008) 907–922

CHILD AND
ADOLESCENT
PSYCHIATRIC CLINICS
OF NORTH AMERICA

Bridging for Success in Autism: Training and Collaboration Across Medical, Educational, and Community Systems

Naomi Swiezy, PhD, HSPP*, Melissa Stuart, MS,
Patricia Korzekwa, MS

*Christian Sarkine Autism Treatment Center, HANDS in Autism Program,
Riley Hospital for Children and the Indiana University School of Medicine,
Indianapolis, IN 46202-5200, USA*

Autism is viewed as more common than Down syndrome and childhood cancer [1]. With increased prevalence rates nationwide [2], it is likely that many care providers not specializing in autism spectrum disorders (ASDs) will encounter an individual along the spectrum. Furthermore, with increased prevalence rates comes a need for more care providers with specialized training in ASDs to address the needs of these individuals and their families. These needs are varied and often involve a multiplicity of care providers, each with their own perspective and philosophy regarding effective intervention. To provide the most effective programming, the team of care providers should be knowledgeable about ASDs and the support for evidence-based practice with individuals with ASD, as well as be able to work in a coordinated and collaborative effort [3].

Many challenges impede the effective implementation of programming. The provision of training and collaboration (across home, medical, educational, and community systems), both essential to effective programming for this special population, is one such challenge and is the focus of this article. When attempting to understand training and collaboration as it relates to working with individuals with an ASD, one must understand the context in which it is most needed. This discussion begins by presenting a contextual background for understanding special education laws and evidence-based

This work was supported by the Division of Exceptional Learners, Indiana Department of Education under Part B of the Individuals with Disabilities Education Improvement Act (P.L. 108-446) and by a grant from the Nina Mason Pulliam Charitable Trust.

* Corresponding author.

E-mail address: nswiezy@iupui.edu (N. Swiezy).

practice for individuals with autism because they are central to issues in effective programming. The second and third sections, respectively, detail current issues surrounding the training of professionals and collaboration across systems. The final section describes the Helping Answer Needs by Developing Specialists (HANDS) in Autism model, a professional training program designed to facilitate more effective training and collaboration across the home, medical, educational, and community settings.

To provide a context for understanding the need for training and collaboration across the home, medical, educational, and community systems, a review of special education laws and the foundation of evidence-based practice as they relate to individuals with ASD is provided. Both guide the development and implementation of interventions and serve to facilitate effective programming.

Special education laws

In considering the needs for effective programming for individuals along the autism spectrum, one must consider the history and complexity of laws relating to special education services. As the largest provider of services to individuals with autism [4], early intervention and educational systems significantly influence practices specific to ASD across several systems.

Until the 1920s, individual programs for disability-specific groups, including the hearing and visually impaired, were able to define their own programming for individuals with special needs [5]. After the passing of the Individuals with Disabilities Education Act (IDEA), other federal mandates were instituted, including Section 504 of the Americans with Disabilities Act [6] and the No Child Left Behind Act [7]. Separately and collectively, the passing of these three laws has helped to shape the current state of educational and public services for individuals with disabilities.

IDEA was designed to ensure that all individuals with disabilities receive a free and appropriate public education that is individualized to meet their unique needs. IDEA has subsequently become reauthorized and, in its current version from 2004, is known as the Individuals with Disabilities Education Improvement Act (IDEIA) [8]. In general, this act has allowed students with identified disabilities that impact their educational performance to be provided with special education services at the expense of the local education agency. These services and the student's progress are then monitored to determine if the programming is effective and the student is receiving services that are beneficial.

Further protection for individuals with disabilities in both educational and community settings occurred in 1990 with the introduction of Section 504 of the Americans with Disabilities Act. Not all individuals with disabilities qualify for special education services under IDEA. If the child's disability does not directly affect his or her ability to be successful in the educational setting, the child may not receive special education services through IDEA but may receive protection under Section 504. Children who receive services under Section 504 are protected from discrimination and may receive accommodations and modifications that are not available to children who are not disabled; however, these children have fewer rights than children receiving services through IDEA [9].

In 2001, the reauthorization of the Elementary and Secondary Education Act, now referred to as No Child Left Behind (NCLB), further impacted how students with disabilities, including those with an ASD, were being educated by the local education agency. NCLB [7] marked the federal government's attempt at improving the academic achievement of the nation's students and a change in how the federal government approached the concept of accountability for all students being educated in public and private classrooms. Although many of the intentions behind NCLB are geared to better the education for all children, the impact has not been entirely positive for students with disabilities. NCLB carries with it the expectation that all students should be able to meet the minimum standards identified by the US Department of Education; however, the expectation that "one size fits all" is not always appropriate for students with an ASD who require an individualized education.

Evidence-based practices

The identification and application of evidence-based guidelines and practices (ie, those demonstrated through systematic research to be effective) is fast becoming standard practice in clinical and medical practice. The United States Department of Education, beginning with the 1997 Amendments to IDEA [10] and further outlined in NCLB [7], has pushed for the identification and use of classroom evidence-based practices whose effectiveness has been proven through rigorous scientific research. Stemming from this federal agenda, several strategies have been identified as promising though there continues to be a gap between research and practice to truly establish an evidence-base for any practice specific to individuals with ASD. Some of this gap may be attributed to the fact that single-case, multifaceted and multicomponent psychosocial interventions appropriate to ASD may not lend themselves to the same rigorous scientific study as appropriate to clinical trial research in medicine. As such, it is possible that alternative criteria need to be identified for establishing an evidence-base in this area [11]. Until such is established we can refer only to interventions that are scientifically or research-based or empirically-supported.

Within this limited scope of empirically-supported practices, the use of methods evolving from the Applied Behavior Analysis (ABA) philosophy has proven to be most effective for individuals with ASD [12].

Several ABA-based strategies and numerous iterations of those strategies are currently used across the home, medical, educational, and community systems. Strategies evolving from this philosophy are the most identified empirically-supported interventions for individuals with an ASD. Although each method individually holds scientific merit, a blended program using several techniques to suit the needs of the individual is ideal [4,13].

Regardless of the strategies used, specific methodologies cannot be required as a blanket treatment for all children. Each intervention needs to be specifically tailored to the individual child for whom no "one size fits all" methodology can address [13,14]. As documented within the literature, there has been a general movement away from reactive programming toward programming that is proactive and informed by ongoing data collection and assessment [13,15]. Overall, professionals must blend a variety of strategies that are best matched to the person's individual learning style, strengths, and needs. Furthermore, these strategies must be consistently evaluated for effectiveness and their contribution to the individual's overall success. Several prominent researchers advocate for an empirically-supported eclectic model as the most appropriate course of intervention [4,13]. Regardless, only 12% of states providing early intervention and educational programming report using an eclectic model incorporating several empirically-supported interventions [4].

Comprehensive programming: guidelines and examples

Several focus groups have offered a list of components ideal for comprehensive programming. A growing literature base has identified a collective list of core components that focus on effective educational practices that are also applicable to other settings [13,15]. In 2001, the National Research Council formed a committee of experts to examine programs and practices aimed at children with autism who were aged 8 years and younger. The outcome of the National Research Council's work identified five characteristics of effective interventions: early entry into intervention programs, active engagement in intensive instructional programming, use of planned teaching opportunities, a sufficient amount of adult attention to meet individualized goals, and active family involvement.

In 2003, Iovannone and coworkers [15] identified six essential themes or components that should be included in effective educational programs for students with ASD. The themes identified reiterated those acknowledged in other literature and guidelines [3,13,16,17]. They included individualized supports and services, systematic instruction, comprehensive and structured learning environments, specialized curriculum content, a functional approach to problem behavior, and family involvement.

As guidelines and standards for effective programming for individuals with an ASD are developed, a mechanism for determining fidelity to those guidelines must be derived to ensure accountability for meeting these standards. To be held accountable, professional and legislative bodies alike indicate that training in effective programming practices and collaboration with other professionals are essential elements.

Issues in training

Who needs training and why

The need for consistent and appropriate training is essential for all care providers working with individuals with an ASD. Each part of the care team needs to be informed about ASDs and the empirically supported interventions noted to be effective for this population beyond his or her basic foundation of practice [1]. In a related vein, persons with more limited contact with individuals with ASD but still having an impact on their programming (eg, administrators, general medical professionals, consultants, and general education teachers) need specialized training to understand the needs of individuals with ASD to effectively educate others, support those providing direct care, and understand when and what resources may be needed [18,19].

Care providers across disciplines and settings are likely to be jointly responsible for the care and programming of an individual with an ASD. A great deal of structure and consistency is needed for individuals with ASD. As such, all care providers should be aware of and adhere to the strategies in place. For example, paraprofessionals often spend the most time with individuals in the class or work setting and need training to be able to apply the various teaching methods while under the supervision of the special education teacher [20,21].

It is not appropriate or correct to suggest that there is one way to educate an individual with an ASD [13,21]. It is best to have a "toolbox" from which several strategies or "tools" may be used based on the individual's needs. To do so effectively, persons providing direct care to individuals with an ASD must be trained in multiple approaches, strategies, and methods. By having knowledge about the many strategies available, the provider can choose the most effective plan for programming and can evaluate or determine other plans when data indicate progress is not being made. Having a consistent philosophy upon which the various strategies and methods are derived is important to provide a solid basis and understanding for problem solving and intervention [22]. When caregivers across all settings have specialized training in both ASDs and empirically supported practices, they will be well equipped to implement effective programming, increasing the potential for positive outcomes for the individual with an ASD [21,23].

Training in the home and community settings

The opportunity for teaching is not restricted to the school day. Parents and care providers outside of the educational environment must learn effective methods to help facilitate maintenance and generalization of skills [21]. Parents are by far the most knowledgeable when it comes to their children; therefore, they are often identified as integral members of the care team responsible for coordinating services and disseminating information across settings. To most effectively assist in their child's programming, parents need to be knowledgeable about the different strategies used for their child. Hume and coworkers [24] identify parent training as the most effective service in child progress, providing an indication for parents as part of the team of care providers. Similarly, parents and other providers need to understand the factors involved in special education service provision so that they have reasonable expectations and requests for programming.

Training in the medical setting

With an increase in prevalence of ASD and the use of guidelines for screening and diagnosis, medical students and practicing physicians must be trained to recognize the core symptoms of ASD as well as be able to make informed recommendations or referrals for appropriate services [25,26]. Many families have found delays in the referral process to appropriate specialists because their physician was not concerned about presenting characteristics. Likewise, the physician, when concerned, often does not know what can be done or to whom the family should be referred [27].

In a survey of agencies administering early identification and intervention services across 46 states, there was an overwhelming lack of uniformity in policies and practices regarding the identification and care of children with autism [4]. Only one fifth of states reported having diagnostic guidelines in place, and only 22% of states required the diagnosing professional to have experience with ASD [4]. This finding is alarming given that early identification and intervention are keys for optimizing long-term positive outcomes for individuals with an ASD.

Training in the educational setting

Teacher training and preparation have received increased attention with the creation of NCLB [7]. As is true for other systems, teachers and others in the educational setting need to be knowledgeable about ASDs and empirically supported practices. Many due process and legal cases have been won by parents due to school personnel not having sufficient training [28]. In addition, an increasing number of parents are requesting empirically supported interventions, and teachers need to have training to be able to assess the appropriateness of the parent's requests [29].

Simpson [28] notes, "preparing qualified teachers and other professionals to educate and support students with ASD is the most significant challenge facing the autism field." Even though many of the empirically supported interventions noted as effective for individuals with an ASD are grounded in generic educational and behavioral science principles, personnel training programs must be designed specifically to prepare educators, related service personnel, and others to individually address the needs of students with an ASD.

Another reason to encourage training for those in the educational setting is to alleviate the potential for burnout and frequent staff turnover. Jennett and coworkers [22] suggest an increased risk of educator burnout in special education and classrooms for students with ASD. Providing proper training and support to these teachers can lead to positive feelings of empowerment and competence, decreasing the risk of burnout.

It is clear that all care providers working with individuals with an ASD need to be knowledgeable about ASDs and empirically supported practices beyond their individual areas of expertise. Less clear are the guidelines and methods for obtaining training and the mechanism for accountability.

Guidelines for training

Although highly qualified and trained individuals provide service delivery to individuals along the autism spectrum, it remains unclear what constitutes training or what the mechanism is to become a qualified and trained individual in ASD [21].

A definition fromdictionary.com indicates that to train is "to *coach* in or *accustom* to a mode of *behavior or performance*; to *make proficient* with *specialized instruction and practice*" [30]. The specification is on more than exposure and awareness through written and lecture materials and includes the component of hands-on learning to gain a skill. Several methods for training professionals have been identified. Turnbell and coworkers [14] suggest the need for on-site training of personnel by experts in the field, whereas several researchers in the field advocate for more training in higher education as well as through staff in-service [14,28]. Simpson [28] maintains that it is essential that the skills needed to work with individuals with an ASD be modeled, taught, practiced, and evaluated in quality field placements with students with ASDs and that ongoing opportunities for skill enhancement and refinement be provided in addition to traditional higher education courses and in-service programs. Furthermore, according to Joyce and Showers [31], individuals improve upon their skills, knowledge, and actual application within the naturalistic environment when coaching and feedback methods are used in training. Fig. 1 illustrates the proposed levels of learning necessary to provide effective training for persons working with individuals with an ASD. For some, the extent to which an individual is trained should be dependent upon their role with the individual and family. Even within these roles, the preparation and certification practices vary within disciplines and across programs and states.

Specific guidelines relating to training

Both NCLB [7] and IDEA [8] require all teachers and paraprofessionals to be "highly qualified" according to uniform and objective state standards. The exact mechanism for training educational staff is not outlined in IDEA and is typically left up to the state educational agency to determine the most

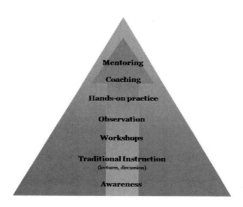

Fig. 1. Levels of learning diagram.

appropriate avenue for staff training. For persons working explicitly with individuals with an ASD, there is no federal or state level requirement for disability-specific training.

Training opportunities

Pre-service (colleges and universities)

To meet the training needs of current and future educators and care providers, several colleges and universities (eg, Arizona State University, West Virginia University, Pennsylvania State University, University of Massachusetts, Portland State University) have developed certificate programs beyond the bachelors or graduate degree that focus specifically on ASDs. These certificates typically require 12 to 15 credit hours of curriculum centered on working specifically with individuals with an ASD. Often, a practicum placement is also required with supervision by a practitioner specializing in ASD. These programs, although still in their infancy, speak to the high demand for training specific to ASD.

In-service

Most notably in the educational setting, staff in-service presentations or workshops are used as a means of providing ASD-specific training. Several state educational agencies have employed an "Autism Specialist" or "Autism Consultant" to facilitate these trainings. The premise behind the use of these specialists is to centralize and focus training efforts and to develop individuals with expertise who can facilitate training at the local level. Nevertheless, the reality is that creating such specialists often fails to suffice due to the limited number of these specialists relative to the number of individuals with an ASD who need support.

These training opportunities provide professionals with one venue for gaining essential knowledge but do not address the components identified for effective integration of information. Each and every person who has hands-on contact or direct influence on the course of programming should be immersed in some comprehensive, cohesive, and coordinated learning opportunities, preferably with the more active hands-on training and experience.

Difficulties in training

Several issues make training professionals in working with individuals with an ASD difficult. Factors such as disagreement as to the content of training (eg, core philosophy and intervention strategies) and territorial issues regarding who should receive training have decreased the number of professionals trained specifically in ASD [21,32]. Often, the training does not provide enough scope or depth. For example, despite the presence of a motivational speaker at a lecture or workshop, this presence does not address the comprehensive skills needed nor does it help with mastery of skills through coaching, practice, and feedback [13,21,29]. Likewise, when individuals gather information from a multiplicity of venues and sources, the potential for information to conflict from one venue to the next could limit the application of skills. Trainings often focus on single strategies or methods, which may unduly convey the message that only one approach will be effective with these individuals. For persons who do gain effective training, not having ongoing support as they attempt to apply the information learned can decrease their motivation to apply the information or to seek further training [33].

Care providers across all settings need specialized training in ASDs and empirically supported interventions to determine effective programming. Furthermore, this training should be comprehensive and include opportunities for interactive learning beyond traditional lecture-based formats. Once all care providers are properly trained, the next important element in providing effective programming for individuals with an ASD is to ensure that there is effective collaboration across all systems.

Issues in collaboration

Who should collaborate and why

The spectrum of abilities and needs of an individual with an ASD requires ongoing integration of the programming across home, medical, educational, and community settings. Collaboration involves good communication, consultation, organization, and case management skills [3,21]. Collaboration not only incorporates several perspectives but also allows for consistency in program implementation and comprehensive evaluation of current programming.

Each individual with an ASD is different. The multiple care providers must coordinate and share expertise relevant to their areas with the entire team to facilitate consistency and maintenance of programming and generalization of skills to other settings [19,34,35].

Ultimately, as Baer and coworkers have [36] indicated, "effectiveness for the future will probably be built primarily on system-wide interventions." We can have great interventions, but their success will likely depend on the consistency with which they are implemented across disciplines [34] (eg, clinicians, clients, administrators, parents, teachers, paraprofessionals).

Through collaboration, data regarding the effectiveness of an individual's current programming can be more adequately assessed. Collecting and sharing information across settings allows for a comprehensive analysis of the individual's behavior and can influence decisions regarding current programming.

Guidelines for collaboration

Resulting from increased due process requests, state and local education agencies have begun to look more closely at providing flexibility in programming, have looked increasingly to better and more frequent staff training, and have worked to improve collaboration among parents, care providers, and school districts [37]. Federal laws and guidelines are also creating the impetus for change [7,8,13]. In addition, programs for training medical and other professionals are recognizing the empiric support, justification in theory, and legal foundation for collaboration across systems and are facilitating the consideration and learning of different perspectives in programming [1,38]. Nevertheless, the laws and guidelines that have been developed specifying the factors relevant to effective programming with individuals along the autism spectrum [13] and the guidelines developed by various disciplines in terms of training and credentialing do not yet adequately address issues relating to collaboration across disciplines.

Difficulties with collaboration

Often, factors including time, knowledge, training, service availability, and the support of collaboration can impede the process [3]; however, working in isolation can result in plans that are not functional or comprehensive for the individual [39]. Given time and other pressures, collaboration is seen as a frivolity rather than a necessity [20]. In addition, conflicts may result among what is desired for the child, what is practical given the resources, and what is ultimately offered [40].

Fostering a collaborative relationship

Service providers across the home, medical, educational, and community settings need to collaborate. Fig. 2 illustrates the proposed interrelationships necessary for effective collaboration.

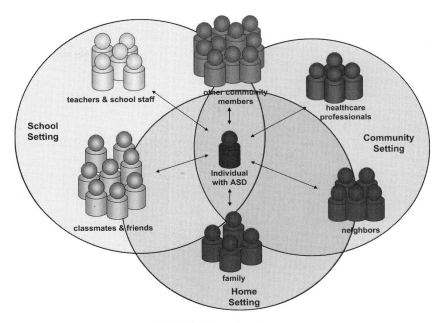

Fig. 2. Collaboration diagram.

Care providers may have differing views, but all views should be accounted for and considered when collaborating [41,42]. For those in the medical field, there is a need for consistent, accurate, and reliable reporting to parents because they are the main vehicles for transporting information across systems. Additionally, there must be open communication between the educational and medical systems to coordinate care and evaluate current programming.

Various collaborative team members will bring different strengths to the individual's care team [43]. The team will most effectively serve the individual and family by having joint knowledge and understanding about each others' roles, expertise, and the policies and guidelines that inform effective programming with an individual with an ASD [7,8,13,43,44].

Similar to the needed training in ASDs and empirically supported practices, care providers need to be trained to collaborate effectively. Although collaboration can be of great benefit if done well, it can also lead to decreased growth and development of the individual with ASD if not done effectively. Unfortunately, training programs have not all kept pace with the changes in the roles of professionals, the needs of students, or general literature base in ASD [18].

The helping answer needs by developing specialists in autism model

Despite the documented need for comprehensive training and collaboration across systems to facilitate effective programming for individuals with

ASDs, the literature is clear about the limitations of this training and collaboration. Difficulties for both are inherent in the definition, content, and practical tools available for those in the field. The HANDS in Autism model, a university and hospital-based professional training program, was developed in response to the needs outlined above. It is described as a model to facilitate professional training and improve systems collaboration efforts.

Informed through practice and literature, focused programming in the areas of training, collaboration, and building of local capacity in the area of ASDs has been a part of the HANDS in Autism program since 2004. Initially, an intensive, hands-on, active learning opportunity for professional training was established to extend beyond more typical didactic trainings otherwise offered. It had been noted that care providers wanting to implement information gained from traditional conferences were not adequately tooled to apply the knowledge they had gained. They became promptly discouraged with the methodologies and processes as they struggled to effectively apply and individualize the principles in their naturalistic settings.

The week-long intensive training program held during the summer months provided for these needs while also allowing participants to learn and apply principles directly to a range of students across the autism spectrum within a laboratory classroom environment. In 2006, the HANDS in Autism program was extended to begin development of collaborative community-based classrooms and programming. The effort was to layer in the HANDS in Autism philosophy (Fig. 3) into existing community programs open to such teaming and collaboration. The HANDS in Autism model is based upon the core philosophy of ABA and the practical integration and blending of specific intervention strategies evolving from that core philosophy. The premise is that no one strategy is effective with all individuals with an ASD. Rather, the specific components (ie, "facets") incorporated into the programming for each individual (ie, "gem") differ, but all evolve from this data-driven philosophy. School staff in the collaborative classroom were trained in the program's philosophy with intensive coaching and mentoring as well as modeling, practice, and feedback. These collaboratives serve as means for demonstrating the practicality and transportability of the philosophy and strategies beyond an intervention or center-based environment to the classroom and educational system as a whole. Ultimately, the goal was not only to integrate empirically-supported practices into the classroom but also to demonstrate the relevance and success in influencing entire educational systems and practices and to prepare the collaborative sites as training sites utilized by local educational agencies to build and broaden the local capacity to serve individuals with an ASD. The model has been successful in training staff on a variety of dimensions and has also successfully served as a model of the effective collaboration and blending among the home, medical, educational, and community systems outlined in Figs. 1 and 2.

The HANDS in Autism program has created a vision that has continued to grow and evolve with the need across the state of Indiana and can serve as

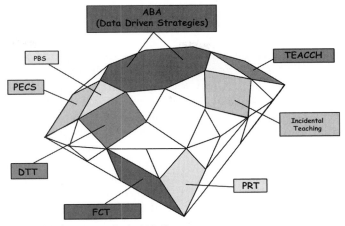

Applied Behavior Analysis (ABA)
Picture Exchange Communication Systems (PECS)
Functional Communication Training (FCT)
Incidental Teaching
Pivotal Response Training (PRT)
Discrete Trial Training (DTT)
Positive Behavioral Support (PBS)
Treatment and Education of Autistic and related
    Communication-handicapped Children (TEACCH)

Fig. 3. HANDS in Autism diamond philosophy.

a model for other states. The programming and development described by this model reflects what has been specified and sought by various guidelines [13], policies [7,8] and current literature pertaining to ASD (eg, the study by Scheuermann and colleagues [21]). The general vision stems from the realization that there needs to be more care providers specialized in ASDs and empirically supported interventions who are open to collaboration across systems.

Summary

Information related to effectively programming for individuals with an ASD has been highlighted. The history of practices and legislation has been presented, particularly from the special education and behavioral literatures; however, the information and issues related to training and collaboration in particular are relevant to all care providers of an individual with an ASD. Training specific to ASD and effective empirically supported intervention is advocated for all care providers influencing an individual's programming. The most effective avenue for training is through an intensive model incorporating hands-on opportunities and feedback. Furthermore, once effective training has occurred, collaboration across systems should be emphasized to facilitate consistency and comprehensive program evaluation.

Care providers across all systems have a shared responsibility in the decision-making and programming processes for these individuals. Ultimately, if care providers across the home, medical, educational, and community settings do not address the advice in the literature and legal guidelines for training and collaboration, individuals may fail to progress, schools may face the expense and challenges of litigation, and parents may struggle with how to best care for their children [21]. The HANDS in Autism program is highlighted as a model to address issues in training and collaboration. The program has been effective not only in expanding services and options provided to individuals with an ASD but also in developing and enhancing the training and collaboration of caregivers and providers across home, medical, educational, and community settings.

References

[1] Sperry LA, Whaley KT, Shaw E, et al. Services for young children with autism spectrum disorder: voices of parents and providers. Infants Young Child 1999;11(4):17–33.

[2] CDC releases new data on autism spectrum disorders (ASDs) from multiple communities in the United States. Centers for Disease Control and Prevention Web site 2007. Available at: http://www.cdc.gov/od/oc/media/pressrel/2007/r070208.htm. Accessed December 20, 2007.

[3] Baker S, Bauman M, Bishop M, et al. Autism spectrum disorders roadmap. Washington, DC: National Institute of Mental Health; 2005. Available at: http://www.nimh.nih.gov/research-funding/scientific-meetings/recurring-meetings/iacc/expert-working-group-on-services-report-to-the-iacc-services-subcommittee.pdf. Accessed October 11, 2007.

[4] Stahmer AC, Mandell DS. State infant/toddler program policies for eligibility and services provision for young children with autism. Adm Policy Ment Health 2007;34(1):29–37.

[5] LaVor M. Federal legislation for exceptional children: implications and a view of the future. In: Kneedler RD, Tarver SG, editors. Changing perspectives in special education. Columbus (OH): Charles E. Merrill; 1977. p. 245–70.

[6] US Department of Justice. Americans with Disabilities Act. 1990. Available at: http://www.ada.gov/pubs/ada.htm. Accessed December 27, 2007.

[7] US Department of Education. No Child Left Behind. 2001. Available at: http://www.ed.gov/policy/elsec/leg/esea02/107-110.pdf. Accessed December 27, 2007.

[8] US Department of Education. Individuals with Disabilities Education Improvement Act. 2004. Available at: http://frwebgate.access.gpo.gov/cgi-bin/getdoc.cgi?dbname=108_cong_public_laws&docid=f:publ446.108. Accessed December 27, 2007.

[9] Wright PWD, Wright PD. Wrights law: special education law. 1st edition. Hartfield (VA): Harbor House Law; 2000.

[10] US Department of Education. Individuals with Disabilities Education Act Amendments. 1997. Available at: http://thomas.loc.gov/cgi-bin/query/z?c105:H.R.5.ENR. Accessed December 27, 2007.

[11] Lonigan CJ, Elbert JC, Johnson SB. Empirically supported psychosocial interventions for children: An overview. Journal of Clinical Child Psychology 1998;27(2):138–45.

[12] Matson JL, Benavidez DA, Compton LS, et al. Behavioral treatment of autistic persons: a review of research from 1980 to the present. Res Dev Disabil 1996;17(6):433–65.

[13] Lord C, McGee JP, editors. Educating children with autism. Washington, DC: National Academy Press; 2001.

[14] Turnbull HR, Wilcox BL, Stowe E, et al. IDEA requirements for use of PBS: guidelines for responsible agencies. Journal of Positive Behavior Support 2001;3(1):11–8.

[15] Iovannone R, Dunlap G, Huber H, et al. Effective educational practices for students with autism spectrum disorders. Focus Autism Other Dev Disabl 2003;18(3):150–65.

[16] Crimmins DB, Durand VM, Theurer-Kaufman K, et al. Autism program quality indicators: a self-review and quality improvement guide for schools and programs serving students with autism spectrum disorders. New York: New York State Education Department, Office of Vocational and Educational Services for Individuals with Disabilities; 2001. Available at: http://www.vesid.nysed.gov/specialed/autism/apqi.htm. Accessed December 19, 2007.

[17] Handleman JS, Harris SL. Preschool education programs for children with autism. Austin (TX): PRO-ED; 1994.

[18] Young B, Simpson RL. An examination of paraprofessional involvement in supporting inclusion of students with autism. Focus Autism Other Dev Disabl 1997;12(1):31–8.

[19] Marks SU, Schrader C, Levine M. Paraeducator experiences in inclusive settings: helping, hovering, or holding their own? Except Child 1999;65(3):315–28.

[20] Giangreco MF, Edelman SW, Luiselli TE, et al. Helping or hovering? Effects of instructional assistant proximity on students with disabilities. Except Child 1997;64(1):7–18.

[21] Scheuermann B, Webber J, Boutot EA, et al. Problems with personnel preparation in autism spectrum disorders. Focus Autism Other Dev Disabl 2003;18(3):197–206.

[22] Jennett HK, Harris SL, Mesibov GB. Commitment to philosophy, teacher efficacy, and burnout among teachers of children with autism. J Autism Dev Disord 2003;33(6): 583–93.

[23] Harrower JK, Dunlap G. Including children with autism in general education classrooms: a review of effective strategies. Behav Modif 2001;25(5):762–84.

[24] Hume K, Bellini S, Pratt C. The usage and perceived outcomes of early intervention and early childhood programs for young children with autism spectrum disorder. Topics in Early Childhood Special Education 2005;25(4):195–207.

[25] Filipek PA, Accardo PJ, Ashwal S, et al. Practice parameter: screening and diagnosis of autism. Report of the Quality Standards Subcommittee of the American Academy of Neurology and the Child Neurology Society. Neurology 2000;55(4):468–79.

[26] Johnson CP, Myers SM. Identification and evaluation of children with autism spectrum disorders. Pediatrics 2007;120(5):1183–215.

[27] Shah K. What do medical students know about autism? Autism 2001;5(2):127–33.

[28] Simpson RL. Policy-related issues and perspectives. Focus on Autism and Other Developmental Disorders 2003;18(3):192–6.

[29] Lerman DC, Vorndran CM, Addison L, et al. Preparing teachers in evidence-based practices for young children with autism. School Psych Rev 2004;33(4):510–26.

[30] Train. Dictionary.com Web site. Available at: http://dictionary.reference.com/browse/train. Accessed December 27, 2007.

[31] Joyce BR, Showers B. Student achievement through staff development. Alexandria (VA): Association for Supervision and Curriculum Development; 2002.

[32] Harris SL, LaRue R, Weiss MJ. Programmatic issues. In: Sturmey P, Fitzer A, editors. Autism spectrum disorders: applied behavior analysis, evidence and practice. Austin (TX): Pro-Ed; 2007. p. 235–64.

[33] Gravois TA, Knotek S, Babinski LM. Educating practitioners as consultants: development and implementation of the instructional consultation team consortium. Journal of Educational and Psychological Consultation 2002;13(1–2):113–32.

[34] McClannahan LE, Krantz PJ. On systems analysis in autism intervention programs. J Appl Behav Anal 1993;26(4):589–96.

[35] Rogers SJ. Intervention for young children with autism: from research to practice. Infants Young Child 1999;12(2):1–16.

[36] Baer DM, Wolf MM, Risley TR. Some still-current dimensions of applied behavior analysis. J Appl Behav Anal 1987;20(4):313–27.

[37] Mandlawitz MR. The impact of the legal system on educational programming for young children with autism spectrum disorder. J Autism Dev Disord 2002;35(5):495–508.

[38] Spann SJ, Kohler FW, Soenksen D. Examining parents' involvement in and perceptions of special education services: an interview with families in a parent support group. Focus Autism Other Dev Disabl 2003;18(4):228–37.

[39] de Clercq H, Peeters T. A partnership between parents and professionals. In: Pérez JM, Martos J, González PM, et al, editors. New developments in autism: the future is today. London: Jessica Kingsley; 2007. p. 310–40.

[40] Hurth J, Shaw E, Izeman SG, et al. Areas of agreement about effective practices among programs serving young children with autism spectrum disorders. Infants Young Child 1999; 12(2):17–26.

[41] Simpson RL. Early intervention with children with autism: the search for best practices. J Assoc Pers Sev Handicaps 1999;24(3):218–21.

[42] Simpson RL, Myles BS. The general education collaboration model: a model for successful mainstreaming. Focus on Exceptional Children 1990;23(4):1–10.

[43] Feinberg E, Vacca J. The drama and trauma of creating policies on autism: critical issues to consider in the new millennium. Focus Autism Other Dev Disabl 2000;15(3):130–7.

[44] Smith SW, Slattery WJ. Beyond the mandate: developing individualized education programs that work for students with autism. Focus on Autistic Behavior 1993;8(3):1–15.

ELSEVIER
SAUNDERS

Child Adolesc Psychiatric Clin N Am
17 (2008) 923–932

CHILD AND
ADOLESCENT
PSYCHIATRIC CLINICS
OF NORTH AMERICA

Index

Note: Page numbers of article titles are in **boldface** type.

1056-4993/08/$ - see front matter © 2008 Elsevier Inc. All rights reserved.
doi:10.1016/S1056-4993(08)00075-8

childpsych.theclinics.com

Moving?

Make sure your subscription moves with you!

To notify us of your new address, find your **Clinics Account Number** (located on your mailing label above your name), and contact customer service at:

E-mail: elspcs@elsevier.com

800-654-2452 (subscribers in the U.S. & Canada)
1-407-563-6020 (subscribers outside of the U.S. & Canada)

Fax number: 407-363-9661

Elsevier Periodicals Customer Service
6277 Sea Harbor Drive
Orlando, FL 32887-4800

*To ensure uninterrupted delivery of your subscription, please notify us at least 4 weeks in advance of move.

United States Postal Service

Statement of Ownership, Management, and Circulation
(All Periodicals Publications Except Requestor Publications)

1. Publication Title	2. Publication Number	3. Filing Date
Child and Adolescent Psychiatric Clinics of North America	0 1 1 1 - 3 6 8 8	9/15/08

4. Issue Frequency	5. Number of Issues Published Annually	6. Annual Subscription Price
Jan, Apr, Jul, Oct	4	$220.00

7. Complete Mailing Address of Known Office of Publication (Not printer) (Street, city, county, state, and ZIP+4)

Elsevier Inc.
360 Park Avenue South
New York, NY 10010-1710

Contact Person
Stephen Bushing

Telephone (Include area code)
215-239-3688

8. Complete Mailing Address of Headquarters or General Business Office of Publisher (Not printer)

Elsevier Inc., 360 Park Avenue South, New York, NY 10010-1710

9. Full Names and Complete Mailing Addresses of Publisher, Editor, and Managing Editor (Do not leave blank)

Publisher (Name and complete mailing address)

John Schrefer, Elsevier, Inc., 1600 John F. Kennedy Blvd. Suite 1800, Philadelphia, PA 19103-2899

Editor (Name and complete mailing address)

Sarah Barth, Elsevier, Inc., 1600 John F. Kennedy Blvd. Suite 1800, Philadelphia, PA 19103-2899

Managing Editor (Name and complete mailing address)

Catherine Bewick, Elsevier, Inc., 1600 John F. Kennedy Blvd. Suite 1800, Philadelphia, PA 19103-2899

10. Owner (Do not leave blank. If the publication is owned by a corporation, give the name and address of the corporation immediately followed by the names and addresses of all stockholders owning or holding 1 percent or more of the total amount of stock. If not owned by a corporation, give the names and addresses of the individual owners. If owned by a partnership or other unincorporated firm, give its name and address as well as those of each individual owner. If the publication is published by a nonprofit organization, give its name and address.)

Full Name	Complete Mailing Address
Wholly owned subsidiary of	4520 East-West Highway
Reed/Elsevier, US holdings	Bethesda, MD 20814

11. Known Bondholders, Mortgagees, and Other Security Holders Owning or Holding 1 Percent or More of Total Amount of Bonds, Mortgages, or Other Securities. If none, check box ☐ None

Full Name	Complete Mailing Address
N/A	

12. Tax Status (For completion by nonprofit organizations authorized to mail at nonprofit rates) (Check one)
The purpose, function, and nonprofit status of this organization and the exempt status for federal income tax purposes:
☐ Has Not Changed During Preceding 12 Months
☐ Has Changed During Preceding 12 Months (Publisher must submit explanation of change with this statement)

PS Form 3526, September 2006 (Page 1 of 3 (Instructions Page 3)) PSN 7530-01-000-9931 **PRIVACY NOTICE:** See our Privacy policy in www.usps.com

---

13. Publication Title		14. Issue Date for Circulation Data Below
Child and Adolescent Psychiatric Clinics of North America		July 2008

15. Extent and Nature of Circulation			Average No. Copies Each Issue During Preceding 12 Months	No. Copies of Single Issue Published Nearest to Filing Date
a. Total Number of Copies (Net press run)			1600	1400
b. Paid Circulation (By Mail and Outside the Mail)	(1)	Mailed Outside-County Paid Subscriptions Stated on PS Form 3541. (Include paid distribution above nominal rate, advertiser's proof copies, and exchange copies)	788	754
	(2)	Mailed In-County Paid Subscriptions Stated on PS Form 3541 (Include paid distribution above nominal rate, advertiser's proof copies, and exchange copies)		
	(3)	Paid Distribution Outside the Mails Including Sales Through Dealers and Carriers, Street Vendors, Counter Sales, and Other Paid Distribution Outside USPS®	116	130
	(4)	Paid Distribution by Other Classes Mailed Through the USPS (e.g. First-Class Mail®)		
c. Total Paid Distribution (Sum of 15b (1), (2), (3), and (4))		▶	904	884
d. Free or Nominal Rate Distribution (By Mail and Outside the Mail)	(1)	Free or Nominal Rate Outside-County Copies Included on PS Form 3541	60	66
	(2)	Free or Nominal Rate In-County Copies Included on PS Form 3541		
	(3)	Free or Nominal Rate Copies Mailed at Other Classes Mailed Through the USPS (e.g. First-Class Mail)		
	(4)	Free or Nominal Rate Distribution Outside the Mail (Carriers or other means)		
e. Total Free or Nominal Rate Distribution (Sum of 15d (1), (2), (3) and (4))		▶	60	66
f. Total Distribution (Sum of 15c and 15e)		▶	964	950
g. Copies not Distributed (See instructions to publishers #4 (page #3))		▶	636	450
h. Total (Sum of 15f and g)		▶	1600	1400
i. Percent Paid (15c divided by 15f times 100)		▶	93.78%	93.05%

16. Publication of Statement of Ownership

☐ If the publication is a general publication, publication of this statement is required. Will be printed in the **October 2008** issue of this publication. ☐ Publication not required

17. Signature and Title of Editor, Publisher, Business Manager, or Owner	Date
[signature] Jay Donucci – Executive Director of Subscription Services	September 15, 2008

I certify that all information furnished on this form is true and complete. I understand that anyone who furnishes false or misleading information on this form or who omits material or information requested on the form may be subject to criminal sanctions (including fines and imprisonment) and/or civil sanctions (including civil penalties).

PS Form 3526, September 2006 (Page 2 of 3)